Cancer Drug Discovery and Development

Series Editor

Beverly A. Teicher
Bethesda, Maryland, USA

Cancer Drug Discovery and Development, the Springer series headed by Beverly A. Teicher, is the definitive book series in cancer research and oncology. Volumes cover the process of drug discovery, preclinical models in cancer research, specific drug target groups, and experimental and approved therapeutic agents. The volumes are current and timely, anticipating areas where experimental agents are reaching FDA approval. Each volume is edited by an expert in the field covered, and chapters are authored by renowned scientists and physicians in their fields of interest.

More information about this series at http://www.springer.com/series/7625

Alister C. Ward

Editor

STAT Inhibitors in Cancer

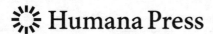 Humana Press

Editor
Alister C. Ward
School of Medicine
Deakin University
Warun Ponds, VIC, Australia

ISSN 2196-9906   ISSN 2196-9914   (electronic)
Cancer Drug Discovery and Development
ISBN 978-3-319-82701-8   ISBN 978-3-319-42949-6   (eBook)
DOI 10.1007/978-3-319-42949-6

Printed on acid-free paper

This Humana Press imprint is published by Springer Nature
The registered company is Springer International Publishing AG
The registered company address is: Gewerbestrasse 11, 6330 Cham, Switzerland

Preface

Signal Transducer and Activator of Transcription (STAT) proteins were discovered over two decades ago as transcription factors mediating the actions of interferons on responsive cells. Over the intervening time period, STATs have become recognized as a paradigm for facilitating rapid changes in gene transcription in response to an array of external factors, with additional 'non-canonical' functions also established. STATs have diverse roles in normal biology, but especially in the development and function of blood and immune cells. However, they also represent important mediators of a number of diseases, especially various cancers, which has led to the development of a variety of direct and indirect inhibitors of relevance to oncology.

In this volume, Liongue et al. provide a broad summary of STATs in normal biology and its perturbation in disease (Chap. 1), with O'Keefe and Grandis extending this to their role in cancer specifically (Chap. 2). Liu and Frank then present an overview of the approaches applicable to STAT inhibition, highlighting the key challenges and most promising strategies (Chap. 3). The next two chapters focus on inhibitors of the most important STAT in cancer, STAT3, with Yu et al. detailing the history of STAT3 inhibitors along with early clinical studies (Chap. 4) and Bharadwaj et al. providing a wide-ranging description of the various STAT3 inhibitors being investigated (Chap. 5). Finally, the last two chapters examine approaches to indirectly inhibit STATs through targeting upstream activators, with Rasighaemi and Ward focusing on Janus kinase inhibitors (Chap. 6) and Kumar detailing inhibitors of receptors and other kinases (Chap. 7). Collectively, this work provides comprehensive and state-of-the-art information about STAT inhibitors in cancer.

Warun Ponds, VIC, Australia   Alister C. Ward

Contents

Chapter 1
STATs in Health and Disease

Clifford Liongue, Rowena S. Lewis, and Alister C. Ward

Abstract Signal Transducers and Activators of Transcription (STATs) represent a central paradigm of cell-cell signaling, providing a rapid and effective mechanism to transfer an external signal into a transcriptional response. They act as core components downstream of a myriad of cytokine and other receptors to mediate a diverse range of functions. This chapter provides an overview of the STAT protein family, their structure, mode of activation, specificity, variants and negative regulation along with their multiple roles in both normal biology as well as the etiology of disease.

Keywords Cytokine receptor • Signaling • JAK-STAT • STAT1 • STAT2 • STAT3 • STAT4 • STAT5 • STAT6

1.1 Introduction

Signal Transducers and Activators of Transcription (STATs) were first identified over 20 years ago in the context of interferon signaling [1]. They are now firmly established as one of the most important signaling modalities, particularly in the context of mediating rapid responses of target cells to specific external factors, with a veritable mountain of studies detailing a variety of functions for these transcription factors in a myriad of cell systems across diverse species. STAT proteins play numerous roles in normal biology, particularly within immune and blood cells, and contribute to the etiology of disease, notably including a range of malignancies.

C. Liongue • R.S. Lewis • A.C. Ward (✉)
School of Medicine, Deakin University, Melbourne, VIC, Australia

Centre for Molecular and Medical Research, Deakin University, Melbourne, VIC, Australia
e-mail: c.liongue@deakin.edu.au; rowena.lewis@onjcri.org.au; alister.ward@deakin.edu.au

© Springer International Publishing Switzerland 2016
A.C. Ward (ed.), *STAT Inhibitors in Cancer*, Cancer Drug
Discovery and Development, DOI 10.1007/978-3-319-42949-6_1

1

1.2 STAT Protein Structure, Regulation and Specificity

Seven STAT proteins are present in humans: STAT1–6, which includes the closely-related STAT5A and STAT5B proteins that are encoded by adjacent but distinct genes [2].

1.2.1 Structure

Each member of the STAT family is composed of several variably conserved domains: the N-terminal, coiled-coil, DNA binding, linker, Src-homology 2 (SH2) and C-terminal domains [3, 4] (Fig. 1.1). The hydrophilic four helix-bundle N-terminal domain has numerous functions, including mediating important protein-protein interactions and controlling nuclear translocation, the coiled-coil domain regulates the activation of STAT proteins and mediates nuclear export, whereas the β-barrel DNA binding domain is responsible for the interaction with specific DNA sequences. This is connected via a helical linker to a highly conserved SH2 domain that facilitates interactions with phosphotyrosine residues on receptor components as well as other STATs [4]. The so-called 'transactivation domain' (TAD) regions at the C-terminus of different STAT proteins show the lowest sequence conservation and contain alternate protein motifs responsible for influencing transcription, either directly or via recruitment of other transcriptional regulators [5].

1.2.2 Activation

One of the defining characteristics of STAT proteins is their ability to be activated rapidly in response to external stimuli. This is a consequence of the pre-formed STATs existing in a latent state in the cytoplasm such that they are able to be readily activated – through tyrosine phosphorylation – following stimulation of different

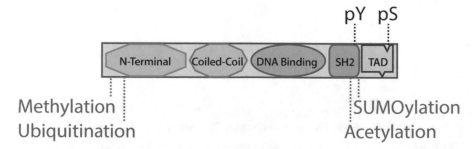

Fig. 1.1 Structure/function of STAT proteins. Schematic representation of the structure of STAT proteins, showing the conserved domains and the sites of post-translational modifications

upstream receptors. The most notable of these are the class I and II cytokine receptors, but they also include receptor tyrosine kinases (RTKs) and G-protein coupled receptors [6].

The basic schema of canonical STAT activation was described long ago [7], although many variations and exceptions have since been noted. But at its core is a mechanism by which an extracellular signal is rapidly transmitted to the nucleus to mediate transcriptional changes. Thus, binding of ligand causes multimerization of the cell-surface receptors and conformational changes that result in activation of intrinsic kinase activity in the case of RTKs, or associated tyrosine kinases in the case of cytokine receptors, particular members of the so-called Janus kinase (JAK) family (Fig. 1.2). This mediates tyrosine phosphorylation of the receptor complex,

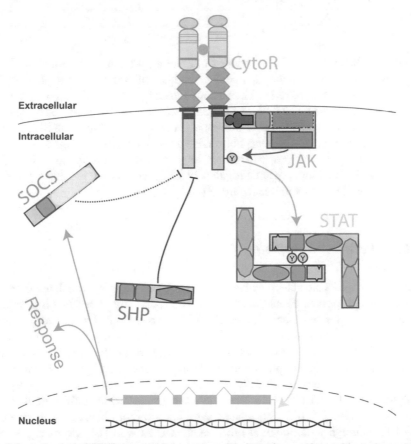

Fig. 1.2 Activation of STATs by cytokine receptors. Binding of a specific cytokine to its receptor leads to conformational changes that activate JAK kinases associated with their intracellular domain. These can then phosphorylate components of the receptor complex in addition to STAT proteins that are recruited by binding to specific phosphotyrosines. The phosphorylated STATs can then form dimers and translocate to the nucleus to induce transcription of responsive genes via specific DNA binding sequences. These include those encoding SOCS proteins that—along with SHPs and other negative regulators—serve to extinguish signaling

Table 1.1 Key activators of individual STAT proteins

STAT protein	Activators		References
	Cytokines	Other factors	
STAT1	IFNα/β, IFNγ, IFNλ	FGF, CCL5	[99, 101, 102, 105, 106, 277]
STAT2	IFNα/β, IFNλ		[101, 113, 277]
STAT3	IL-6, IL-11, IL-21, IL-23, OSM, LIF, LEP, G-CSF, IL-10, IL-22, IFNλ	EGF, PDGF, VEGF TSH, CCL5, TLR-ligands, catecholamines, nicotine	[103, 106, 116–128]
STAT4	IL-12, IL-23		[139]
STAT5 A/B	IL-2, IL-7, IL-9, IL-15, IL-21, IL-3, IL-5, GM-CSF, EPO, TPO, PRL, GH, G-CSF	PDGF, CSF-1, NRG	[21, 141–149, 278]
STAT6	IL-4, IL-13		[169]

generating docking sites for a variety of signaling proteins. These include STAT proteins, which associate via their SH2 domains, with other kinases such as SRC family members also recruited. The various kinases are then able to phosphorylate a conserved tyrosine residue at the C-termini of the STAT proteins. Subsequently, the STATs are able to form stable dimers by interactions between the SH2 domain of one STAT protein and the phosphotyrosine of another. These dimers are then able to translocate to the nucleus, where they impact on the transcription of important target genes by binding to specific regulatory sequences in their promoter, generally exerting a positive effect in this regard [8].

1.2.3 Receptor Specificity

Different receptors are able to activate different STAT proteins, which are then able to mediate appropriate cellular responses. The specificity in activation profiles is largely a consequence of the ability of the STAT to be recruited to the receptor complex via its SH2 domain (Table 1.1). Recruitment is typically facilitated by direct binding of a STAT to specific tyrosine (Y) residues within the cytoplasmic domain of the receptor that become phosphorylated following receptor ligation. For instance, STAT1 is able to dock specifically to Y440 of the interferon gamma (IFNγ) R1 receptor chain [9]. STAT3 is recruited via a consensus Y××Q motif present in several glycoprotein 130 (GP130)-related cytokine receptor chains as well as RTKs [10–13], although it can dock at other sequences as well [14]. Similarly, STAT5 docks to activated receptors at consensus Y××V/L/M motifs [15, 16]. Furthermore, STAT6 can dock to Y578 and Y606 of the interleukin-4 (IL-4) receptor α chain [17].

However, activation of STAT proteins is not reliant on direct docking to receptor phosphotyrosine residues. For example, STAT1 molecules are able to be recruited by binding to STAT2 molecules docked at Y466 of IFNαR1 [18]. In addition, it has been shown that STAT1 activation by growth hormone [19], STAT3 activation by granulocyte colony-stimulating factor (G-CSF) [20] and STAT5 activation by granulocyte-macrophage colony-stimulating factor (GM-CSF) [21], erythropoietin (EPO) [15] and G-CSF [22] can occur in the total absence of receptor tyrosines. In these cases, phosphotyrosine residues present on other components of the receptor components are utilized. Thus, STAT1 and STAT5 can be recruited via docking to activated JAK proteins [23, 24], while STAT3 can dock to phosphotyrosines on other receptor-associated kinases [25]. STAT specificity is therefore determined by recruitment to all components of a receptor complex, rather than just the receptor cytoplasmic domain.

The repertoire of STATs activated by specific receptors can also be affected by the particular cell-type and/or its differentiation state, reflecting differential expression of the STATs themselves or other essential signaling components [26, 27]. Additional modulation of STAT activation can be facilitated by receptor "cross-talk". For instance, interleukin (IL)-4 stimulation can suppress IL-2-mediated STAT5 activation in the same cell [28], IL-10 can similarly suppress IFN-mediated STAT1/2 activation [29], whereas prostaglandin E2 and other cyclic adenosine monophosphate (cAMP)-elevating agents can dampen IL-2-dependent signaling by down-regulating levels of the critical JAK3 protein [30].

1.2.4 Gene Specificity

STATs are able to affect transcription of specific target genes by binding directly to DNA response elements in their promoters. The core recognition site is $TTCN_{2-4}GAA$, but this varies between different STATs [31–33], and so different genes are targeted for induction by different STATs (Table 1.2). For example, STAT1 homodimers act via the so-called gamma interferon activated site (GAS), a regulatory element in the promoter of interferon γ-inducible genes [34]. In contrast, the heterotrimeric STAT1/STAT2/p48 complex utilizes the interferon stimulated response element (ISRE) found upstream of genes induced by IFNs [35]. Moreover, many responsive genes contain closely adjacent tandem sites, with STAT dimer-dimer (tetramer) interactions required to induce maximal transcriptional stimulation, as has been described for STAT5 [36].

The effects of STATs on transcription are mediated, at least in part, through direct association with components of basal transcriptional machinery, including the helicase MCM5 [37] and the histone transacetylase CBP/p300 [38]. In addition, STATs can interact with a range of other transcription factors bound at neighboring sites: for example, STAT1 and Sp1 associate on the ICAM promoter [39], STAT3, c-Jun and the glucocorticoid receptor (GR) form a complex on the α2-macroglobulin promoter [40], STAT5, CEBP/β and GR interact on the β-casein promoter [41], while STAT1 and STAT5 associate with N-myc interacting (Nmi) protein on many promoters [42].

Table 1.2 Selected genes induced by STAT proteins

STAT	Gene function	Genes encoding	References
STAT1	Th1 promoting	TBX21; IL-12; CD40; CD80; IRF-1; 2',3' dioxygenase	[34, 265, 279, 280]
	Anti-viral	ISG54; CIITA	
	Negative regulatory	p21^{Cip}; SOCS1	
	Pro-apoptotic	Caspases	
STAT1/STAT2/p48 (ISGF3)	Th1 promoting	2',3'-dioxygenase	[34, 265]
	Anti-viral	2',5' oligoadenylate synthetase; ISG15; ISG54	
STAT3	Th17 promoting	IL-17; IL-21/22; IL-2Rα	[235, 244, 252, 258, 260, 271, 280–283]
	Anti-apoptotic	BCL2; BCL-x$_L$; Survivin	
	Pro-proliferative	JUNB; c-MYC; Cyclin D	
	Differentiation	Integrins	
	Acute phase	SAA3; CRP	
	Negative regulatory	p19^{Ink4D}; p21^{Cip1}; p27^{Kip1}; SOCS3	
	Angiogenesis	VEGF	
	Metastasis	MMPs; Twist; Snail	
STAT4	Th1 promoting	IFNγ; IL-18 R1	[280, 284]
	Differentiation	FcγRI; IRF-1; MHC class II; CD23	
STAT5 A/B	Treg promoting	FoxP3; IL-2Rα	[83, 152, 154, 241, 250, 285–287]
	Anti-apoptotic	BCL-x$_L$	
	Pro-proliferative	Pim1; Cyclin D1; IGF-1; OSM	
	Differentiation	α-lactalbumin; MUP	
	Negative regulatory	p21^{Cip1}; SOCS2; CISH	
	Metabolic	Adiponectin; PDK4; LPL; AOX	
STAT6	Th2 promoting	GATA3; IL-24; GFI1; IL-4Rα	[48, 238, 245, 288]
	Differentiation	MHC; CD86; FcεRIIa; Cε; Cγ1; Cγ4	
	Anti-apoptotic	Bcl-x$_L$; Bcl-2	

1.2.5 Alternate STAT Isoforms

Naturally-occurring splice variants exist for several STATs, including STAT1β, STAT3β, STAT4β, and STAT5β, which lack a C-terminal activation domain, and so function as a dominant-negative in some, although not all, cell types [43–47]. Similarly, mast cells express a specific STAT6 isoform that appears to act as a repressor of IL-4 transcription [48]. Other isoforms are produced through specific proteolysis, such as STAT3γ [49], STAT3δ [50] and STAT5 p80 [51]. Furthermore, while STATs typically form homodimers, they can also heterodimerize to extend the range of DNA site specificities [52]. For example, G-CSF signaling mediates activation of STAT3, STAT5 and some STAT1 homodimers, but also STAT1/STAT3 and STAT3/STAT5 heterodimers [53, 54]. Similarly, STAT4 is able to form a heterodimer with STAT1 downstream of IL-35R [55], and with STAT3 downstream of IL-23R [56]. Finally, the duration of STAT activation can significantly affect the transcriptional response [54].

1.2.6 Additional Post-Translational Modification

Several mechanisms exist to control STAT activation to either modify or extinguish the response (Fig. 1.1). In addition to tyrosine phosphorylation, STATs are able to undergo serine phosphorylation that affects transcriptional activity. For example, phosphorylation of Ser (S) residues – S708 and S727 on STAT1 and S727 on STAT3 – facilitates an altered transcriptional response that can represent an enhanced or a reduced response depending on the setting [57–60], and is mediated through effects on co-activator recruitment [37] or homodimerization [61]. Specific STATs can also be modified by methylation [62], acetylation [63], SUMOylation [64] and ubiquitination [65, 66] that impacts on their activity. Methylation appears to be a mechanism that enables STAT3 to integrate signals related to energy balance [67], SUMOylation inhibits STAT1 activity via several mechanisms [64, 68], ubiquitination plays a similar inhibitory role for several STATs [65], while acetylation appears to be important for non-canonical functions of STAT3 [69, 70].

1.2.7 Negative Regulators

There are a number of mechanisms by which STATs are negatively regulated (Fig. 1.2). Activated STATs are able to be dephosphorylated to return them to an inactive state. This can occur via the transmembrane protein tyrosine phosphatase receptor-type (PTPRT) [71], or cytoplasmic proteins such as SH2 domain-containing protein tyrosine phosphatase (SHP) proteins that are recruited to activated receptor complexes to dampen signaling [72, 73], or nuclear proteins such as T cell PTP (TC-PTP) [74]. The mechanistic details of serine dephosphorylation remain to be elucidated, although protein phosphatase 2A has been implicated [75]. STATs also induce the transcription of genes encoding the Suppressor of Cytokine Signaling (SOCS) family of negative regulators [76]. SOCS proteins suppress STAT activation by directly blocking JAK activity, competing for docking sites on the receptor complex or targeting receptor components for degradation [77]. Protein inhibitor of activated STATs (PIAS) proteins, in contrast, interact with specific STATs to block their nuclear activity [78], which is due – at least in part – to their ability to SUMOylate STATs [79]. A variety of other mechanism exist to modulate transcriptional responses. For example, STAT5 and BCL6 have antagonistic functions, showing reciprocal occupancy of DNA binding sites due to overlapping binding specificity [80].

There are several layers of specificity with regard to these negative regulatory mechanisms. Firstly, at the level expression. Thus, the expression of SHP-1 [81] and TC-PTP [82] is restricted to hematopoietic and immune cells, and so can only act on STAT activation in these lineages, whereas SHP-2 is more broadly expressed and so has a wider range of influence [81]. Amongst the SOCS proteins, CISH is principally induced by STAT5 [83], whereas SOCS3 is largely induced by STAT3 [77]. Secondly, at the level of protein-protein interactions. For, SHP and SOCS proteins, SH2 domain specificity is a major determinant. For example, the effects of SHP-1 on STAT5 activation is mainly due to its ability to associate with upstream receptors, such as EPO receptor [84], whereas SHP-2 can dock directly to STAT5A [85]. Finally, several of these regulators can act indirectly to promote STAT activation, such as via the ability of SHPs to block the action of SOCS proteins [86].

1.2.8   Non-Canonical STAT Signaling

While STATs participate in an enormous range of biological roles as part of the canonical signaling outlined above, it is clear that they exert numerous effects outside of this paradigm. Perhaps the most widespread of these is the ability of STATs to mediate transcriptional repression at specific promoters, such as described for STAT5 on the promoters for IRF8 [87] and Igk [88]. Certain STATs can also be activated independent of JAKs and receptors. For example, STAT6 can be activated by tyrosine and serine phosphorylation in the endoplasmic reticulum via the protein STING induced by viral infection [89], whereas STAT3 can be phosphorylated in the nucleus by pyruvate kinase M2 in response to changes in glucose metabolism [90]. Amongst the most profound variations from the canonical pathway, however, are the biological roles that have been attributed to unphosphorylated STATs, namely controlling the function of mitochondria and other organelles [91], chromatin remodeling [92] and the modulation of transcriptional responses [93–96]. Interestingly, many of these functions still relate to cytokine signaling since this is one of the mechanisms by which the levels of STAT proteins are up-regulated, which serves to increase the levels of unphosphorylated STATs [97]. Importantly, several of these non-canonical roles are conserved in the single STAT found in *Drosophila* [98].

1.3   Role of STATs in Normal Biology

The collective results from a raft of studies point to critical roles for STAT proteins in development, particularly of immune and blood cells, and as part of various homeostatic and defense processes (Table 1.3).

Table 1.3 STAT functions phenotypes of selected mouse knockouts

STAT	KO type	Relevant phenotypes	Factors affected	References
STAT1	Global	• ↓ innate immune responses/↑ sensitivity to infection	IFNs α/β, γ, λ	[107–109, 289]
		• ↓ chondrocyte proliferation	FGF	[105]
	Myeloid-specific	• ↑ microbial sensitivity	IFNs	[111]
	T cell-specific	• ↑ microbial sensitivity (partial)/↓ protective immunity	IFNs	[111]
	DC-specific	• ↓ protective immunity	IFNs	[111, 112]
STAT2	Global	• ↓ innate immune responses/↑ sensitivity to infection	IFNα/β	[114]
STAT3	Global	• Embryonic lethality	LIF	[129]
	T cell-specific	• ↑ lymphocyte proliferation/↓ apoptosis	IL-2, IL-6	[130]
	Myeloid-specific	• ↑ inflammation/Th1 responses	IL-10	[133]
	Skin-specific	• Impaired wound healing/ disorganized hair cycle	IL-6, EGF	[135]
	Liver-specific	• Impaired acute-phase response	IL-6	[12]
	Thymic epi.-specific	• Disruption of post-natal thymus architecture	?	[138]
	Neuron-specific	• ↓ sensory neuron survival	LIF, CNTF	[136]
	Mammary-specific	• Delayed mammary gland involution	PRL	[137, 290]
	Myocardium-specific	• ↑ susceptibility to heart failure	IL-6 family	[134]
	CD4⁺-specific	• ↓ Th17 cells	IL-6, IL-23	[131]
	Treg-specific	• Lethal auto-immune syndrome	IL-6	[132]
	Uterus-specific	• Embryo implantation failure	LIF, Progesterone	[291]
STAT4	Global	• ↓ Th1 cells/↑ Th2 cell/↓ NK cell-mediated cytotoxicity	IL-12	[140]
		• ↓ obesity-induced insulin resistance/inflammation	IL-12?	[292]
STAT5A	Global	• ↓ mammary gland development/lactogenesis	PRL	[150]
		• ↓ T cell proliferation	IL-2	[151]
STAT5B	Global	• ↓ postnatal growth	GH	[152]
		• ↓ NK proliferation/activity	IL-2, IL-15	[153]

(continued)

Table 1.3 (continued)

STAT	KO type	Relevant phenotypes	Factors affected	References
STAT5A/B	ΔN/Global	• ↓ mammary gland development/↓ postnatal growth	PRL/GH	[154]
		• ↓ T cell proliferation/NK cell deficiency	IL-2	[156]
		• Fetal anemia	EPO	[155]
		• ↓ B cells	IL-7	[157]
	Global	• ↓ T cell proliferation & survival/B cell differentiation block	IL-7	[158]
	Mammary-specific	• ↓ mammary gland development	PRL	[164]
	Liver-specific	• Hepatosteatosis/impaired liver regeneration/↓ growth	GH	[165–167]
	Skeletal muscle-specific	• ↓ postnatal growth	GH	[168]
	CD4+-specific	• Th17 cells	IL-2	[161]
		• Tfh cells	IL-2	[160]
	Hematopoietic-specific	• Impaired erythropoiesis	EPO	[162, 163]
		• Impaired granulopoiesis	GM-CSF	[293]
	Pro B-specific	• ↑V(H) recombination/↓ B cell survival	IL-7	
STAT6	Global	• ↓ Th2 cells/block in B cell IgE class-switching	IL-4, IL-13	[129, 170]
		• Resistance to diet-induced obesity	IL-4	[294]

1.3.1 STAT1

STAT1 is strongly activated via the receptors for IFNα/β, IFNγ and the IFNλs to form STAT1 homodimers [99–101], with IFNα/β and IFNλs also stimulating the formation of the unique STAT1/STAT2/p48 heterodimer [101, 102], called interferon-stimulated gene factor 3 (ISGF3) [35]. STAT1 is also stimulated by other cytokine receptors such as G-CSF receptor and growth hormone (GH) receptor, but typically at lower levels compared to other STATs, generating homodimers as well as heterodimers such as with STAT3 in response to G-CSF [103, 104]. Several other receptor types can also activate STAT1, such as those for fibroblast growth factor (FGF) and the chemokine CCL5 [105, 106].

STAT1-deficient mice exhibit almost complete abrogation of IFN signalling, resulting in ineffective innate immunity against viral and microbial pathogens [107–109]. However, STAT1 also exerts roles outside of the immune system, with defective FGF-dependent chondrocyte proliferation observed in STAT1-deficient embryos [105], but no other overt developmental defects. However, STAT1-deficient mice developed spontaneous tumors, which was exacerbated in the absence of p53, indicating a tumor suppressor role [110]. Specific ablation in myeloid and T cells resulted in enhanced microbial sensitivity [111], whereas ablation in T cells and dendritic cells (DCs) resulted in decreased protective immunity [111, 112].

1.3.2 STAT2

STAT2 is activated by IFNα/β and IFNλs and principally forms the STAT1/STAT2/p48 heterodimeric complex [101, 102, 113]. STAT2-deficient mice exhibit phenotypes that largely overlapped those observed in STAT1-deficient mice, being unresponsive to IFNα/β with high susceptibility to viral infections, although they are still able to respond to IFNγ [114]. Mice in which both STAT1 and STAT2 had been ablated were not responsive to IFNs and showed enhanced susceptibility to infection compared with either single knock-outs, indicating that STAT2 exerts some STAT1-independent effects [115].

1.3.3 STAT3

STAT3 is activated by a broad range of cytokine receptors, particular members of the IL-6R family and related receptors, including IL-6R, IL-11R, oncostatin M receptor (OSMR), leukemia inhibitory factor receptor (LIFR), G-CSFR and leptin receptor (LEPR) as well as the immunomodulatory IL-10R, IL-21R, IL-22R and IL-23R [103, 106, 116–128]. STAT3 is also robustly activated by a variety of other receptors, such as epidermal growth factor receptor (EGFR), platelet-derived growth factor receptor (PDGFR), vascular endothelial growth factor receptor (VEGFR), thyroid stimulating hormone receptor (TSHR), chemokine receptors, Toll-like receptors (TLR), as well as the adrenergic and nicotinic receptors [103, 106, 116–128].

STAT3-deficient mice exhibited embryonic lethality prior to gastrulation, a result of ineffective embryo implantation due to defective LIFR signaling [129]. Numerous tissue-specific STAT3-deficient mice have subsequently been produced that have identified a myriad of roles for this protein later in development. Loss of STAT3 in T cells resulted in reduced T lymphocytes as a consequence of increased apoptosis due to impaired IL-6-induced survival signals and decreased IL-2-mediated proliferation [130], and reduced T helper (Th)17 cells due to impaired responsiveness to both IL-6 and IL-23 [131]. In constrast, ablation in regulatory T (Treg) cells resulted in a lethal auto-immune syndrome due to loss of IL-6 signals [132]. Myeloid cell-specific STAT3 loss also resulted in increased inflammatory responses, including enhanced susceptibility to chronic enterocolitis and endotoxic shock, but this was due to loss of IL-10 signals that caused increased Th1 responses [133]. Liver-specific STAT3 ablation impaired the acute-phase response, also largely attributable to disruption of IL-6R signaling [12], with myocardium-specific ablation leading to increased susceptibility to drug-induced heart failure due to disruption of signals from IL-6 and related cytokines [134]. Other tissue-specific lines have revealed diverse other roles such as various epidermal and follicular functions mediated by IL-6 and EGF, including hair cycle and wound healing [135], sensory neuronal survival via LIF and ciliary neurotropic factor (CNTF) [136], prolactin (PRL)-mediated mammary gland involution [137], and maintenance of thymic function [138].

1.3.4   STAT4

STAT4 is activated exclusively in response to IL-12 and IL-23 [139]. As a consequence, STAT4-deficient mice showed similar phenotypes to IL-12-deficient mice, with lymphocyte development skewed toward T_H2 cells at the expense of T_H1 cells. This was principally due to the inability of natural killer (NK) cells to respond to IL-12 to produce the T_H1-inducing cytokine IFNγ [140].

1.3.5   STAT5 Proteins

The STAT5A and STAT5B proteins are encoded by adjacent genes and are highly homologous, with around 96 % amino acid identity [21, 141]. The STAT5 proteins are activated by a large number of upstream receptors [6]. These include a wide range of cytokine receptors as a result of recruitment to several common signaling chains, including $β_C$ (shared by IL-3R, IL-5R and GM-CSFR) and $γ_C$ (shared by IL-2R, IL-7R, IL-9R, IL-15R and IL-21R), but also through recruitment to several single chain receptors, including EPO receptor, thrombopoietin (TPO) receptor PRL receptor and GH receptor, as well as being activated to a lesser extent by other receptors such as G-CSFR [21, 141–149]. Additionally, several RTKs strongly activate STAT5 including EGFR, PDGFR and colony stimulating factor-1 (CSF-1) receptor [21, 141–149].

A variety of different STAT5-deficient mouse lines have been generated. Surprisingly, ablation of individual STAT5 proteins resulted in distinct and specific phenotypes. STAT5A-deficient mice were principally defective in mammary gland development and lactogenesis attributable to loss of PRL signals, with STAT5B unable to compensate [150], and also showed reduced IL-2-mediated T cell proliferation [151]. STAT5B-deficient mice, on the other, exhibited loss of sexually-dimorphic post-natal growth defect due to ablated growth hormone signals [152], as well as reduced NK cell prolifereation and activation due to abrogated IL-2 and IL-15 signals [153].

The initial mouse line in which both STAT5A and STAT5B were targeted was subsequently demonstrated to possess some functional N-terminally truncated STAT5 protein. Despite this, these so-called 'ΔN' mice showed a combination of the phenotypes that were observed with the respective single knockouts, including reduced PRL-mediated mammary gland development and GH-mediated post-natal growth, as well as female infertility due to a block in PRL-induced development of the corpora lutea [154]. Further analysis of these mice revealed fetal anemia as a result of abrogated EPO signaling [155], a block in IL-2R-mediated T cell proliferation [156], and reduced B cell precursors due to disrupted IL-7R signals [157]. Subsequently, a new doubly-deficient mouse line was generated in which no STAT5 proteins were produced [158]. These mice showed >99 % perinatal lethality, with the fetuses displaying severe hematopoietic defects, with anemia comparable to EPOR deficient mice, a reduction in thymocytes similar to IL-7R and γ_c deficient mice and in splenocytes even more severe than γ_c deficient mice, suggesting the involvement of other receptors [158]. The small number of mice surviving weaning had significantly reduced thymocytes and B cells due to defective IL-7 signaling [158].

Lineage-specific STAT5 knockouts have revealed additional details, including defective IL-2 signals leading to increased Th17 and follicular T helper (Tfh) cells [159, 160] and perturbed IL-7 signals leading to inceased V(H) recombination and decreased B cell survival [161]. They have also confirmed roles in EPO-mediated erythropoiesis [162] and GM-CSF-mediated emergency granulopoiesis [163], PRL-mediated mammopoiesis [164] as well as GH-mediated growth and liver regeneration [165, 166], with distinct roles for STAT5 in GH signaling between liver and skeletal muscle [167, 168].

1.3.6   STAT6

STAT6 is activated principally by IL-4 and IL-13 via specific recruitment to the common receptor chain shared by their respective receptor complexes [169]. STAT6-deficient mice were defective in lymphocyte proliferation and Th2 cell differentiation, showing a more profound defect than that of IL-4R deficient mouse, due to the additional loss of IL-13 signals [129, 170].

1.4   Role of STATs in Disease

Given the important roles played by STATs, it is not surprising that dysregulation and mutation of STATs are associated with significant pathological outcomes, with a particularly important etiological role in immune and inflammatory disorders as well as cancer [171].

1.4.1 Immunodeficiencies

Several STAT mutations have been described that impact on the immune system such that they exacerbate the consequence of microbial exposure. Patients harboring loss-of-function mutations in STAT1 exhibited increased susceptibility to mycobacterial and viral infections, consistent with defective IFN signaling [172–174]. Dominant-negative STAT3 mutations underpin hyper IgE syndrome in which T cell memory defects result in enhanced susceptibility to viral infection [175], and mutations in STAT5B are also associated with immune deficiency [176]. In other disorders, abrogated STAT activation downstream of other mutations appears to represent one of the key mediators of disease, such as defective STAT5 activation downstream of IL-7R and JAK3 mutations in SCID [177] and G-CSFR mutations in severe congenital neutropenia [178].

1.4.2 Immune Disorders

In contrast, a number of immune and inflammatory disorders are associated with enhanced STAT activation. Patients with asthma exhibited increased levels of activated STAT1 that correlated with T cell accumulation [179], and those with gain-of-function STAT1 mutations were susceptible to fatal viral infections due to hyper-responsiveness to IFNs and other cytokines [180, 181]. STAT3 polymorphisms have been linked to autoimmune disorders such as multiple sclerosis [182], whereas STAT4 polymorphisms were associated with the chronic inflammatory disease rheumatoid arthritis as well as systemic lupus erythematosus [183]. Constitutive activation of STAT3 and STAT4 was also observed in intestinal T cells in Crohn's disease [184]. Chronic obstructive pulmonary disease patients exhibited elevated levels of STAT4 activation that skewed T cells to a Th1 phenotype that exacerbated lung injury [183, 185], and constitutive activation of STAT5 was also observed in immune cells of primary Sjogren's syndrome patients [186]. Finally, polymorphisms in STAT6 have been associated with several allergic diseases [187].

1.4.3 Microbial Pathogenesis

As a corollary of their role in immune deficiencies, STAT proteins have been identified as common targets for viruses to augment their infection. For example, paramyxoviruses target STAT1 and STAT2 for degradation to evade IFN signaling [188], such that STAT2 has been shown to serve as a key determinant of host range amongst specific virus strains [189]. Herpes virus can also evade IFN signaling but this is achieved via inhibition of STAT1 nuclear entry [190]. Infection with HIV caused similar impairment of nuclear access, but via action on STAT5 to disrupt IL-7 signaling and potentially contribute to loss of CD4+ T cells [191].

1.4.4   Myeloproliferative Neoplasms/Leukemias/Lymphomas

Constitutive activation of a variety of STATs has been reported in a large number of hematopoietic disorders characterized by increased proliferation at the expense of maturation, specifically myeloproliferative neoplasms (MPNs), leukemias and lymphomas.

In MPNs, constitutive STAT5 activation appears to play the most important etiological role. This is often mediated by hyperactivating mutations in the upstream JAK2 most commonly in polycythemia vera [192], the BCR-ABL translocation in chronic myelogenous leukemia (CML) [193], as well as activating mutations in several cytokine receptors, including erythropoietin receptor in erythrocytosis [194] and thrombopoietin receptor in thrombocythemia [195]. In several cases, the pivotal role of STAT5 has been formally demonstrated [196–198].

In hematological malignancies, constitutive STAT1 activation has been observed in acute myeloid leukemia (AML), various forms of acute lymphoblastic leukemia (ALL) erythroleukemia and Epstein-Barr virus related lymphomas [199, 200], STAT3 in AML, Hodgkins lymphoma, human T cell lymphotropic virus (HTLV) dependent T cell leukemia and multiple myeloma [184, 199–204], STAT5 in AML, megakaryocytic leukemia, and ALL, including HTLV-dependent [199, 200] and STAT6 in Hodgkin's lymphoma [205]. This can be due to activating mutations in the upstream JAKs, including point mutations in JAK1, JAK2 and JAK3 [206–208] translocations such as ETV6-JAK2 [209], as well as overexpression and/or activating mutations of cytokine receptors, including IL-3R components [210, 211] and G-CSFR [212], autocrine secretion of cytokines [213] or by mutations in other genes that cause activation by as yet unknown mechanisms [214]. Alternatively, gain-of-function mutations of both STAT3 and STAT5 have been reported in Sezary syndrome lymphomas [215]. Animal models have confirmed the hyperproliferative effects mediated by STAT5 in myeloid and lymphoid cells [216, 217].

1.4.5   Solid Tumors

Constitutive activation of STATs is also a common observation in a variety of solid tumors, especially of STAT3 and to lesser extent STAT5. For STAT3 this includes squamous cell carcinoma [218], prostate cancer [219], gastric cancer [220], pancreatic cancer [221], lung cancer [222] and ovarian cancer [223], while both STAT3 and STAT5 have been implicated in breast cancer [203, 224] and glioblastoma [225]. This can be mediated by activation of upstream oncogenes, such as EGFR [11] and SRC [226, 227], enhanced secretion of cytokines and growth factors, including as a result of inflammation or infection [228] or disruption or suppression of key negative regulators [229, 230]. Importantly, constitutive STAT3 and STAT5 activation is typically associated with increased tumor proliferation, survival and invasion [231], with several studies confirming the key role for these STATs in several cancer types [220, 232]. In contrast, STAT1 activation often correlates negatively with tumor progression [228, 233].

1.4.6   Other Diseases

STAT proteins have also been implicated in an ever-increasing array of other diseases. For example, loss-of-function STAT5B mutations lead to growth defects associated with growth hormone insensitivity and insulin-like growth factor deficiency [176], while in contrast increased STAT5 activation has been observed in cardiovascular disease [234]. However, these are beyond the scope of this chapter.

1.5   Mechanisms of STAT Action

It is apparent from the studies described in Sects 1.3 and 1.4 that STAT proteins exert pleiotropic functions across diverse cell types participating in a vast range of biological processes. However, closer analysis reveals that many of the underlying mechanisms of STAT action can be grouped into distinct categories that are applicable to both normal biology and disease states. This section summarizes these mechanisms, noting that the same mechanism can be employed by different STAT proteins, different mechanisms can be utilized by the same STAT in different cells, and that more than one may operate concurrently in the same cell.

1.5.1   Proliferation

STATs are able to directly contribute to cell proliferation. This can be mediated by inducing key mediators of cell cycle progression. For example, STAT1, STAT3 and STAT5 can stimulate proliferation by inducing c-MYC [235–237], STAT3 and STAT5 can induce the cell cycle regulator cyclin D1 [238–240], while STAT5 can induce PIM-1 [237]. STATs can also induce pro-proliferative cytokines, such as STAT3-mediated IL-6 production [228] and STAT5-mediated OSM production [238].

1.5.2   Differentiation

STAT proteins can also facilitate various aspects of cell differentiation. This can be at the level of influencing lineage commitment, such as the ability of STAT6 to induce GATA-3 and c-MAF to promote Th2 differentiation and function [238], of STAT4 to induce IFNγ to skew T cell differentiation toward the Th1 subtype by [140], or STAT5 to induce ELF5 to stimulate the development of mammalian epithelium [241]. Repression can also play a role, with STAT5 repressing BCL6A to promote B cell differentiation [242] and IRF8 to block plasmacytoid DC development [87]. As an additional mode of regulation, unphosphorylated STAT5 has been shown to elicit a transcriptional program inhibitory for megakaryocyte differentiation, with STAT5 activation relieving this inhibitory effect to allow differentiation to proceed [96]. STATs can be antagonistic with regard to differentiation, such as STAT3 and STAT5 in Th9 cell development [243]. In addition, STAT proteins can stimulate the production of key proteins that represent the final and often defining stages of differentiation. For example, G-CSFR-mediated STAT3 can induce integrins and promote cell adhesion during granulocytic maturation [244], while IL-4 acts via STAT6 to induce key B cell proteins, such as CD86, MHC molecules and Fc receptors [245]. Finally, PRLR-mediated STAT5 induces hundreds of genes in the mammary gland, many related to the production of milk proteins [246].

1.5.3 Survival

Another key action of STAT proteins is to enhance survival. This is typically mediated through induction of anti-apoptotic genes, including members of the BCL-2 family [247]. Thus, BCL-2 itself is induced by GP130-mediated STAT3 activation [248], the BCL-2-like gene A1 by GM-CSF induced STAT5A [249]. BCL-x_L is induced by STAT3 activated downstream of IL-6R [202], by STAT5 proteins activated downstream of IL-3R [250] or EPOR [251] and by STAT6 downstream of IL-4R [245]. Other pro-survival proteins can also be induced, including as Survivin by STAT3 [252] and Akt by STAT5 [253], or alternatively pro-apoptotic genes can be suppressed, such as Fas and Bad by STAT1 [254]. The enhanced survival mediated by STAT proteins can indirectly augment effects on both proliferation and differentiation.

1.5.4 Negative Regulatory Functions

STAT proteins are also able to exert negative regulatory effects. Indeed, for STAT1 such negative effects represent a major function, with STAT1-deficient mice showing propensity to develop spontaneous tumors, identifying STAT1 as a tumor suppressor [110]. These can be subtle affects to dampen signaling, including via induction of negative regulators such as the SOCS family of proteins; for example, IFNγ-mediated STAT1 induced SOCS1 to limit the potentially pathologic effects of this cytokine [255]. Alternatively, STATs can regulate the cell cycle. Thus, IFN-mediated activation of STAT1 induced the cell-cycle inhibitors p27[kip1] [256] and p21[cip] [257]. Moreover, G-CSF-mediated STAT3 activation similarly induced p27[kip1] in myeloid cells [244, 258], and TPOR-mediated STAT5 activation induced p21[cip] in megakaryocytes [259], whereas IL-6-mediated STAT3 activation induced the alternate cell cycle inhibitor p19[INK4B] [260]. Conversely, essential cell cycle components can be repressed. For example, IFN-mediated STAT1 activatin repressed c-MYC [261] and led to degradation of Cyclin D [262], with IL-6R-mediated STAT3 activation able to repress expression of both c-MYB and c-MYC [263, 264]. These effects on the cell cycle can also represent major drivers for differentiation, the terminal stages of which require cell cycle exit. For example, STAT5-mediated p21^{cip} induction is sufficient for megakaryocyte differentiation [259].

1.5.5 Immune Modulation

Another core property for STAT proteins is their ability to modulate immune responses, which is very relevant in the context of cancer. For example, STAT1 and STAT2 were shown to be important in the polarization of macrophages toward an M1 phenotype [265], and both STAT2 and STAT4 promoted Th1 polarization [266, 267], which collectively contribute to anti-tumor immune responses. In contrast, STAT3 was demonstrated to drive M2 polarization, suppress DC maturation and promote Th17 development, STAT5 contributed to Treg development [268], while STAT6 promoted M2 and Th2 polarization [269, 270]. As a result, STAT3, STAT5 and STAT6 contribute to a tumor-promoting microenvironment that can play an important role in both tumor initiation and malignant progression [228].

1.5.6 Other Mechanisms

STATs can exert their actions via several additional mechanisms, especially in the context of cancer, as investigated in most details with respect to STAT3. These include the stimulation of angiogenesis [271] and metastasis [272], the latter due to increased motility and invasion [273]. This is often concurrent with induction of epithelial-to-mesenchymal transition [274], as well as maintenance of stem cell-ness [275] and induction of chemoresistance [276].

1.6 Conclusion

STAT proteins are clearly pivotal in mediating a range of biological processes through their actions on key genes. A strong illustration of their critical nature is the multiple layers of control that govern their activity, being selectively activated by an array of factors and regulated by diverse mechanisms including phosphorylation status, alternative splicing, specific proteolysis, receptor "cross-talk" and negative feedback loops. Together, this complex control of specificity enables individual cells to instigate the appropriate transcriptional program, and hence biological response, to the myriad of signals it receives at any given time. However, as a result of these pivotal functions, perturbations in STAT activation represent a key mechanism underpinning a wide range of diseases, especially including cancer, as detailed in the next chapter. Moreover, the effects on health and disease often utilize similar underlying mechanisms that must be considered when engineering therapeutic approaches to target STAT proteins.

Acknowledgements The authors recognize the support of an Alfred Deakin Postdoctoral Research Fellowship (CL) from Deakin University.

References

1. Stark GR, Darnell JE Jr (2012) The JAK-STAT pathway at twenty. Immunity 36:503–514
2. O'Sullivan LA, Liongue C, Lewis RS et al (2007) Cytokine receptor signaling through the Jak/Stat/Socs pathway in disease. Mol Immunol 44:2497–2506
3. Kisseleva T, Bhattacharya S, Schroeder-Braunstein J et al (2002) Signaling through the JAK-STAT pathway: recent advances and future challenges. Gene 285:1–24
4. Neculai D, Neculai AM, Verrier S et al (2005) Structure of the unphosphorylated Stat5a dimer. J Biol Chem 280:40782–40787
5. Schindler C, Levy DE, Decker T (2007) JAK-STAT signaling: from interferons to cytokines. J Biol Chem 282:20059–20063
6. Bromberg JF (2001) Activation of STAT proteins and growth control. Bioessays 23:161–169
7. Darnell JE Jr, Kerr IM, Stark GR (1994) JAK-STAT pathways and transcriptional activation in response to interferons and other extracellular signalling proteins. Science 264:1415–1421
8. Horvath CM, Darnell JE Jr (1997) The state of the STATs: recent developments in the study of signal transduction to the nucleus. Curr Opin Cell Biol 9:233–239
9. Heim MII, Kerr IM, Stark GR et al (1995) Contribution of STAT SH2 groups to specific interferon signaling by the Jak-STAT pathway. Science 267:1347–1349
10. Stahl N, Farruggella TJ, Bolton TG et al (1995) Choice of STATs and other substrates specified by modular tyrosine-based motifs in cytokine receptors. Science 267:1349–1353
11. Grandis JR, Drenning SD, Chakraborty A et al (1998) Requirement of Stat3 but not Stat1 activation for epidermal growth factor receptor- mediated cell growth in vitro. J Clin Invest 102:1385–1392
12. Alonzi T, Maritano D, Gorgoni B et al (2001) Essential role of STAT3 in the control of the acute-phase response as revealed by inducible gene inactivation in the liver. Mol Cell Biol 21:1621–1632
13. Floss DM, Mrotzek S, Klocker T et al (2013) Identification of canonical tyrosine-dependent and non-canonical tyrosine-independent STAT3 activation sites in the intracellular domain of the interleukin 23 receptor. J Biol Chem 288:19386–19400
14. Chakraborty A, Dyer KF, Cascio M et al (1999) Identification of a novel Stat3 recruitment and activation motif within the granulocyte colony-stimulating factor receptor. Blood 93:15–24
15. Klingmuller U, Bergelson S, Hsiao JG et al (1996) Multiple tyrosine residues in the cytosolic domain of the erythropoietin receptor promote activation of STAT5. Proc Natl Acad Sci USA 93:8324–8328
16. Osborne LC, Duthie KA, Seo JH et al (2010) Selective ablation of the YxxM motif of IL-7Rα suppresses lymphomagenesis but maintains lymphocyte development. Oncogene 29:3854–3864
17. Hou J, Schindler U, Henzel WJ et al (1994) An interleukin-4-induced transcription factor: IL-4 Stat. Science 265:1701–1706
18. Yan H, Krishnan K, Greenlund AC et al (1996) Phosphorylated interferon-alpha receptor 1 subunit (IFNaR1) acts as a docking site for the latent form of the 113 kDa STAT2 protein. EMBO J 15:1064–1074

19. Wang YD, Wong K, Wood WI (1995) Intracellular tyrosine residues of the human growth hormone receptor are not required for the signaling of proliferation or Jak-STAT activation. J Biol Chem 270:7021–7024
20. Ward AC, Hermans MHA, Smith L et al (1999) Tyrosine-dependent and independent mechanisms of STAT3 activation by the human granulocyte colony-stimulating factor (G-CSF) receptor are differentially utilized depending on G-CSF concentration. Blood 93:113–124
21. Mui AL-F, Wakao H, O'Farrell A-M et al (1995) Interleukin-3, granulocyte-macrophage colony stimulating factor and interleukin-5 transduce signals through two STAT5 homologs. EMBO J 14:1166–1175
22. Dong F, Liu X, de Koning JP et al (1998) Stimulation of Stat5 by granulocyte colony-stimulating factor (G-CSF) is modulated by two distinct cytoplasmic regions of the G-CSF receptor. J Immunol 161:6503–6509
23. Barahmand-Pour F, Meinke A, Groner B et al (1998) Jak2-Stat5 interactions analyzed in yeast. J Biol Chem 273:12567–12575
24. Ali MS, Sayeski PP, Bernstein KE (2000) Jak2 acts as both a STAT1 kinase and as a molecular bridge linking STAT1 to the angiotensin II AT1 receptor. J Biol Chem 275:15586–15593
25. Cao X, Tay A, Guy GR et al (1996) Activation and association of Stat3 with Src in v-Src-transformed cell lines. Mol Cell Biol 16:1595–1603
26. Caldenhoven E, Buitenhuis M, van Dijk TB et al (1999) Lineage-specific activation of STAT3 by interferon-gamma in human neutrophils. J Leukoc Biol 65:391–396
27. Caldenhoven E, van Dijk TB, Raaijmakers JAM et al (1999) Activation of a functionally distinct 80-kDa STAT5 isoform by IL-5 and GM-CSF in human eosinophils and neutrophils. Mol Cell Biol Res Commun 1:95–101
28. Castro A, Sengupta TK, Ruiz DC et al (1999) IL-4 selectively inhibits IL-2-triggered Stat5 activation, but not proliferation, in human T cells. J Immunol 162:1261–1269
29. Ito S, Ansari P, Sakatsume M et al (1999) Interleukin-10 inhibits expression of both interferon alpha- and interferon gamma-induced genes by suppressing tyrosine phosphorylation of STAT1. Blood 93:1456–1463
30. Kolenko V, Rayman P, Roy B et al (1999) Downregulation of JAK3 protein levels in T lymphocytes by prostaglandin E_2 and other cyclic adenosine monophosphate-elevating agents: impact on interleukin-2 receptor signaling pathway. Blood 93:2308–2318
31. Lamb P, Seidel HM, Haslam J et al (1995) STAT protein complexes activated by interferon-γ and gp130 signaling molecules differ in their sequence preferences and transcriptional induction properties. Nucleic Acids Res 23:3283–3289
32. Seidel HM, Milocco LH, Lamb P et al (1995) Spacing of palindromic half sites as a determinant of selective STAT (signal transducers and activators of transcription) DNA binding and transcriptional activity. Proc Natl Acad Sci USA 92:3041–3045
33. Basham B, Sathe M, Grein J et al (2008) In vivo identification of novel STAT5 target genes. Nucleic Acids Res 36:3802–3818
34. Decker T, Kovarik P, Meinke A (1997) GAS elements: a few nucleotides with a major impact on cytokine-induced gene expression. J Interferon Cytokine Res 17:121–134
35. Qureshi SA, Salditt-Georgieff M, Darnell JE Jr (1995) Tyrosine-phosphorylated Stat1 and Stat2 plus a 48-kDa protein all contact DNA in forming interferon-stimulated-gene factor 3. Proc Natl Acad Sci USA 92:3829–3833
36. Bunting KD, Bradley HL, Hawley TS et al (2002) Reduced lymphomyeloid repopulating activity from adult bone marrow and fetal liver of mice lacking expression of STAT5. Blood 99:479–487
37. Zhang JJ, Zhao Y, Chait BT et al (1998) Ser727-dependent recruitment of MCM5 by Stat1α in IFN-γ-induced transcriptional activation. EMBO J 17:6963–6971
38. Zhang JJ, Vinkemeier U, Gu W et al (1996) Two contact regions between Stat1 and CBP/p300 in interferon gamma signaling. Proc Natl Acad Sci USA 93:15092–15096
39. Look DC, Pelletier MR, Tidwell RM et al (1995) Stat1 depends on transcriptional synergy with Sp1. J Biol Chem 270:30264–30267

40. Zhang X, Wrzeszczynska MH, Horvath CM et al (1999) Interacting regions in Stat3 and c-Jun that participate in cooperative transcriptional activation. Mol Cell Biol 19:7138–7146
41. Wyszomierski SL, Rosen JM (2001) Cooperative effects of STAT5 (signal transducer and activator of transcription 5) and C/EBPbeta (CCAAT/enhancer-binding protein-beta) on beta-casein gene transcription are mediated by the glucocorticoid receptor. Mol Endocrinol 15:228–240
42. Zhu M-h, John S, Berg M et al (1999) Functional association of Nmi with Stat5 and Stat1 in IL-2- and IFNγ-mediated signaling. Cell 96:121–130
43. Mui AL-F, Wakao H, Kinoshita T et al (1996) Suppression of interleukin-3-induced gene expression by a C-terminal truncated Stat5: role of Stat5 in proliferation. EMBO J 15:2425–2433
44. Moriggl R, Gouilleux-Gruart V, Jahne R et al (1996) Deletion of the carboxyl terminal trans-activation domain of MGF-Stat5 results in sustained DNA binding and a dominant negative phenotype. Mol Cell Biol 16:6141–6148
45. Caldenhoven E, van Dijk TB, Solari R et al (1996) STAT3 beta, a splice variant of transcription factor STAT3, is a dominant-negative regulator of transcription. J Biol Chem 271:13221–13227
46. de Koning JP, Ward AC, Caldenhoven E et al (2000) STAT3beta does not interfere with granulocyte colony-stimulating factor-induced neutrophilic differentiation. Hematol J 1:220–225
47. Hoey T, Zhang S, Schmidt N et al (2003) Distinct requirements for the naturally occurring splice forms Stat4α and Stat4β in IL-12 responses. EMBO J 22:4237–4248
48. Sherman MA (2001) The role of STAT6 in mast cell IL-4 production. Immunol Rev 179:48–56
49. Chakraborty A, Tweardy DJ (1998) Granulocyte colony-stimulating factor activates a 72-kDa isoform of STAT3 in human neutrophils. J Leukoc Biol 64:675–680
50. Hevehan DL, Miller WM, Papoutsakis ET (2002) Differential expression and phosphorylation of distinct STAT3 proteins during granulocytic differentiation. Blood 99:1627–1637
51. Chakraborty A, Dyer KF, Tweardy DJ (2000) Delineation and mapping of Stat5 isoforms activated by granulocyte colony-stimulating factor in myeloid cells. Blood Cells Mol Dis 26:320–330
52. Darnell JE Jr (1997) STATs and gene regulation. Science 277:1630–1635
53. de Koning JP, Dong F, Smith L et al (1996) The membrane-distal cytoplasmic region of human granulocyte colony-stimulating factor receptor is required for STAT3 but not STAT1 homodimer formation. Blood 87:1335–1342
54. Ward AC, van Aesch YM, Schelen AM et al (1999) Defective internalization and sustained activation of truncated granulocyte colony-stimulating factor receptor found in severe congenital neutropenia/acute myeloid leukemia. Blood 93:447–458
55. Collison LW, Delgoffe GM, Guy CS et al (2012) The composition and signaling of the IL-35 receptor are unconventional. Nat Immunol 13:290–299
56. Trinchieri G, Pflanz S, Kastelein RA (2003) The IL-12 family of heterodimeric cytokines: new players in the regulation of T cell responses. Immunity 19:641–644
57. Zhang X, Blenis J, Li H-C et al (1995) Requirement of serine phosphorylation for formation of STAT-promoter complexes. Science 267:1990–1994
58. Wen Z, Zhong Z, Darnell JE Jr (1995) Maximal activation of transcription by Stat1 and Stat3 requires both tyrosine and serine phosphorylation. Cell 82:241–250
59. Jain N, Zhang T, Fong SL et al (1998) Repression of Stat3 activity by activation of mitogen-activated protein kinase. Oncogene 17:3157–3167
60. Tenoever BR, Ng SL, Chua MA et al (2007) Multiple functions of the IKK-related kinase IKKepsilon in interferon-mediated antiviral immunity. Science 315:1274–1278
61. Ng SL, Friedman BA, Schmid S et al (2011) IkappaB kinase epsilon (IKK(epsilon)) regulates the balance between type I and type II interferon responses. Proc Natl Acad Sci U S A 108:21170–21175

62. Yang J, Huang J, Dasgupta M et al (2010) Reversible methylation of promoter-bound STAT3 by histone-modifying enzymes. Proc Natl Acad Sci USA 107:21499–21504

63. Yuan ZL, Guan YJ, Chatterjee D et al (2005) Stat3 dimerization regulated by reversible acetylation of a single lysine residue. Science 307:269–273

64. Ungureanu D, Vanhatupa S, Gronholm J et al (2005) SUMO-1 conjugation selectively modulates STAT1-mediated gene responses. Blood 106:224–226

65. Ungureanu D, Silvennoinen O (2005) SLIM trims STATs: ubiquitin E3 ligases provide insights for specificity in the regulation of cytokine signaling. Sci STKE 304:pe9

66. Ray S, Zhao Y, Jamaluddin M et al (2014) Inducible STAT3 NH2 terminal mono-ubiquitination promotes BRD4 complex formation to regulate apoptosis. Cell Signal 26:1445–1455

67. Iwasaki H, Kovacic JC, Olive M et al (2010) Disruption of protein arginine N-methyltransferase 2 regulates leptin signaling and produces leanness in vivo through loss of STAT3 methylation. Circ Res 107:992–1001

68. Droescher M, Begitt A, Marg A et al (2011) Cytokine-induced paracrystals prolong the activity of signal transducers and activators of transcription (STAT) and provide a model for the regulation of protein solubility by small ubiquitin-like modifier (SUMO). J Biol Chem 286:18731–18746

69. Nie Y, Erion DM, Yuan Z et al (2009) STAT3 inhibition of gluconeogenesis is downregulated by SirT1. Nat Cell Biol 11:492–500

70. Sestito R, Madonna S, Scarponi C et al (2011) STAT3-dependent effects of IL-22 in human keratinocytes are counterregulated by sirtuin 1 through a direct inhibition of STAT3 acetylation. FASEB J 25:916–927

71. Zhang X, Guo A, Yu J et al (2007) Identification of STAT3 as a substrate of receptor protein tyrosine phosphatase T. Proc Natl Acad Sci USA 104:4060–4064

72. Andersen JN, Mortensen OH, Peters GH et al (2001) Structural and evolutionary relationships among protein tyrosine phosphatase domains. Mol Cell Biol 21:7117–7136

73. Poole AW, Jones ML (2005) A SHPing tale: perspectives on the regulation of SHP-1 and SHP-2 tyrosine phosphatases by the C-terminal tail. Cell Signal 17:1323–1332

74. ten Hoeve J, de Jesus I-SM, Fu Y et al (2002) Identification of a nuclear Stat1 protein tyrosine phosphatase. Mol Cell Biol 22:5662–5668

75. Woetmann A, Nielsen M, Christensen ST et al (1999) Inhibition of protein phosphatase 2A induces serine/threonine phosphorylation, subcellular redistribution, and functional inhibition of STAT3. Proc Natl Acad Sci USA 96:10620–10625

76. Wormald S, Hilton DJ (2004) Inhibitors of cytokine signal transduction. J Biol Chem 279:821–824

77. Trengove MC, Ward AC (2013) SOCS proteins in development and disease. Am J Exp Clin Immunol 2:1–29

78. Shuai K, Liu B (2005) Regulation of gene-activation pathways by PIAS proteins in the immune system. Nat Rev Immunol 5:593–605

79. Palvimo JJ (2007) PIAS proteins as regulators of small ubiquitin-related modifier (SUMO) modifications and transcription. Biochem Soc Trans 35:1405–1408

80. Lin G, LaPensee CR, Qin ZS et al (2014) Reciprocal occupancy of BCL6 and STAT5 on Growth Hormone target genes: contrasting transcriptional outcomes and promoter-specific roles of p300 and HDAC3. Mol Cell Endocrinol 395:19–31

81. Neel BG, Gu H, Pao L (2003) The 'Shp'ing news: SH2 domain-containing tyrosine phosphatases in cell signaling. Trends Biochem Sci 28:284–293

82. Neel BG, Tonks NK (1997) Protein tyrsosine phosphatases in signal transduction. Curr Opin Cell Biol 9:193–204

83. Yoshimura A, Ohkubo T, Kiguchi T et al (1995) A novel cytokine-inducible gene CIS encodes an SH2-containing protein that binds to tyrosine-phosphorylated interleukin 3 and erythropoietin receptors. EMBO J 14:2816–2826

84. Klingmuller U, Lorenz U, Cantley LC et al (1995) Specific recruitment of SH-PTP1 to the erythropoietin receptor causes inactivation of JAK2 and termination of proliferative signals. Cell 80:729–739

85. Chen Y, Wen R, Yang S et al (2003) Identification of Shp-2 as a Stat5A phosphatase. J Biol Chem 278:16520–16527
86. Nicholson SE, De Souza D, Fabri LJ et al (2000) Suppressor of cytokine signaling-3 preferentially binds to the SHP-2-binding site on the shared cytokine receptor subunit gp130. Proc Natl Acad Sci USA 97:6493–6498
87. Esashi E, Wang YH, Perng O et al (2008) The signal transducer STAT5 inhibits plasmacytoid dendritic cell development by suppressing transcription factor IRF8. Immunity 28:509–520
88. Mandal M, Powers SE, Maienschein-Cline M et al (2011) Epigenetic repression of the Igk locus by STAT5-mediated recruitment of the histone methyltransferase Ezh2. Nat Immunol 12:1212–1220
89. Chen H, Sun H, You F et al (2011) Activation of STAT6 by STING is critical for antiviral innate immunity. Cell 147:436–446
90. Gao X, Wang H, Yang JJ et al (2012) Pyruvate kinase M2 regulates gene transcription by acting as a protein kinase. Mol Cell 45:598–609
91. Lee JE, Yang YM, Liang FX et al (2012) Nongenomic STAT5-dependent effects on Golgi apparatus and endoplasmic reticulum structure and function. Am J Physiol Cell Physiol 302:C804–C820
92. Christova R, Jones T, Wu PJ et al (2007) P-STAT1 mediates higher-order chromatin remodelling of the human MHC in response to IFNgamma. J Cell Sci 120:3262–3270
93. Yang J, Chatterjee-Kishore M, Staugaitis SM et al (2005) Novel roles of unphosphorylated STAT3 in oncogenesis and transcriptional regulation. Cancer Res 65:939–947
94. Yang J, Liao X, Agarwal MK et al (2007) Unphosphorylated STAT3 accumulates in response to IL-6 and activates transcription by binding to NFkappaB. Genes Dev 21:1396–1408
95. Morrow AN, Schmeisser H, Tsuno T et al (2011) A novel role for IFN-stimulated gene factor 3II in IFN-gamma signaling and induction of antiviral activity in human cells. J Immunol 186:1685–16893
96. Park HJ, Li J, Hannah R et al (2016) Cytokine-induced megakaryocytic differentiation is regulated by genome wide loss of a uSTAT transcriptional program. EMBO J 35(6):580–594
97. Cheon H, Yang J, Stark GR (2011) The functions of signal transducers and activators of transcriptions 1 and 3 as cytokine-inducible proteins. J Interferon Cytokine Res 31:33–40
98. Yan SJ, Lim SJ, Shi S et al (2011) Unphosphorylated STAT and heterochromatin protect genome stability. FASEB J 25:232–241
99. Shuai K, Schindler C, Prezioso VR et al (1992) Activation of transcription by IFN-gamma: tyrosine phosphorylation of a 91-kD DNA binding protein. Science 258:1808–1812
100. Shuai K, Stark GR, Kerr IM et al (1993) A single phosphotyrosine residue of Stat91 required for gene activation by interferon-gamma. Science 261:1744–1746
101. Kotenko SV, Gallagher G, Baurin VV et al (2003) IFN-lambdas mediate antiviral protection through a distinct class II cytokine receptor complex. Nat Immunol 4:69–77
102. Shuai K, Ziemiecki A, Wilks AF et al (1993) Polypeptide signalling to the nucleus through tyrosine phosphorylation of Jak and Stat proteins. Nature 366:580–583
103. Nicholson SE, Novak U, Ziegler SF et al (1995) Distinct regions of the granulocyte colony-stimulating factor receptor are required for tyrosine phosphorylation of the signaling molecules JAK2, Stat3, and p42, p44 MAPK. Blood 86:3698–3704
104. Freeth JS, Silva CM, Whatmore AJ et al (1998) Activation of the signal transducers and activators of transcription signaling pathway by growth hormone (GH) in skin fibroblasts from normal and GH binding protein-positive Laron syndrome children. Endocrinology 139:20–28
105. Sahni M, Ambrosetti DC, Mansukhani A et al (1999) FGF signaling inhibits chondrocyte proliferation and regulates bone development through the STAT-1 pathway. Genes Dev 13:1361–1366
106. Wong M, Uddin S, Majchrzak B et al (2001) Rantes activates Jak2 and Jak3 to regulate engagement of multiple signaling pathways in T cells. J Biol Chem 276:11427–11431
107. Durbin JE, Hackenmiller R, Simon MC et al (1996) Targeted disruption of the mouse Stat1 gene results in compromised innate immunity to viral disease. Cell 85:443–450

108. Meraz MA, White JM, Sheehan KCF et al (1996) Targeted disruption of the Stat1 gene in mice reveals unexpected physiologic specificity in the JAK-STAT signaling pathway. Cell 84:431–442

109. Dickensheets H, Sheikh F, Park O et al (2013) Interferon-lambda (IFN-lambda) induces signal transduction and gene expression in human hepatocytes, but not in lymphocytes or monocytes. J Leukoc Biol 93:377–385

110. Kaplan DH, Shankaran V, Dighe AS et al (1998) Demonstration of an interferon gamma-dependent tumor surveillence system in immunocompetent mice. Proc Natl Acad Sci USA 95:7556–7561

111. Kernbauer E, Maier V, Stoiber D et al (2012) Conditional Stat1 ablation reveals the importance of interferon signaling for immunity to Listeria monocytogenes infection. PLoS Pathog 8:e1002763

112. Johnson LM, Scott P (2007) STAT1 expression in dendritic cells, but not T cells, is required for immunity to Leishmania major. J Immunol 178:7259–7266

113. Schindler C, Fu XY, Improta T et al (1992) Proteins of transcription factor ISGF-3: one gene encodes the 91-and 84-kDa ISGF-3 proteins that are activated by interferon alpha. Proc Natl Acad Sci USA 89:7836–7839

114. Park C, Li S, Cha E et al (2000) Immune response in Stat2 knockout mice. Immunity 13:795–804

115. Perry ST, Buck MD, Lada SM et al (2011) STAT2 mediates innate immunity to Dengue virus in the absence of STAT1 via the type I interferon receptor. PLoS Pathog 7:e1001297

116. Zhong Z, Wen Z, Darnell JE Jr (1994) Stat3: a STAT family member activated by tyrosine phosphorylation in response to epidermal growth factor and interleukin-6. Science 264:95–98

117. Akira S, Nishio Y, Inoue M et al (1994) Molecular cloning of APRF, a novel IFN-stimulated gene factor 3 p91-related transcription factor involved in the gp130-mediated signalling pathway. Cell 77:63–71

118. Heinrich PC, Behrmann I, Muller-Newen G et al (1998) Interleukin-6-type cytokine signalling through the gp130/Jak/STAT pathway. Biochem J 334:297–314

119. Donnelly RP, Dickensheets H, Finbloom DS (1999) The interleukin-10 signal transduction pathway and regulation of gene expression in mononuclear phagocytes. J Interferon Cytokine Res 19:563–573

120. Park ES, Kim H, Suh JM et al (2000) Involvement of JAK/STAT (Janus kinase/signal transducer and activator of transcription) in the thyrotropin signaling pathway. Mol Endocrinol 14:662–670

121. Yanagisawa M, Nakashima K, Arakawa H et al (2000) Astrocyte differentiation of fetal neuroepithelial cells by interleukin-11 via activation of a common cytokine signal transducer, gp130, and a transcription factor, STAT3. J Neurochem 74:1498–1504

122. Bowman T, Broome MA, Sinibaldi D et al (2001) Stat3-mediated Myc expression is required for Src transformation and PDGF-induced mitogenesis. Proc Natl Acad Sci USA 98:7319–7324

123. Bartoli M, Platt D, Lemtalsi T et al (2003) VEGF differentially activates STAT3 in microvascular endothelial cells. FASEB J 17:1562–1564

124. Arredondo J, Chernyavsky AI, Jolkovsky DL et al (2006) Receptor-mediated tobacco toxicity: cooperation of the Ras/Raf-1/MEK1/ERK and JAK-2/STAT-3 pathways downstream of alpha7 nicotinic receptor in oral keratinocytes. FASEB J 20:2093–2101

125. Landen CN Jr, Lin YG, Armaiz Pena GN et al (2007) Neuroendocrine modulation of signal transducer and activator of transcription-3 in ovarian cancer. Cancer Res 67:10389–10396

126. Caprioli F, Sarra M, Caruso R et al (2008) Autocrine regulation of IL-21 production in human T lymphocytes. J Immunol 180:1800–1807

127. Kortylewski M, Kujawski M, Herrmann A et al (2009) Toll-like receptor 9 activation of signal transducer and activator of transcription 3 constrains its agonist-based immunotherapy. Cancer Res 69:2497–2505

128. Sonnenberg GF, Fouser LA, Artis D (2011) Border patrol: regulation of immunity, inflammation and tissue homeostasis at barrier surfaces by IL-22. Nat Immunol 12:383–390

129. Takeda K, Tanaka T, Shi W et al (1996) Essential role of Stat6 in IL-4 signalling. Nature 380:627–630

130. Takeda K, Kaisho T, Yoshida N et al (1998) Stat3 activation is responsible for IL-6-dependent T cell proliferation through preventing apoptosis: generation and characterization of T cell-specific Stat3-deficient mice. J Immunol 161:4652–4660

131. Yang XO, Panopoulos AD, Nurieva R et al (2007) STAT3 regulates cytokine-mediated generation of inflammatory helper T cells. J Biol Chem 282:9358–9363

132. Chaudhry A, Rudra D, Treuting P et al (2009) CD4+ regulatory T cells control TH17 responses in a Stat3-dependent manner. Science 326:986–991

133. Takeda K, Clausen BE, Kaisho T et al (1999) Enhanced Th1 activity and development of chronic enterocolitis in mice devoid of Stat3 in macrophages and neutrophils. Immunity 10:39–49

134. Jacoby JJ, Kalinowski A, Liu MG et al (2003) Cardiomyocyte-restricted knockout of STAT3 results in higher sensitivity to inflammation, cardiac fibrosis, and heart failure with advanced age. Proc Natl Acad Sci U S A 100:12929–12934

135. Sano S, Itami S, Takeda K et al (1999) Keratinocyte-specific ablation of Stat3 exhibits impaired skin remodeling, but does not affect skin morphogenesis. EMBO J 18:4657–4668

136. Alonzi T, Middleton G, Wyatt S et al (2001) Role of STAT3 and PI 3-kinase/Akt in mediating the survival actions of cytokines on sensory neurons. Mol Cell Neurosci 18:270–282

137. Chapman RS, Lourenco PC, Tonner E et al (1999) Suppression of epithelial apoptosis and delayed mammary gland involution in mice with a conditional knockout of Stat3. Genes Dev 13:2604–2616

138. Sano S, Takahama Y, Sugawara T et al (2001) Stat3 in thymic epithelial cells is essential for postnatal maintenance of thymic architecture and thymocyte survival. Immunity 15:261–273

139. Jacobson NG, Szabo SJ, Weber-Nordt RM et al (1995) Interleukin 12 signaling in T helper type 1 (Th1) cells involves tyrosine phosphorylation of signal transducer and activator of transcription (Stat)3 and Stat4. J Exp Med 181:1755–1762

140. Kaplan MH, Sun YL, Hoey T et al (1996) Impaired IL-12 responses and enhanced development of Th2 cells in Stat4-deficient mice. Nature 382:174–177

141. Azam M, Erdjument-Bromage H, Kreider BL et al (1995) Interleukin-3 signals through multiple isoforms of Stat5. EMBO J 14:1402–1411

142. Gouilleux F, Wakao H, Mundt M et al (1994) Prolactin induces phosphorylation of Tyr694 of Stat5 (MGF), a prerequisite for DNA binding and induction of transcription. EMBO J 13:4361–4369

143. Liu X, Robinson GW, Gouilleux F et al (1995) Cloning and expression of Stat5 and an additional homologue (Stat5b) involved in prolactin signal transduction in mouse mammary tissue. Proc Natl Acad Sci U S A 92:8831–8835

144. Pallard C, Gouilleux F, Benit L et al (1995) Thrombopoietin activates a STAT5-like factor in hematopoietic cells. EMBO J 14:2847–2856

145. Demoulin JB, Uyttenhove C, Van Roost E et al (1996) A single tyrosine of the interleukin-9 (IL-9) receptor is required for STAT activation, antiapoptotic activity, and growth regulation by IL-9. Mol Cell Biol 16:4710–4716

146. Tian S-S, Tapley P, Sincich C et al (1996) Multiple signaling pathways induced by granulocyte colony-stimulating factor involving activation of JAKs, STAT5, and/or STAT3 are required for regulation of three distinct classes of immediate early genes. Blood 88:4435–4444

147. Novak U, Mui A, Miyajima A et al (1996) Formation of STAT5-containing DNA binding complexes in response to colony-stimulating factor-1 and platelet-derived growth factor. J Biol Chem 271:18350–18354

148. Valgeirsdottir S, Paukku K, Silvennoinen O et al (1998) Activation of Stat5 by platelet-derived growth factor (PDGF) is dependent on phosphorylation sites in PDGF beta-receptor juxtamembrane and kinase insert domains. Oncogene 16:505–515

149. Lin JX, Leonard WJ (2000) The role of Stat5a and Stat5b in signaling by IL-2 family cytokines. Oncogene 19:2566–2576

150. Liu X, Robinson GW, Wagner K-U et al (1997) Stat5a is mandatory for adult mammary gland development and lactogenesis. Genes Dev 11:179–186
151. Nakajima H, Liu XW, Wynshaw-Boris A et al (1997) An indirect effect of Stat5a in IL-2-induced proliferation: a critical role for Stat5a in IL-2-mediated IL-2 receptor alpha chain induction. Immunity 7:691–701
152. Udy GB, Towers RP, Snell RG et al (1997) Requirement of STAT5b for sexual dimorphism of body growth rates and liver gene expression. Proc Natl Acad Sci USA 94:7239–7244
153. Imada K, Bloom ET, Nakajima H et al (1998) Stat5b is essential for natural killer cell-mediated proliferation and cytolytic activity. J Exp Med 188:2067–2074
154. Teglund S, McKay C, Schuetz E et al (1998) Stat5a and Stat5b proteins have essential and nonessential, or redundant, roles in cytokine responses. Cell 93:841–850
155. Socolovasky M, Fallon AEJ, Wang S et al (1999) Fetal anemia and apoptosis of red cell progenitors in Stat5a-/-5b-/- mice: a direct role for Stat5 in Bcl-XL induction. Cell 98:181–191
156. Moriggl R, Topham DJ, Teglund S et al (1999) Stat5 is required for IL-2-induced cell cycle progression of peripheral T cells. Immunity 10:249–259
157. Sexl V, Piekorz R, Moriggl R et al (2000) Stat5a/b contribute to interleukin 7-induced B-cell precursor expansion, but ABL- and BCR/ABL-induced transformation are independent of Stat5. Blood 96:2277–2283
158. Yao Z, Cui Y, Watford WT et al (2006) Stat5a/b are essential for normal lymphoid development and differentiation. Proc Natl Acad Sci USA 104:1000–1004
159. Hoelbl A, Kovavic B, Kerenyi MA et al (2006) Clarifying the role of Stat5 in lymphoid development and Abelson induced transformation. Blood 107:4898–4906
160. Laurence A, Tato CM, Davidson TS et al (2007) Interleukin-2 signaling via STAT5 constrains T helper 17 cell generation. Immunity 26:371–381
161. Johnston RJ, Choi YS, Diamond JA et al (2012) STAT5 is a potent negative regulator of TFH cell differentiation. J Exp Med 209:243–250
162. Zhu BM, McLaughlin SK, Na R et al (2008) Hematopoietic-specific Stat5-null mice display microcytic hypochromic anemia associated with reduced transferrin receptor gene expression. Blood 112(5):2071–2080
163. Kimura A, Rieger MA, Simone JM et al (2009) The transcription factors STAT5A/B regulate GM-CSF-mediated granulopoiesis. Blood 114:4721–4728
164. Cui Y, Riedlinger G, Miyoshi K et al (2004) Inactivation of Stat5 in mouse mammary epithelial during pregancy reveals distinct functions in cell proliferation, survival and differentiation. Mol Cell Biol 24:8037–8047
165. Engblom D, Kornfeld JW, Schwake L et al (2007) Direct glucocorticoid receptor-Stat5 interaction in hepatocytes control body size and maturation-related gene expression. Genes Dev 21:1157–1162
166. Cui Y, Hosui A, Sun R et al (2007) Loss of signal transducer and activator of transcription 5 leads to hepatosteatosis and impaired liver regeneration. Hepatology 46:504–513
167. Holloway MG, Cui Y, Laz EV et al (2007) Loss of sexually dimorphic liver gene expression upon hepatocyte-specific deletion of Stat5a-Stat5b locus. Endocrinology 148:1977–1986
168. Klover P, Hennighausen L (2007) Postnatal body growth is dependent on the transcription factors signal transducers and activators of transcription 5a/b in muscle: a role for autocrine/paracrine insulin-like growth factor 1. Endocrinology 148:1489–1497
169. Lin J-X, Migone TS, Tsang M et al (1995) The role of shared receptor motifs and common STAT proteins in the generation of cytokine pleiotropy and redundancy by IL-2, IL-4, IL-7, IL-13 and IL-15. Immunity 2:331–339
170. Kaplan MH, Schindler U, Smiley ST et al (1996) Stat6 is required for mediating responses to IL-4 and for the development of Th2 cells. Immunity 4:313–319
171. O'Shea JJ, Holland SM, Staudt LM (2013) JAKs and STATs in immunity, immunodeficiency, and cancer. N Engl J Med 368:161–170
172. Dupuis S, Dargemont C, Fieschi C et al (2001) Impairment of mycobacterial but not viral immunity by a germline human STAT1 mutation. Science 293:300–303

173. Dupuis S, Jouanguy E, Al-Hajjar S et al (2003) Impaired response to interferon-gamma/beta and lethal viral disease in human STAT1 deficiency. Nat Genet 33:388–391
174. Sharfe N, Nahum A, Newell A et al (2014) Fatal combined immunodeficiency associated with heterozygous mutation in STAT1. J Allergy Clin Immunol 133:807–817
175. Minegishi Y, Saito M, Tsuchiya S et al (2007) Dominant-negative mutations in the DNA-binding domain of STAT3 cause hyper-IgE syndrome. Nature 448:1058–1062
176. Kofoed EM, Hwa V, Little B et al (2003) Growth hormone insensitivity associated with a STAT5b mutation. N Engl J Med 349:1139–1147
177. Yao Z, Cui Y, Watford WT et al (2006) Stat5a/b are essential for normal lymphoid development and differentiation. Proc Natl Acad Sci USA 103(4):1000–1005
178. Liongue C, Wright C, Russell AP et al (2009) Granulocyte colony-stimulating factor receptor: stimulating granulopoiesis and much more. Int J Biochem Cell Biol 41:2372–2375
179. Sampath D, Castro M, Look DC et al (1999) Constitutive activation of an epithelial signal transducer and activator of transcription (STAT) pathway in asthma. J Clin Invest 103:1353–1361
180. Liu L, Okada S, Kong XF et al (2011) Gain-of-function human STAT1 mutations impair IL-17 immunity and underlie chronic mucocutaneous candidiasis. J Exp Med 208:1635–1648
181. Sampaio EP, Hsu AP, Pechacek J et al (2013) Signal transducer and activator of transcription 1 (STAT1) gain-of-function mutations and disseminated coccidioidomycosis and histoplasmosis. J Allergy Clin Immunol 131:1624–1634
182. Jakkula E, Leppa V, Sulonen AM et al (2010) Genome-wide association study in a high-risk isolate for multiple sclerosis reveals associated variants in STAT3 gene. Am J Hum Genet 86:285–291
183. Remmers EF, Plenge RM, Lee AT et al (2007) STAT4 and the risk of rheumatoid arthritis and systemic lupus erythematosus. N Engl J Med 357:977–986
184. Lovato P, Brender C, Agnholt J et al (2003) Constitutive STAT3 activation in intestinal T cells from patients with Crohn's disease. J Biol Chem 278:16777–16781
185. Di Stefano A, Caramori G, Capelli A et al (2004) STAT4 activation in smokers and patients with chronic obstructive pulmonary disease. Eur Respir J 24:78–85
186. Pertovaara M, Silvennoinen O, Isomaki P (2015) STAT-5 is activated constitutively in T cells, B cells and monocytes from patients with primary Sjogren's syndrome. Clin Exp Immunol 181:29–38
187. Murata K, Kumagai H, Kawashima T et al (2003) Selective cytotoxic mechanism of GTP-14564, a novel tyrosine kinase inhibitor in leukemia cells expressing a constitutively active Fms-like tyrosine kinase 3 (FLT3). J Biol Chem 278:32892–32898
188. Andrejeva J, Young DF, Goodbourn S et al (2002) Degradation of STAT1 and STAT2 by the V proteins of simian virus 5 and human parainfluenza virus type 2, respectively: consequences for virus replication in the presence of alpha/beta and gamma interferons. J Virol 76:2159–2167
189. Parisien JP, Lau JF, Horvath CM (2002) STAT2 acts as a host range determinant for species-specific paramyxovirus interferon antagonism and simian virus 5 replication. J Virol 76:6435–6441
190. Afroz S, Brownlie R, Fodje M et al (2016) VP8, the major tegument protein of bovine herpesvirus-1, interacts with cellular STAT1 and inhibits interferon-beta signaling. J Virol 90:4889–4904
191. Landires I, Bugault F, Lambotte O et al (2011) HIV infection perturbs interleukin-7 signaling at the step of STAT5 nuclear relocalization. AIDS 25:1843–1853
192. James C, Ugo V, Le Couédic J-P et al (2005) A unique clonal JAK2 mutation leading to constitutive signalling causes polycythaemia vera. Nature 434:1144–1148
193. Shuai K, Halpern J, ten Hoeve J et al (1996) Constitutive activation of STAT5 by the BCR-ABL oncogene in chronic myelogenous leukemia. Oncogene 13:247–254
194. Arcasoy MO, Harris KW, Forget BG (1999) A human erythropoietin receptor gene mutant causing familial erythrocytosis is associated with deregulation of the rates of Jak2 and Stat5 inactivation. Exp Hematol 27:63–74

195. Gibson SE, Schade AE, Szpurka H et al (2008) Phospho-STAT5 expression pattern with the MPL W515L mutation is similar to that seen in chronic myeloproliferative disorders with JAK2 V617F. Hum Pathol 39:1111–1114

196. de Groot RP, Raaijmakers JAM, Lammers J-WJ et al (1999) STAT5 activation by BCR-Abl contributes to transformation of K562 leukemia cells. Blood 94:1108–1112

197. Funakoshi-Tago M, Tago K, Abe M et al (2010) STAT5 activation is critical for the transformation mediated by myeloproliferative disorder-associated JAK2 V617F mutant. J Biol Chem 285:5296–5307

198. Bar-Natan M, Nelson EA, Walker SR et al (2012) Dual inhibition of Jak2 and STAT5 enhances killing of myeloproliferative neoplasia cells. Leukemia 26:1407–1410

199. Weber-Nordt RM, Egen C, Wehinger J et al (1996) Constitutive activation of STAT proteins in primary lymphoid and myeloid leukemia cells and in Epstein-Barr virus (EBV)-related lymphoma cell lines. Blood 88:809–816

200. Gouilleux-Gruart B, Gouilleux F, Desaint C et al (1996) STAT-related transcription factors are constitutively activated in peripheral blood cells from acute leukemia patients. Blood 87:1692–1697

201. Hayakawa F, Towatari M, Iida H et al (1998) Differential constitutive activation between STAT-related proteins and MAP kinase in primary acute myelogenous leukaemia. Br J Haematol 101:521–528

202. Catlett-Falcone R, Landowski TH, Oshiro MM et al (1999) Constitutive activation of Stat3 signaling confers resistance to apoptosis in human U266 myeloma cells. Immunity 10:105–115

203. Dolled-Filhart M, Camp RL, Kowalski DP et al (2003) Tissue microarray analysis of signal transducers and activators of transcription 3 (Stat3) and phospho-Stat3 (Tyr705) in node-negative breast cancer shows nuclear localization is associated with a better prognosis. Clin Cancer Res 9:594–600

204. Calo V, Migliavacca M, Bazan V et al (2003) STAT proteins: from normal control of cellular events to tumorigenesis. J Cell Physiol 197:157–168

205. Skinnider BF, Elia AJ, Gascoyne RD et al (2002) Signal transducer and activator of transcription 6 is frequently activated in Hodgkin and Reed-Sternberg cells of Hodgkin lymphoma. Blood 99:618–626

206. Hornakova T, Staerk J, Royer Y et al (2009) Acute lymphoblastic leukemia-associated JAK1 mutants activate the Janus kinase/STAT pathway via interleukin-9 receptor alpha homodimers. J Biol Chem 284:6773–6781

207. Lee JW, Kim YG, Soung YH et al (2006) The JAK2 V617F mutation in de novo acute myelogenous leukemias. Oncogene 25:1434–1436

208. Yin C, Sandoval C, Baeg GH (2015) Identification of mutant alleles of JAK3 in pediatric patients with acute lymphoblastic leukemia. Leuk Lymphoma 56:1502–1506

209. Schwaller J, Parganas E, Wang D et al (2000) Stat5 is essential for the myelo- and lymphoproliferative disease induced by TEL/JAK2. Mol Cell 6:693–704

210. Gale RE, Freeburn RW, Khwaja A et al (1998) A truncated isoform of the human beta chain common to the receptors for granulocyte-macrophage colony-stimulating factor, interleukin-3 (IL-3), and IL-5 with increased mRNA expression in some patients with acute leukemia. Blood 91:54–63

211. Testa U, Riccioni R, Diverio D et al (2004) Interleukin-3 receptor in acute leukemia. Leukemia 18:219–226

212. Gits J, van Leeuwen D, Carroll HP et al (2006) Multiple pathways contribute to the hyperproliferative responses from truncated granulocyte colony-stimulating factor receptors. Leukemia 20:2111–2118

213. Scheeren FA, Diehl SA, Smit LA et al (2008) IL-21 is expressed in Hodgkin lymphoma and activates STAT5: evidence that activated STAT5 is required for Hodgkin lymphomagenesis. Blood 111:4706–4715

214. Klampfl T, Gisslinger H, Harutyunyan AS et al (2013) Somatic mutations of calreticulin in myeloproliferative neoplasms. N Engl J Med 369:2379–2390

215. Kiel MJ, Sahasrabuddhe AA, Rolland DC et al (2015) Genomic analyses reveal recurrent mutations in epigenetic modifiers and the JAK-STAT pathway in Sezary syndrome. Nat Commun 6:8470

216. Moriggl R, Sexl V, Kenner L et al (2005) Stat5 tetramer formation is associated with leukemogenesis. Cancer Cell 7:87–99

217. Lewis RS, Stephenson SEM, Ward AC (2006) Constitutive activation of zebrafish stat5 expands hematopoietic cell populations in vivo. Exp Hematol 34:179–187

218. Grandis JR, Drenning SD, Zeng Q et al (2000) Constitutive activation of Stat3 signaling abbrogates apoptosis in squamous cell carcinogenesis in vivo. Proc Natl Acad Sci U S A 97:4227–4232

219. Campbell CL, Jiang Z, Savarese DM et al (2001) Increased expression of the interleukin-11 receptor and evidence of STAT3 activation in prostate carcinoma. Am J Pathol 158:25–32

220. Burke WM, Jin X, Lin HJ et al (2001) Inhibition of constitutively active Stat3 suppresses growth of human ovarian and breast cancer cells. Oncogene 20:7925–7934

221. Baumgart S, Chen NM, Siveke JT et al (2014) Inflammation-induced NFATc1-STAT3 transcription complex promotes pancreatic cancer initiation by KrasG12D. Cancer Discov 4:688–701

222. Errico A (2015) Lung cancer: Driver-mutation-dependent stratification: learning from STAT3. Nat Rev Clin Oncol 12:251

223. Campbell CL, Guardiani R, Ollari C et al (2001) Interleukin-11 receptor expression in primary ovarian carcinomas. Gynecol Oncol 80:121–127

224. Reynolds C, Montone KT, Powell CM et al (1997) Expression of prolactin and its receptor in human breast carcinoma. Endocrinology 138:5555–5560

225. Fan QW, Cheng CK, Gustafson WC et al (2013) EGFR phosphorylates tumor-derived EGFRvIII driving STAT3/5 and progression in glioblastoma. Cancer Cell 24:438–449

226. Bromberg JF, Horvath CM, Besser D et al (1998) Stat3 activation is required for cellular transformation by v-*src*. Mol Cell Biol 18:2553–2558

227. Xi S, Zhang Q, Dyer KF et al (2003) Src kinases mediate STAT growth pathways in squamous cell carcinoma of the head and neck. J Biol Chem 278:31574–31583

228. Yu H, Pardoll D, Jove R (2009) STATs in cancer inflammation and immunity: a leading role for STAT3. Nat Rev Cancer 9:798–809

229. Costa-Pereira AP, Bonito NA, Seckl MJ (2011) Dysregulation of janus kinases and signal transducers and activators of transcription in cancer. Am J Cancer Res 1:806–816

230. Peyser ND, Du Y, Li H et al (2015) Loss-of-function PTPRD mutations lead to increased STAT3 activation and sensitivity to STAT3 inhibition in head and neck cancer. PLoS One 10:e0135750

231. Frank DA (2003) STAT signaling in cancer: insights into pathogenesis and treatment strategies. Cancer Treat Res 115:267–291

232. Iavnilovitch E, Cardiff RD, Groner B et al (2004) Deregulation of Stat5 expression and activation causes mammary tumors in transgenic mice. Int J Cancer 112:607–619

233. Sica A, Mantovani A (2012) Macrophage plasticity and polarization: in vivo veritas. J Clin Invest 122:787–795

234. Mascareno E, El-Shafei M, Maulik N et al (2001) JAK/STAT signaling is associated with cardiac dysfunction during ischemia and reperfusion. Circulation 104:325–329

235. Kiuchi N, Nakajima K, Ichiba M et al (1999) STAT3 is required for the gp130-mediated full activation of the c-myc gene. J Exp Med 189:63–73

236. Nosaka T, Kawashima T, Misawa K et al (1999) STAT5 as a molecular regulator of proliferation, differentiation and apoptosis in hematopoietic cells. EMBO J 18:4754–4765

237. Shirogane T, Fukada T, Muller JM et al (1999) Synergistic roles for Pim-1 and c-Myc in STAT3-mediated cell cycle progression and antiapoptosis. Immunity 11:709–719

238. Ouyang W, Ranganath S, Weindel K et al (1998) Inhibition of Th1 development mediated by GATA-3 through an IL-4 independent mechanism. Immunity 9:745–755

239. Matsumura I, Kitamura T, Wakao H et al (1999) Transcriptional regulation of the cyclin D1 promoter by STAT5: its involvement in cytokine-dependent growth of hematopoietic cells. EMBO J 18:1367–1377

240. Sakamoto K, Creamer BA, Triplett AA et al (2007) The Janus kinase 2 is required for expression and nuclear accumulation of cyclin D1 in proliferating mammary epithelial cells. Mol Endocrinol 21:1877–1892
241. Harris J, Stanford PM, Sutherland KD et al (2006) Socs2 and Elf5 mediate prolactin-induced mammary gland development. Mol Endocrinol 20:1177–1187
242. Walker SR, Nelson EA, Frank DA (2007) STAT5 represses BCL6 expression by binding to a regulatory region frequently mutated in lymphomas. Oncogene 26:224–233
243. Olson MR, Verdan FF, Hufford MM et al (2016) STAT3 impairs STAT5 activation in the development of IL-9-secreting T cells. J Immunol 196(8):3297–3304
244. Wooten DK, Xie X, Bartos D et al (2000) Cytokine signaling through Stat3 activates integrins, promotes adhesion, and induces growth arrest in the myeloid cell line 32D. J Biol Chem 275:26566–26575
245. Goenka S, Kaplan MH (2011) Transcriptional regulation by STAT6. Immunol Res 50:87–96
246. Yamaji D, Kang K, Robinson GW et al (2013) Sequential activation of genetic programs in mouse mammary epithelium during pregnancy depends on STAT5A/B concentration. Nucleic Acids Res 41:1622–1636
247. Grad JM, Zeng XR, Boise LH (2000) Regulation of Bcl-xL: a little bit of this and a little bit of STAT. Curr Opin Oncol 12:543–549
248. Fukada T, Hibi M, Yamanaka Y et al (1996) Two signals are necessary for cell proliferation induced by a cytokine receptor gp130: involvement of STAT3 in anti-apoptosis. Immunity 5:449–460
249. Feldman GM, Rosenthal LA, Liu X et al (1997) STAT5A-deficient mice demonstrate a defect in granulocyte-macrophage colony-stimulating factor-induced proliferation and gene expression. Blood 90:1768–1776
250. Dumon S, Santos SC, Debierre-Grockiego F et al (1999) IL-3 dependent regulation of Bcl-xL gene expression by STAT5 in a bone marrow derived cell line. Oncogene 18:4191–4199
251. Silva M, Benito A, Sanz C et al (1999) Erythropoietin can induce the expression of bcl-x(L) through Stat5 in erythropoietin-dependent progenitor cell lines. J Biol Chem 274:22165–22169
252. Gritsko T, Williams A, Turkson J et al (2006) Persistent activation of Stat3 signaling induces survivin gene expression and confers resistance to apoptosis in human breast cancer cells. Clin Cancer Res 12:11–19
253. Creamer BA, Sakamoto K, Schmidt JW et al (2010) Stat5 promotes survival of mammary epithelial cells through transcriptional activation of a distinct promoter in Akt1. Mol Cell Biol 30:2957–2970
254. Zimmerman MA, Rahman NT, Yang D et al (2012) Unphosphorylated STAT1 promotes sarcoma development through repressing expression of Fas and bad and conferring apoptotic resistance. Cancer Res 72:4724–4732
255. Alexander WS, Starr R, Fenner JE et al (1999) SOCS1 is a critical inhibitor of interferon gamma signaling and prevents the potentially fatal neonatal actions of this cytokine. Cell 98:597–608
256. Wang S, Raven JF, Durbin JE et al (2008) Stat1 phosphorylation determines Ras oncogenicity by regulating p27 kip1. PLoS One 3, e3476
257. Lee CK, Smith E, Gimeno R et al (2000) STAT1 affects lymphocyte survival and proliferation partially independent of its role downstream of IFN-gamma. J Immunol 164:1286–1292
258. de Koning JP, Soede-Bobok AA, Ward AC et al (2000) STAT3-mediated differentiation and survival of myeloid cells in response to granulocyte colony-stimulating factor: role for the cyclin-dependent kinase inhibitor p27Kip1. Oncogene 19:3290–3298
259. Matsumura I, Ishikawa J, Nakajima K et al (1997) Thrombopoietin-induced differentiation of a human megakaryoblastic leukemia cell line, CMK, involves transcriptional activation of p21(WAF1/Cip1) by STAT5. Mol Cell Biol 17:2933–2943
260. Narimatsu M, Nakajima K, Ichiba M et al (1997) Association of Stat3-dependent transcriptional activation of p19INK4D with IL-6-induced growth arrest. Biochem Biophys Res Commun 238:764–768

261. Ramana CV, Grammatikakis N, Chernov M et al (2000) Regulation of c-Myc expression by IFN-gamma through Stat1-dependent and -independent pathways. EMBOJ 19:263–272
262. Dimco G, Knight RA, Latchman DS et al (2010) STAT1 interacts directly with cyclin D1/ Cdk4 and mediates cell cycle arrest. Cell Cycle 9:4638–4649
263. Nakajima K, Yamanaka Y, Nakae K et al (1996) A central role for Stat3 in IL-6-induced regulation of growth and differentiation in M1 leukemia cells. EMBO J 15:3651–3658
264. Minami M, Inoue M, Wei S et al (1996) STAT3 activation is a critical step in GP130-mediated terminal differentiation and growth arrest of a myeloid cell line. Proc Natl Acad Sci U S A 93:3963–3966
265. Rauch I, Muller M, Decker T (2013) The regulation of inflammation by interferons and their STATs. JAKSTAT 2:e23820
266. Han G, Zhao W, Wang L et al (2014) Leptin enhances the invasive ability of glioma stem-like cells depending on leptin receptor expression. Brain Res 1543:1–8
267. Nakayamada S, Kanno Y, Takahashi H et al (2011) Early Th1 cell differentiation is marked by a Tfh cell-like transition. Immunity 35:919–931
268. Zorn E, Nelson EA, Mohseni M et al (2006) IL-2 regulates FOXP3 expression in human CD4+CD25+ regulatory T cells through a STAT-dependent mechanism and induces the expansion of these cells in vivo. Blood 108:1571–1579
269. Maier E, Duschl A, Horejs-Hoeck J (2012) STAT6-dependent and -independent mechanisms in Th2 polarization. Eur J Immunol 42:2827–2833
270. Kapoor N, Niu J, Saad Y et al (2015) Transcription factors STAT6 and KLF4 implement macrophage polarization via the dual catalytic powers of MCPIP. J Immunol 194:6011–6023
271. Niu G, Wright KL, Huang M et al (2002) Constitutive Stat3 activity up-regulates VEGF expression and tumor angiogenesis. Oncogene 21:2000–2008
272. Devarajan E, Huang S (2009) STAT3 as a central regulator of tumor metastases. Curr Mol Med 9:626–633
273. Teng Y, Ross JL, Cowell JK (2014) The involvement of JAK-STAT3 in cell motility, invasion, and metastasis. JAKSTAT 3:e28086
274. Wendt MK, Balanis N, Carlin CR et al (2014) STAT3 and epithelial–mesenchymal transitions in carcinomas. JAKSTAT 3:e28975
275. Kim E, Kim M, Woo DH et al (2013) Phosphorylation of EZH2 activates STAT3 signaling via STAT3 methylation and promotes tumorigenicity of glioblastoma stem-like cells. Cancer Cell 23:839–852
276. Lee HJ, Zhuang G, Cao Y et al (2014) Drug resistance via feedback activation of Stat3 in oncogene-addicted cancer cells. Cancer Cell 26:207–221
277. Kotenko SV, Pestka S (2000) Jak-Stat signal transduction pathway through the eyes of cytokine class II receptor complexes. Oncogene 19:2557–2565
278. Long W, Wagner KU, Lloyd KC et al (2003) Impaired differentiation and lactational failure of Erbb4-deficient mammary glands identify ERBB4 as an obligate mediator of STAT5. Development 130:5257–5268
279. Ramana CV, Gil MP, Schreiber RD et al (2002) Stat1-dependent and -independent pathways in IFN-gamma-dependent signaling. Trends Immunol 23:96–101
280. Adamson AS, Collins K, Laurence A et al (2009) The Current STATus of lymphocyte signaling: new roles for old players. Curr Opin Immunol 21:161–166
281. Cheng GZ, Zhang WZ, Sun M et al (2008) Twist is transcriptionally induced by activation of STAT3 and mediates STAT3 oncogenic function. J Biol Chem 283:14665–14673
282. Fukuda A, Wang SC, Morris JP et al (2011) Stat3 and MMP7 contribute to pancreatic ductal adenocarcinoma initiation and progression. Cancer Cell 19:441–455
283. Yadav A, Kumar B, Datta J et al (2011) IL-6 promotes head and neck tumor metastasis by inducing epithelial-mesenchymal transition via the JAK-STAT3-SNAIL signaling pathway. Mol Cancer Res 9:1658–1667
284. Thieu VT, Yu Q, Chang HC et al (2008) Signal transducer and activator of transcription 4 is required for the transcription factor T-bet to promote T helper 1 cell-fate determination. Immunity 29:679–690

285. Matsumoto A, Masuhara M, Mitsui K et al (1997) CIS, a cytokine inducible SH2 protein, is a target of the JAK-STAT5 pathway and modulates STAT5 activation. Blood 89:3148–3154

286. Matsumoto A, Seki Y, Kubo M et al (1999) Suppression of STAT5 functions in liver, mammary glands, and T cells in cytokine-inducible SH2 protein-1 (CIS1) transgenic mice. Mol Cell Biol 19:6396–6407

287. Zhao P, Stephens JM (2013) Identification of STAT target genes in adipocytes. JAKSTAT 2:e23092

288. Wei L, Vahedi G, Sun HW et al (2010) Discrete roles of STAT4 and STAT6 transcription factors in tuning epigenetic modifications and transcription during T helper cell differentiation. Immunity 32:840–851

289. Kaplan MH, Grusby MJ (1998) Regulation of T helper cell differentiation by STAT molecules. J Leukoc Biol 64:2–5

290. Humphreys RC, Bierie B, Zhao L et al (2002) Deletion of Stat3 blocks mammary gland involution and extends functional competence of the secretory epithelium in the absence of lactogenic stimuli. Endocrinology 143:3641–3650

291. Lee JH, Kim TH, Oh SJ et al (2013) Signal transducer and activator of transcription-3 (Stat3) plays a critical role in implantation via progesterone receptor in uterus. FASEB J 27:2553–2563

292. Dobrian AD, Galkina EV, Ma Q et al (2013) STAT4 deficiency reduces obesity-induced insulin resistance and adipose tissue inflammation. Diabetes 62:4109–4121

293. Malin S, McManus S, Cobaleda C et al (2010) Role of STAT5 in controlling cell survival and immunoglobulin gene recombination during pro-B cell development. Nat Immunol 11:171–179

294. Ricardo-Gonzalez RR, Red Eagle A, Odegaard JI et al (2010) IL-4/STAT6 immune axis regulates peripheral nutrient metabolism and insulin sensitivity. Proc Natl Acad Sci U S A 107:22617–22622

Chapter 2
STAT Proteins in Cancer

Rachel A. O'Keefe and Jennifer R. Grandis

Abstract The seven members of the signal transducer and activator of transcription (STAT) family of proteins are transcription factors that are activated in response to, and mediate signaling downstream of, growth factors and cytokines. STATs are dysregulated in a broad range of cancer types. Although the genes that encode STATs are rarely mutated in cancer, constitutive phosphorylation and hence activation of STATs, particularly STAT3, is a common alteration in cancer. STAT3 and STAT5 are considered to play primarily pro-tumorigenic roles in tumor cells and within the tumor microenvironment (TME), while STAT1 has been described as a tumor suppressor (although recent publications have also revealed pro-tumorigenic functions of STAT1). In this chapter, we survey STATs in cancer, providing a general overview of STAT function and regulation in tumor cells and in immune cells within the TME.

Keywords STAT1 • STAT3 • STAT5 • JAK/STAT • Cancer • Tumor microenvironment

2.1 Introduction

The signal transducer and activator of transcription (STAT) family comprises seven structurally similar proteins (STAT1, STAT2, STAT3, STAT4, STAT5A, STAT5B, and STAT6) that can function as both signaling proteins and transcription factors. STAT5A and STAT5B are encoded by two different genes that generate highly homologous proteins [1, 2]. Although STAT5A and STAT5B are distinct proteins with overlapping but non-redundant functions, they are often referred to collectively as STAT5.

Each STAT protein consists of six functionally conserved domains, including an SH2 domain and the C-terminal transactivation domain (TAD), which can be

R.A. O'Keefe • J.R. Grandis (✉)
Helen Diller Family Comprehensive Cancer Center, University of California, San Francisco, 1450 3rd Street, San Francisco, CA 94158, USA
e-mail: rachel.okeefe@ucsf.edu; jennifer.grandis@ucsf.edu

© Springer International Publishing Switzerland 2016   33
A.C. Ward (ed.), *STAT Inhibitors in Cancer*, Cancer Drug
Discovery and Development, DOI 10.1007/978-3-319-42949-6_2

phosphorylated on a conserved tyrosine residue (Tyr705 in STAT3) [3–6]. Tyrosine phosphorylation of STATs often occurs downstream of cytokine and growth factor receptors. STAT protein phosphorylation leads to STAT dimerization and translocation into the nucleus, where the STAT dimers can activate or repress transcription. Thus, phosphorylation of STATs links growth factor and cytokine signaling to gene expression.

Tyrosine phosphorylation of the TAD domain is the most well-characterized post-translational modification of STAT proteins. Serine phosphorylation of STATs also occurs and has been shown to be dysregulated in cancer [1, 4, 7–12]. Additional STAT regulatory mechanisms include ubiquitination, sumoylation, acetylation, and interactions with protein inhibitor of activated STAT (PIAS) proteins, which block STAT-DNA binding. This chapter will focus on the regulation of tyrosine phosphorylation of STATs in cancer. Recent reviews have addressed alternative STAT regulatory mechanisms [1, 3, 13–15].

2.2 Tyrosine Phosphorylation of STAT Proteins

In normal (non-transformed) cells, tyrosine phosphorylation of STAT proteins is triggered by the binding of growth factors and cytokines to their cognate receptors. Though the precise mechanism of activation is specific to each ligand/receptor complex, a common mechanism of STAT phosphorylation downstream of these receptors is by members of the Janus kinase (JAK) family of non-receptor tyrosine kinases (JAK1, JAK2, JAK3, and TYK2) [4–7, 13, 16, 17] (Fig. 2.1).

Following receptor dimerization, JAKs are recruited to and phosphorylate intracellular tyrosine residues on these receptors [4–7, 13, 16, 17]. For some receptors, phosphorylation of these sites can also be accomplished by autophosphorylation. This creates docking sites for STAT proteins, as the SH2 domains of STATs can bind the phosphorylated residues and, in turn, become phosphorylated by JAKs at the conserved tyrosine residue within the TAD. Phosphorylation at this site promotes STAT homo- or heterodimerization via reciprocal interactions between the SH2 domain of one STAT molecule and the tyrosine-phosphorylated TAD of its dimerization partner. Phosphorylated STAT dimers can be recognized by importins and transported into the nucleus [3, 7, 18], where they can activate or repress gene expression. It should be noted that, while JAKs are the primary mediators of STAT tyrosine phosphorylation downstream of cytokine and growth factor receptors, other kinases have also been shown to phosphorylate STATs.

Given the importance of tyrosine phosphorylation for STAT function and the involvement of STATs in cellular processes that are often dysregulated in cancer, it is not surprising that aberrant phosphorylation of STATs has been observed in many cancer types. Constitutive phosphorylation of STAT proteins often occurs downstream of oncogenic proteins and/or as a result of increased secretion of cytokines or growth factors in the TME. Oncogenic proteins can drive STAT phosphorylation independent of extracellular ligands, uncoupling STAT protein phosphorylation

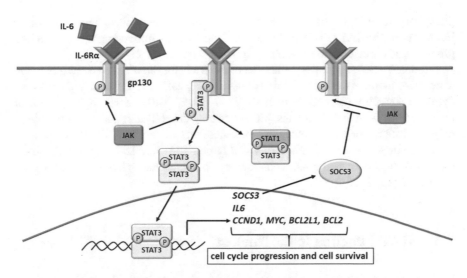

Fig. 2.1 IL-6-induced activation of JAK/STAT3 signaling and gene expression. STAT proteins are important mediators of signal transduction downstream of cytokine and growth factor receptors. Depicted here is STAT3-mediated IL-6 signaling. Binding of IL-6 to IL-6 receptor α (IL-6Rα) induces formation of the IL-6 receptor complex. This leads to activation of JAK family kinases (often JAK1, but also JAK2 or TYK2), which can subsequently phosphorylate several tyrosine residues on gp130. The SH2 domain of STAT3 can then bind to phosphorylated gp130, positioning STAT3 for phosphorylation by JAKs. This promotes STAT3 dimerization, which occurs via reciprocal interactions between the SH2 domain of one STAT3 molecule and the tyrosine-phosphorylated transactivation domain (TAD) of another STAT. STAT3 homodimers can be transported into the nucleus and promote expression of many genes. Shown are examples of STAT3 target genes that promote tumor cell proliferation (*CCND1*, *MYC*), protection from apoptosis (*BCL2L1*, *BCL2*), and immunosuppression in the TME (*IL6*). Notably, STAT3 induction of *IL6* gene expression generates a feed-forward loop that further drives IL-6/JAK/STAT3 signaling. On the other hand, STAT3 also promotes expression of the gene encoding SOCS3 (an inhibitor of JAK1, JAK2, and TYK2). This generates a negative feedback loop that can be disrupted by hypermethylation of the *SOCS3* promoter, which has been detected in several cancer types. IL-6 signaling can also lead to activation of STAT1, which can reduce STAT3 homodimerization by sequestering STAT3 molecules in STAT1:STAT3 heterodimers

from growth factor/cytokine signaling, while increased secretion of cytokines or growth factors in the TME can elicit STAT protein hyperphosphorylation by activating receptors upstream of these STATs [4, 7, 13, 19–22]. Notably, these secreted factors can induce phosphorylation of STATs not only in tumor cells, but also in stromal cells and tumor-infiltrating immune cells.

2.3 Negative Regulators of STAT Signaling

Spatial and temporal regulation of STAT protein phosphorylation is coordinated by a number of phosphatases. While some of these phosphatases act directly on STATs, phosphatases targeting upstream molecules can also elicit downregulation of STAT phosphorylation. Loss of expression or function of these phosphatases or other inhibitors of the JAK/STAT pathway can lead to constitutive activation of STAT proteins and contribute to the malignant phenotype [6, 19, 23–25].

Among the STAT pathway inhibitors that have been shown to be dysregulated in cancer are members of the protein tyrosine phosphatase (PTP) and suppressor of cytokine signaling (SOCS) families [3–6, 17, 19, 23–28]. Interestingly, several of the genes encoding SOCS proteins, which downregulate STAT signaling via inhibition of growth factor/cytokine receptors and members of the JAK family of protein tyrosine kinases, are STAT transcriptional targets [28–30]. This negative feedback loop is disrupted in malignant cells that exhibit hypermethylation of *SOCS* gene promoters [19, 25, 31].

2.4   STAT Function in the Nucleus

STAT protein dimers are transported into the nucleus by importins [3, 7, 18]. Once inside, STAT proteins can either promote or downregulate gene expression, often by cooperating with co-activators and co-repressors of transcription [1, 3, 12, 15]. Thus, STAT target gene expression can be shaped by not only the expression, phosphorylation, and nuclear translocation of STAT proteins themselves, but also by a cadre of transcriptional co-regulators.

It should be noted that, although tyrosine phosphorylation of STAT proteins plays a major role in STAT function, dimerization can occur independent of tyrosine phosphorylation, and unphosphorylated STAT proteins have also been shown to enter the nucleus and activate gene transcription, often in cooperation with other transcription factors [15, 19, 32, 33]. For example, unphosphorylated STAT3 can promote transcription of the oncogene *MET* in cooperation with nuclear factor kappa B (NF-KB) [32, 34].

2.5   STAT Proteins in Tumor-Infiltrating Immune Cells

The mechanisms that regulate STATs within tumor cells also govern their functions in immune cells, wherein STATs have been shown to play diverse roles in innate and adaptive immune cells in the TME. While STAT2 and STAT4 promote the anti-tumor immune response, STAT3 and STAT6 mediate immunosuppression in the TME, and STAT1 and STAT5 have been implicated in both activation and suppression of the anti-tumor immune response (Table 2.1). Thus, the roles of STAT proteins in cancer extend beyond their functions in tumor cells themselves. It is now well-established that immunosuppression in the TME contributes to tumor progression, and therapies that activate the anti-tumor immune response have demonstrated efficacy in a number of cancer types. The functions of STATs in tumor-infiltrating immune cells will be discussed alongside their tumor cell-intrinsic roles in the following sections.

Table 2.1 Diverse roles of STAT proteins in immune cells in the TME

STAT protein	Effects on immune cells in the TME		References
	Anti-tumorigenic	Pro-tumorigenic	
STAT1	• Promotion of Th1 response	• Expansion of MDSCs	[2, 9, 13, 16, 27, 33, 40–47]
	• M1 polarization of macrophages	• M2 polarization of macrophages	
	• Promotion of anti-tumor functions of DCs	• Expression of PD-L1	
STAT2	• Promotion of Th1 response		[16, 81]
STAT3		• Expansion of and immunosuppression by MDSCs	[2, 13, 16, 21, 42, 72–75, 78]
		• M2 polarization of macrophages	
		• Inhibition of DC maturation	
		• Differentiation of Th17 cells	
		• Differentiation and expansion of T_{regs}	
STAT4	• Promotion of Th1 response		[16, 80]
STAT5 A/B	• Promotion of cytotoxic CD8$^+$ T cells	• Differentiation and expansion of T_{regs}	[13, 16, 78, 79]
STAT6		• Expansion of MDSCs	[16, 42, 82, 84–86]
		• M2 polarization of macrophages	
		• Inhibition of tumor infiltration by CD8$^+$ T cells	

2.6   STAT1

STAT1 was initially considered to function primarily as a tumor suppressor. Though studies continue to demonstrate tumor suppressive roles of STAT1, pro-tumorigenic roles of STAT1 have also been identified.

2.6.1   *STAT1 Opposes Tumor Cell Proliferation and Survival*

STAT1 can oppose cell proliferation through the activation of genes that promote growth arrest and through mechanisms independent of its role as a transcription factor. Several STAT1 target genes encode proteins that negatively regulate cell cycle progression, including the cyclin-dependent kinase (CDK) inhibitors p21$^{Cip1/Waf1}$ (gene name: *CDKN1A*) and p27^{Kip1} (*CDKN1B*) [11, 27]. STAT1 can also promote stabilization of p27^{Kip1} through transcriptional repression of the gene encoding

S-phase kinase-associated protein 2 (Skp2), a ubiquitin ligase that tags p27^{Kip1} for proteasomal degradation [35]. In addition, serine-phosphorylated STAT1 can block progression through G1 by interacting with the cyclin D1/CDK4 complex and inducing proteasome-mediated degradation of cyclin D1 [9].

STAT1 can inhibit proliferation by repressing transcription of the proto-oncogene *MYC* [12, 27]. It should be noted, however, that STAT1 was recently identified as a positive regulator of *MYC* transcription in serous papillary endometrial cancer (SPEC) and thus acted as a driver of tumor progression in this cancer type [36]. STAT1 can promote apoptosis by activating the expression of pro-apoptotic genes and inhibiting expression of pro-survival genes [27]. On the other hand, unphosphorylated STAT1 has been shown to protect cells from apoptosis by suppressing the expression of Fas and Bad [37].

2.6.2 STAT1 Can Promote or Inhibit the Anti-Tumor Immune Response

Additional pro- and anti-tumorigenic roles of STAT1 have emerged from studies on STAT1 in tumor-infiltrating immune cells and in modulation of the anti-tumor immune response by tumor cells (Table 2.1, Fig. 2.2). Many functions of STAT1 in cancer are linked to its role as a mediator of type I and type III interferon signaling.

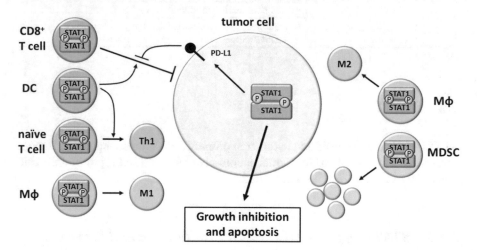

Fig. 2.2 Roles of STAT1 in tumor cells and immune cells within the TME. STAT1 is thought to act primarily as a tumor suppressor through its ability to inhibit growth and promote apoptosis of tumor cells and through its promotion of Th1-type anti-tumor immune responses (left side of figure). STAT1 can promote the activation of tumor cell-targeting Th1 cells by DCs and mediate type I interferon-induced activation of anti-tumor (M1) macrophages (MΦ) and CD8⁺ T cells. However, STAT1 can also promote expansion of immunosuppressive MDSCs and M2 polarization of MΦ (right side of figure), and can induce expression of PD-L1 on tumor cells, protecting them from T cell-mediated lysis

T helper 1 (Th1) immune responses are characterized by the activation of the Th1 subset of CD4$^+$ T cells, which can drive anti-tumor immune responses by releasing pro-inflammatory cytokines such as interferon gamma (IFN-γ) that can mobilize anti-tumor macrophages and cytotoxic CD8$^+$ T cells [13, 16, 38]. STAT1 is an important mediator of the Th1 immune response, as it promotes the expression of IL-12 (a cytokine that induces the polarization of naïve CD4$^+$ T cells into Th1 cells) and mediates the expression of many IFN-γ-inducible genes [13, 16, 39]. Among these genes are those encoding class I major histocompatibility complex (MHC) and co-stimulatory molecules, which are required for effective antigen presentation to and activation of anti-tumor T cells by dendritic cells (DCs) [2, 7, 33]. This implicates STAT1 in the anti-tumor immune response.

STAT1 can antagonize the anti-tumor immune response by inducing expression of the gene encoding programmed death-ligand 1 (PD-L1), an immune checkpoint molecule [8, 40, 41]. PD-L1 expressed on tumor cells engages the inhibitory receptor programmed death-1 (PD-1) on activated natural killer (NK) and T cells in the tumor microenvironment, thereby protecting tumor cells from NK- and T-cell-mediated destruction [8, 41]. A recent study identified activation of the JAK2/STAT1 axis in response to epidermal growth factor (EGF) and interferon gamma (IFN-γ) in head and neck cancer cells [8]. In this system, inhibition of JAK2 abrogated STAT1-dependent expression of PD-L1 and enhanced the ability of NK cells to lyse tumor cells [8].

An additional mechanism by which STAT1 promotes tumor immune evasion is through the induction of myeloid-derived suppressor cells (MDSCs) [27, 42, 43]. MDSCs are a heterogeneous class of immature myeloid cells that share the ability to suppress both innate and adaptive immune cells, thereby impeding the anti-tumor immune response [42]. Immunosuppressive cytokines trigger the expansion of MDSCs, and STAT1 has been shown to promote their accumulation within tumors [27, 43].

STAT1 has also been implicated in immune suppression mediated by another subset of cells of the myeloid lineage: tumor-associated macrophages (TAMs). Macrophages in the tumor microenvironment tend to be polarized toward the immunosuppressive type 2 (M2) phenotype. These TAMs oppose the anti-tumor immune response and are associated with poor prognosis in cancer [44–46]. STAT1 has been implicated in the expansion of M2-polarized macrophages in mouse mammary tumors [44] and in the immunosuppressive functions of M2 TAMs [47]. STAT1 has also been shown to promote M1 macrophage polarization, which is thought to promote the anti-tumor immune response [45, 46].

Overall, the evidence suggests that whether STAT1 functions as a tumor promoter or suppressor is context-specific [27, 33]; i.e., while STAT1 functions as a tumor suppressor by inhibiting tumor cell proliferation and survival in many cancer types, tumor-promoting roles of STAT1 have also been identified (for example, in serous papillary endometrial cancer) [36]. In addition, while STAT1 is a critical mediator of the Th1 response and thereby promotes anti-tumor immunity, it can also effect immunosuppression through expansion of MDSCs and upregulation of the immune checkpoint molecule PD-L1 on tumor cells.

2.7   STAT3

In contrast to STAT1, the functions of STAT3 identified in cancer thus far have been almost exclusively pro-tumorigenic. STAT3 is well-established as a proto-oncogene [3, 48], and constitutive activation of STAT3 has been observed in a broad range of cancer types. In addition, ample evidence implicates STAT3 in suppression of the anti-tumor immune response.

2.7.1   STAT3 Promotes Tumor Cell Proliferation, Survival, Invasion, and Metastasis

Like the other STAT proteins, STAT3 is rarely mutated in cancer. However, STAT3 is phosphorylated downstream of a number of oncogenes, including EGFR [49–51], Src [19, 51, 52], and c-MET [19, 51]. Secretion of STAT3-activating growth factors and cytokines, such as IL-6, and hypermethylation of or loss-of-function mutations in the genes encoding negative regulators of STAT3 signaling, such as SOCS3 or the phosphatases PTPRD and PTPRT, are additional mechanisms by which STAT3 can be constitutively phosphorylated in cancer [4, 23, 24, 31].

The pro-tumorigenic functions of STAT3 stem in part from its ability to activate genes that promote proliferation, protect cells from apoptosis, stimulate angiogenesis, and drive invasion and metastasis [3, 13, 22, 33]. STAT3 target genes that induce cell proliferation include those encoding cyclin D1 (*CCND1*) and c-Myc (*MYC*) [4, 13, 15, 32, 33, 48, 53, 54]. Tumor cell survival can be enhanced by STAT3-mediated expression of the genes *BCL2*, *BCL2L1*, and *BIRC5*, which encode the anti-apoptotic proteins Bcl-2, Bcl-xL and Survivin, respectively [4, 5, 10, 13, 15, 16, 32, 33, 54]. STAT3 promotes angiogenesis in part by activating transcription of the gene encoding vascular endothelial growth factor (VEGF). VEGF, in turn, can promote activation of STAT3 [4, 10, 15, 55, 56]. Additional mediators of STAT3-induced angiogenesis are the matrix metalloproteinases MMP-2, MMP-7, and MMP-9, which degrade the extracellular matrix and basement membrane, facilitating angiogenesis and tumor cell invasion and metastasis [13, 16, 33, 56, 57]. STAT3 also induces epithelial–mesenchymal transition (EMT), a transdifferentiation program that has been shown to enable metastasis, by promoting expression of the EMT-associated transcription factors Snail (*SNAI1*), Twist (*TWIST1*), and ZEB1 (*ZEB1*) [56, 58–62].

Another key function of STAT3 is mediating resistance to cancer therapy, including, but certainly not limited to, the EGFR-targeted monoclonal antibody cetuximab [63], the Src-family kinase inhibitor dasatinib [64], and chemotherapy [20, 65]. In a recent paper, feedback activation of STAT3 was found to mediate resistance to a number of oncogene-targeted therapies [66]. The authors first identified a STAT3-activating feedback loop in an EGFR-mutant non-small cell lung cancer (NSCLC) cell line (PC-9) treated with the EGFR tyrosine kinase inhibitor (TKI) erlotinib. In these cells, erlotinib treatment led to the secretion of molecules that induced tyrosine phosphorylation of STAT3. Exposing erlotinib-naïve PC-9 cells to conditioned medium from erlotinib-treated cells could induce resistance to erlotinib, and knockdown of STAT3 abrogated this effect, demonstrating that inhibition of EGFR could paradoxically drive STAT3 activation and induce STAT3-mediated drug resistance through secretion of STAT3-activating factors. Feedback activation of STAT3 via this mechanism was subsequently observed in many other oncogene-addicted cancer cell lines treated with an inhibitor targeting their driver oncogene. Thus, cumulative evidence supports activation of STAT3 as a common mechanism of resistance to cancer therapy and suggests that targeting STAT3 is a rational strategy to overcome resistance, as has been suggested previously [63, 65, 66].

The STAT3-activating feedback loop reported by Lee and colleagues was identified in the absence of immune cells, but highlights the paradigm of secreted factors in the tumor microenvironment inducing STAT3 phosphorylation within tumor cells [25, 67]. These secreted factors, which may be tumor-, stroma-, and/or immune cell-derived, can also effect STAT3 activation in tumor-infiltrating immune cells, thereby promoting tumor immune evasion.

2.7.2 Activation of STAT3 in Immune Cells in the TME Dampens the Anti-Tumor Immune Response

Activation of STAT3 in tumor cells can promote expression of the genes encoding the immunosuppressive cytokines IL-6, IL-10, and vascular endothelial growth factor (VEGF), which can promote the continued activation of STAT3 in tumor cells in an autocrine or paracrine manner [16, 55, 68]. These cytokines can also drive activation of STAT3 within tumor-infiltrating innate and adaptive immune cells, thereby promoting immunosuppression in the TME [16, 68] (Table 2.1, Fig. 2.3).

Like STAT1, STAT3 can promote the expansion of MDSCs in the TME [16, 42, 68]. Tumor-derived S100A9 protein, the expression of which is promoted by STAT3, drives accumulation of MDSCs [42, 69]. Moreover, STAT3 mediates the immunosuppressive functions of MDSCs by inducing their production of the T cell-suppressive enzymes arginase-I and indoleamine 2,3-dioxygenase (IDO) [70, 71]. STAT3 has also been shown to mediate the secretion of pro-angiogenic factors by MDSCs [16, 22].

STAT3 further promotes immunosuppression in the TME by driving M2 polarization of TAMs and inhibiting dendritic cell (DC) maturation. Activation of STAT3 in TAMs inhibits secretion of pro-inflammatory cytokines and promotes secretion of immunosuppressive cytokines (such as IL-6 and IL-10) that activate STAT3 in DCs [13, 16, 21, 45, 68, 72–74]. STAT3 inhibits the functional maturation of DCs, impeding their ability to activate T cells to mount an effective anti-tumor immune response [13, 21, 45, 68, 72–75].

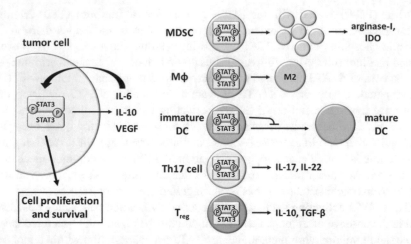

Fig. 2.3 Roles of STAT3 in tumor cells and immune cells within the TME. Activation of STAT3 in tumor cells promotes proliferation, survival, and secretion of the immunosuppressive cytokines IL-6, IL-10, and VEGF. These cytokines can feed back to tumor cells in an autocrine or paracrine manner to further activate STAT3 in tumor cells. In addition, these cytokines can induce phosphorylation of STAT3 in innate and adaptive immune cells in the TME. Activation of STAT3 in MDSCs promotes their expansion and their ability to secrete immunosuppressive enzymes such as arginase-I and IDO. STAT3 promotes M2 polarization of macrophages (MΦ) and inhibits maturation of DCs. STAT3 can also promote differentiation of Th17 and T_{reg} cells and mediate their secretion of IL-17 and IL-22, and IL-10 and TGF-β, respectively. Collectively, activation of STAT3 in tumor-infiltrating immune cells facilitates immunosuppression in the TME

Activation of STAT3 in naïve CD4+ T cells can promote their differentiation into Th17 cells, a T-cell population associated with tumor progression [33, 68, 76, 77]. In addition, STAT3 is implicated in the expansion and immunosuppressive functions of regulatory T cells (T_{regs}) [78]. STAT3 mediates expression of immunosuppressive cytokines in both T_{regs} (which produce IL-10 and transforming growth factor (TGF)-β) and Th17 cells (IL-17 and IL-22) [16, 77]. Secretion of these cytokines can further facilitate immunosuppression in the TME [16].

2.8 STAT5

STAT5 is often implicated in hematologic malignancies, where it is activated downstream of the oncogenic fusion protein BCR-ABL (in chronic myelogenous leukemia (CML)) and as a result of activating mutations in JAK proteins [1, 16, 18, 19]. In solid tumors, cytokines often drive activation of STAT5 [19].

Compared to STAT3, relatively little is known about the role of STAT5 in the anti-tumor immune response. While expression of a constitutively active STAT5 mutant in CD8+ T cells was shown to promote their ability to lyse tumor cells in an immunocompetent mouse model of melanoma [79], suggesting that STAT5 can promote the anti-tumor immune response, STAT5 can also mediate IL-2-induced differentiation of T_{regs}, known antagonists of the anti-tumor immune response [13, 16, 78].

2.9   STAT2, STAT4 and STAT6

The remaining STAT proteins (STAT2, STAT4, and STAT6) have not been as extensively studied in the context of cancer, but functions for each of these proteins in tumor cells and/or immune cells in the TME have nonetheless been identified.

STAT2 and STAT4 participate in Th1 anti-tumor immune responses. STAT4 mediates IL-12-induced expression of IFN-γ [16, 80], while STAT2, operating as a heterodimer with STAT1, promotes expression of IFN-γ-stimulated genes [16, 81].

Evidence suggests that STAT6 primarily mediates pro-tumorigenic functions through its promotion of tumor cell proliferation and survival, particularly in hematologic malignancies [16, 82, 83], and through suppression of the anti-tumor immune response. STAT6 is activated in response to the cytokines IL-4 and IL-13 and mediates the immunosuppressive effects of these cytokines [82]. STAT6 promotes M2 polarization of macrophages and the expansion of MDSCs in the TME [16, 42, 84, 85]. In addition, STAT6 impairs CD8$^+$ T cell tumor infiltration by inducing downregulation of very late antigen-4 (VLA-4, or integrin $\alpha_4\beta_1$), which mediates migration of T cells into tumors [16, 86].

2.10   Conclusion

STAT biology is complex, and both pro- and anti-tumorigenic effects have been described for each STAT protein. STATs play roles in tumor cells as well as other cells in the TME, including tumor-infiltrating immune cells. As such, any attempt to utilize STAT inhibitors must consider the effects of these inhibitors on immune cells as well as on the tumor cells. Modulation of STAT activity in tumor-infiltrating immune cells does not appear to be a side effect of STAT inhibitors; rather, this may be critical for their anti-tumor efficacy. For example, STAT3 inhibitors would be predicted to exert their anti-tumor effects by both abrogating expression of STAT3-regulated genes in tumor cells themselves and antagonizing STAT3-mediated immunosuppression in the TME. Indeed, the anti-tumor efficacy of the STAT3 antisense oligonucleotide AZD9150 is currently thought to stem primarily from its ability to enhance the anti-tumor immune response [87]. STAT5 inhibitors are also in development for cancer treatment, and the bromodomain and extra-terminal (BET) family bromodomain inhibitor JQ1, which inhibits STAT5, has been shown to impact both tumor and immune cells [88–90]. Thus, administering STAT inhibitors, particularly inhibitors of STAT3, may be a promising way to target both tumor cells and the TME and elicit an effective anti-tumor therapeutic response.

References

1. Rani A, Murphy JJ (2015) STAT5 in cancer and immunity. J Interferon Cytokine Res 36(4):226–237
2. Li HS, Watowich SS (2013) Diversification of dendritic cell subsets: emerging roles for STAT proteins. JAKSTAT 2:e25112
3. Santos CI, Costa-Pereira AP (2011) Signal transducers and activators of transcription—from cytokine signalling to cancer biology. Biochim Biophys Acta—Rev Cancer 1816:38–49
4. Costa-Pereira AP, Bonito NA, Seckl MJ (2011) Dysregulation of Janus kinases and Signal transducers and activators of transcription in cancer. Am J Cancer Res 1:806–816
5. Dorritie KA, Redner RL, Johnson DE (2014) STAT transcription factors in normal and cancer stem cells. Adv Biol Regul 56:30–44
6. Xu D, Qu C-K (2008) Protein tyrosine phosphatases in the JAK/STAT pathway. Front Biosci 13:4925–4932
7. Yang J, Stark GR (2008) Roles of unphosphorylated STATs in signaling. Cell Res 18:443–451
8. Concha-Benavente F, Srivastava RM, Trivedi S et al (2016) Identification of the cell-intrinsic and extrinsic pathways downstream of EGFR and IFN that induce PD-L1 expression in head and neck cancer. Cancer Res 76:1031–1043
9. Dimco G, Knight RA, Latchman DS, Stephanou A (2010) STAT1 interacts directly with cyclin D1/Cdk4 and mediates cell cycle arrest. Cell Cycle 9:4638–4649
10. Quesnelle KM, Boehm AL, Grandis JR (2007) STAT-mediated EGFR signaling in cancer. J Cell Biochem 102:311–319
11. Wang S, Raven JF, Durbin JE, Koromilas AE (2008) Stat1 phosphorylation determines Ras oncogenicity by regulating p27Kip1. PLoS One 3:1–14
12. Ramana CV, Grammatikakis N, Chernov M et al (2000) Regulation of c-myc expression by IFN-gamma through Stat1-dependent and -independent pathways. EMBO J 19:263–272
13. Yu H, Kortylewski M, Pardoll D (2007) Crosstalk between cancer and immune cells: role of STAT3 in the tumour microenvironment. Nat Rev Immunol 7:41–51
14. Abroun S, Saki N, Ahmadvand M et al (2015) STATs: an old story, yet mesmerizing. Cell J 17:395–411
15. Timofeeva OP, Tarasova NI (2012) Alternative ways of modulating JAK-STAT pathway: looking beyond phosphorylation. JAKSTAT 1:274–284
16. Yu H, Pardoll D, Jove R (2009) STATs in cancer inflammation and immunity: a leading role for STAT3. Nat Rev Cancer 9:798–809
17. Böhmer F-D, Friedrich K (2014) Protein tyrosine phosphatases as wardens of STAT signaling. JAKSTAT 3:e28087
18. Berger A, Sexl V, Valent P, Moriggl R (2014) Inhibition of STAT5: a therapeutic option in BCR-ABL1-driven leukemia. Oncotarget 5:9564–9576
19. Buchert M, Burns CJ, Ernst M (2016) Targeting JAK kinase in solid tumors: emerging opportunities and challenges. Oncogene 35(8):939–951
20. Barré B, Vigneron A, Perkins N et al (2007) The STAT3 oncogene as a predictive marker of drug resistance. Trends Mol Med 13:4–11
21. Albesiano E, Davis M, See AP et al (2010) Immunologic consequences of signal transducers and activators of transcription 3 activation in human squamous cell carcinoma. Cancer Res 70:6467–6476
22. Kujawski M, Kortylewski M, Lee H et al (2008) Stat3 mediates myeloid cell-dependent tumor angiogenesis in mice. J Clin Invest 118:3367–3377
23. Peyser ND, Du Y, Li H et al (2015) Loss-of-function PTPRD mutations lead to increased STAT3 activation and sensitivity to STAT3 inhibition in head and neck cancer. PLoS One 10:e0135750
24. Peyser ND, Freilino M, Wang L et al (2016) Frequent promoter hypermethylation of PTPRT increases STAT3 activation and sensitivity to STAT3 inhibition in head and neck cancer. Oncogene 35(9):1163–1169

25. Chang Q, Bournazou E, Sansone P et al (2013) The IL-6/JAK/Stat3 feed-forward loop drives tumorigenesis and metastasis. Neoplasia 15:848–862
26. Yoshikawa H, Matsubara K, Qian GS et al (2001) SOCS-1, a negative regulator of the JAK/STAT pathway, is silenced by methylation in human hepatocellular carcinoma and shows growth-suppression activity. Nat Genet 28:29–35
27. Meissl K, Macho-Maschler S, Müller M, Strobl B (2015) The good and the bad faces of STAT1 in solid tumours. Cytokine (in press: doi:10.1016/j.cyto.2015.11.011)
28. Babon JJ, Varghese LN, Nicola NA (2014) Inhibition of IL-6 family cytokines by SOCS3. Semin Immunol 26:13–19
29. Lesina M, Kurkowski MU, Ludes K et al (2011) Stat3/Socs3 activation by IL-6 transsignaling promotes progression of pancreatic intraepithelial neoplasia and development of pancreatic cancer. Cancer Cell 19:456–469
30. Croker BA, Krebs DL, Zhang J-G et al (2003) SOCS3 negatively regulates IL-6 signaling in vivo. Nat Immunol 4:540–545
31. Inagaki-Ohara K, Kondo T, Ito M, Yoshimura A (2013) SOCS, inflammation, and cancer. JAKSTAT 2:e24053
32. Yang J, Liao X, Agarwal MK et al (2007) Unphosphorylated STAT3 accumulates in response to IL-6 and activates transcription by binding to NFkB. Genes Dev 21:1396–1408
33. Avalle L, Pensa S, Regis G et al (2012) STAT1 and STAT3 in tumorigenesis. JAKSTAT 1:65–72
34. Yang J, Chatterjee-Kishore M, Staugaitis SM et al (2005) Novel roles of unphosphorylated STAT3 in oncogenesis and transcriptional regulation. Cancer Res 65:939–947
35. Wang S, Raven JF, Koromilas AE (2010) STAT1 represses Skp2 gene transcription to promote p27Kip1 stabilization in Ras-transformed cells. Mol Cancer Res 8:798–805
36. Kharma B, Baba T, Matsumura N et al (2014) STAT1 drives tumor progression in serous papillary endometrial cancer. Cancer Res 74:6519–6530
37. Zimmerman MA, Rahman N-T, Yang D et al (2012) Unphosphorylated STAT1 promotes sarcoma development through repressing expression of Fas and Bad and conferring apoptotic resistance. Cancer Res 72:4724–4732
38. Knutson KL, Disis ML (2005) Tumor antigen-specific T helper cells in cancer immunity and immunotherapy. Cancer Immunol Immunother 54:721–728
39. Ramana CV, Gil MP, Schreiber RD, Stark GR (2002) Stat1-dependent and -independent pathways in IFN-gamma-dependent signaling. Trends Immunol 23:96–101
40. Loke P, Allison JP (2003) PD-L1 and PD-L2 are differentially regulated by Th1 and Th2 cells. Proc Natl Acad Sci U S A 100:5336–5341
41. Bellucci R, Martin A, Bommarito D et al (2015) Interferon-γ-induced activation of JAK1 and JAK2 suppresses tumor cell susceptibility to NK cells through upregulation of PD-L1 expression. Oncoimmunology 4:e1008824
42. Ostrand-Rosenberg S, Sinha P (2009) Myeloid-derived suppressor cells: linking inflammation and cancer. J Immunol 182:4499–4506
43. Hix LM, Karavitis J, Khan MW et al (2013) Tumor STAT1 transcription factor activity enhances breast tumor growth and immune suppression mediated by myeloid-derived suppressor cells. J Biol Chem 288:11676–11688
44. Tymoszuk P, Evens H, Marzola V et al (2014) In situ proliferation contributes to accumulation of tumor-associated macrophages in spontaneous mammary tumors. Eur J Immunol 44:2247–2262
45. Sica A, Bronte V (2007) Altered macrophage differentiation and immune dysfunction in tumor development. J Clin Invest 117:1155–1166
46. Sica A, Mantovani A (2012) Macrophage plasticity and polarization: in vivo veritas. J Clin Invest 122:787–795
47. Kusmartsev S, Gabrilovich DI (2005) STAT1 signaling regulates tumor-associated macrophage-mediated T cell deletion. J Immunol 174:4880–4891
48. Bromberg JF, Wrzeszczynska MH, Devgan G et al (1999) Stat3 as an oncogene. Cell 98:295–303

49. Grandis JR, Drenning SD, Chakraborty A et al (1998) Requirement of Stat3 but not Stat1 activation for epidermal growth factor receptor-mediated cell growth in vitro. J Clin Invest 102:1385–1392
50. Grandis JR, Drenning SD, Zeng Q et al (2000) Constitutive activation of Stat3 signaling abrogates apoptosis in squamous cell carcinogenesis in vivo. Proc Natl Acad Sci U S A 97:4227–4232
51. Harada D, Takigawa N, Kiura K (2014) The role of STAT3 in non-small cell lung cancer. Cancers (Basel) 6:708–722
52. Xi S, Zhang Q, Dyer KF et al (2003) Src kinases mediate STAT growth pathways in squamous cell carcinoma of the head and neck. J Biol Chem 278:31574–31583
53. Kiuchi N, Nakajima K, Ichiba M et al (1999) STAT3 is required for the gp130-mediated full activation of the c-myc gene. J Exp Med 189:63–73
54. Yu H, Lee H, Herrmann A et al (2014) Revisiting STAT3 signalling in cancer: new and unexpected biological functions. Nat Rev Cancer 14:736–746
55. Niu G, Wright KL, Huang M et al (2002) Constitutive Stat3 activity up-regulates VEGF expression and tumor angiogenesis. Oncogene 21:2000–2008
56. Devarajan E, Huang S (2009) STAT3 as a central regulator of tumor metastases. Curr Mol Med 9:626–633
57. Fukuda A, Wang SC, Morris JP et al (2011) Stat3 and MMP7 contribute to pancreatic ductal adenocarcinoma initiation and progression. Cancer Cell 19:441–455
58. Teng Y, Ross JL, Cowell JK (2014) The involvement of JAK-STAT3 in cell motility, invasion, and metastasis. JAKSTAT 3:e28086
59. Wendt MK, Balanis N, Carlin CR, Schiemann WP (2014) STAT3 and epithelial–mesenchymal transitions in carcinomas. JAKSTAT 3:e28975
60. Xiong H, Hong J, Du W et al (2012) Roles of STAT3 and ZEB1 proteins in E-cadherin down-regulation and human colorectal cancer epithelial–mesenchymal transition. J Biol Chem 287:5819–5832
61. Cheng GZ, Zhang W, Sun M et al (2008) Twist is transcriptionally induced by activation of STAT3 and mediates STAT3 oncogenic function. J Biol Chem 283:14665–14673
62. Yadav A, Kumar B, Datta J et al (2011) IL-6 promotes head and neck tumor metastasis by inducing epithelial–mesenchymal transition via the JAK-STAT3-SNAIL signaling pathway. Mol Cancer Res 9:1658–1667
63. Sen M, Joyce S, Panahandeh M et al (2012) Targeting Stat3 abrogates EGFR inhibitor resistance in cancer. Clin Cancer Res 18:4986–4996
64. Byers LA, Sen B, Saigal B et al (2009) Reciprocal regulation of c-Src and STAT3 in non-small cell lung cancer. Clin Cancer Res 15:6852–6861
65. Poli V, Camporeale A (2015) STAT3-mediated metabolic reprograming in cellular transformation and implications for drug resistance. Front Oncol 5:1–9
66. Lee HJ, Zhuang G, Cao Y et al (2014) Drug resistance via feedback activation of Stat3 in oncogene-addicted cancer cells. Cancer Cell 26:207–221
67. Wan S, Zhao E, Kryczek I et al (2014) Tumor-associated macrophages produce interleukin 6 and signal via STAT3 to promote expansion of human hepatocellular carcinoma stem cells. Gastroenterology 147:1393–1404
68. Lee H, Kumar Pal S, Reckamp K et al (2011) STAT3: a target to enhance antitumor immune response. Curr Top Microbiol Immunol 344:41–59
69. Cheng P, Corzo CA, Luetteke N et al (2008) Inhibition of dendritic cell differentiation and accumulation of myeloid-derived suppressor cells in cancer is regulated by S100A9 protein. J Exp Med 205:2235–2249
70. Vasquez-Dunddel D, Pan F (2013) STAT3 regulates arginase-I in myeloid-derived suppressor cells from cancer patients. J Clin Invest 123:1580–1589
71. Yu J, Wang Y, Yan F et al (2014) Noncanonical NF-kB activation mediates STAT3-stimulated IDO upregulation in myeloid-derived suppressor cells in breast cancer. J Immunol 193:2574–2586

72. Kortylewski M, Kujawski M, Wang T et al (2005) Inhibiting Stat3 signaling in the hematopoietic system elicits multicomponent antitumor immunity. Nat Med 11:1314–1321
73. Park S-J, Nakagawa T, Kitamura H et al (2004) IL-6 regulates in vivo dendritic cell differentiation through STAT3 activation. J Immunol 173:3844–3854
74. Nefedova Y, Huang M, Kusmartsev S et al (2004) Hyperactivation of STAT3 Is involved in abnormal differentiation of dendritic cells in cancer. J Immunol 172:464–474
75. Wang T, Niu G, Kortylewski M et al (2004) Regulation of the innate and adaptive immune responses by Stat-3 signaling in tumor cells. Nat Med 10:48–54
76. Kryczek I, Wei S, Zou L et al (2007) Cutting edge: Th17 and regulatory T cell dynamics and the regulation by IL-2 in the tumor microenvironment. J Immunol 178:6730–6733
77. Kortylewski M, Xin H, Kujawski M et al (2009) Regulation of the IL-23 and IL-12 balance by Stat3 signaling in the tumor microenvironment. Cancer Cell 15:114–123
78. Zorn E, Nelson EA, Mohseni M et al (2006) IL-2 regulates FOXP3 expression in human CD4+CD25+ regulatory T cells through a STAT-dependent mechanism and induces the expansion of these cells in vivo. Blood 108:1571–1579
79. Grange M, Buferne M, Verdeil G et al (2012) Activated STAT5 promotes long-lived cytotoxic CD8+ T cells that induce regression of autochthonous melanoma. Cancer Res 72:76–87
80. Morinobu A, Gadina M, Strober W et al (2002) STAT4 serine phosphorylation is critical for IL-12-induced IFN-gamma production but not for cell proliferation. Proc Natl Acad Sci U S A 99:12281–12286
81. Yue C, Xu J, Tan Estioko MD et al (2014) Host STAT2/type I interferon axis controls tumor growth. Int J Cancer 126:117–126
82. Bruns HA, Kaplan MH (2006) The role of constitutively active Stat6 in leukemia and lymphoma. Crit Rev Oncol Hematol 57:245–253
83. Skinnider BF, Kapp U, Mak TW (2002) The role of interleukin 13 in classical Hodgkin lymphoma. Leuk Lymphoma 43:1203–1210
84. Sinha P, Clements VK, Ostrand-Rosenberg S (2005) Reduction of myeloid-derived suppressor cells and induction of M1 macrophages facilitate the rejection of established metastatic disease. J Immunol 174:636–645
85. Kapoor N, Niu J, Saad Y et al (2015) Transcription factors STAT6 and KLF4 implement macrophage polarization via the dual catalytic powers of MCPIP. J Immunol 194:1–13
86. Sasaki K, Zhao X, Pardee AD et al (2008) Stat6 signaling suppresses VLA-4 expression by CD8+ T cells and limits their ability to infiltrate tumor lesions in vivo. J Immunol 181:104–108
87. McCoon PE, Woessner R, Grosskurth S et al. (2015) Clinical and pre-clinical evidence of an immune modulating role for STAT3-targeting ASO AZD9150 and potential to enhance clinical responses to anti-PDL1 therapy. In: AACR 106th Annual Meeting, Philadelphia, PA, 18–22 April 2015
88. Liu S, Walker SR, Nelson EA et al (2014) Targeting STAT5 in hematologic malignancies through inhibition of the bromodomain and extra-terminal (BET) bromodomain protein BRD2. Mol Cancer Ther 13:1194–1205
89. Toniolo PA, Liu S, Yeh JE et al (2015) Inhibiting STAT5 by the BET bromodomain inhibitor JQ1 disrupts human dendritic cell maturation. J Immunol 194:3180–3190
90. Filippakopoulos P, Qi J, Picaud S et al (2010) Selective inhibition of BET bromodomains. Nature 468:1067–1073

Chapter 3
Translating STAT Inhibitors from the Lab to the Clinic

Suhu Liu and David Frank

Abstract Oncogenic transcription factors represent unique and potentially high value targets for cancer therapy. Proteins like STAT3 and STAT5 are generally not mutated themselves. However, oncogenic signals arising from a wide array of upstream mutations and signaling events converge on a small number of these transcription factors to regulate expression of key genes involved in critical processes including proliferation, survival and invasion. While cancer cells frequently show a high dependency on continued activation of these proteins, normal cells are largely tolerant to interruption of these pathways due to redundancies in transcriptional regulators. Consequently, inhibition of STATs holds the potential to have a very high therapeutic index. The challenge has been to develop strategies to inhibit these proteins that lack domains that are easily amenable to antagonism by small molecules. In recent years, a number of promising strategies have emerged, and now clinical trials of approaches to directly inhibit activated STATs have been developed. The success of these studies, both in terms of clinical efficacy and understanding the molecular effects of STAT inhibitors in humans, may open a new front in the rational, targeted eradication of cancer.

Keywords Cancer • Drug discovery • Gene expression • Signal transduction • STAT transcription factors • Targeted therapy • Clinical trials

3.1 Introduction

Cancer therapy has evolved greatly since its advent in the 1940s, progressing from non-specifically cytotoxic anti-metabolites and alkylating agents to the targeted agents, like kinase inhibitors, that are now available. With the introduction of imatinib (Gleevec), an inhibitor of the Bcr/Abl1 fusion kinase found essentially universally in chronic myeloid leukemia (CML), the treatment of CML was revolutionized.

S. Liu • D. Frank (✉)
Department of Medical Oncology, Dana-Farber Cancer Institute, and Department of Medicine, Brigham and Women's Hospital and Harvard Medical School, Boston, MA, USA
e-mail: suhu_liu@dfci.harvard.edu; david_frank@dfci.harvard.edu

© Springer International Publishing Switzerland 2016
A.C. Ward (ed.), *STAT Inhibitors in Cancer*, Cancer Drug
Discovery and Development, DOI 10.1007/978-3-319-42949-6_3

However, for most other cancers it has proven difficult to identify activated kinases that provide the same therapeutic opportunity. This has raised the question of whether there are common downstream mediators of cancer-driving mutations, which may not be mutated themselves, but which are critical convergence points of oncogenic signaling. In particular, transcription factors, which tightly choreograph the expression of genes under physiologic conditions, can become activated inappropriately in most cancers. While a single transcription factor can often be deleted from normal cells without deleterious consequences to an organism, typically due to redundancies in physiologic signaling, the same transcription factor may represent a critical dependency to a cancer cell. Transcription factors are difficult targets from a medicinal chemistry standpoint. However, the opportunity presented by the fact that they may provide a high therapeutic index has attracted increased attention. The key questions that emerge are whether they are truly critical targets, and whether they can successfully be inhibited in human clinical trials.

3.2 STAT Activation in Cancer

Signal transducers and activators of transcription (STATs) are a family of transcription factors that play important roles in a range of cellular functions. STATs reside in the cytoplasm under basal conditions. Upon activation by tyrosine phosphorylation, STATs form active dimers, translocate to the nucleus, bind to DNA, and regulate transcription of target genes [1]. Under physiological conditions, STATs are activated only transiently. By contrast, in many forms of cancer, STAT family members are activated constitutively and drive the expression of genes underlying malignant cellular behavior. Two family members in particular, STAT3 and STAT5, are activated most commonly in a range of human cancers. Constitutive activation of these transcription factors can directly lead to cancer pathogenesis [2].

3.2.1 Hematologic Malignancies

The transcription factor STAT5 encompasses two highly homologous proteins, STAT5A and STAT5B. In hematological malignancies in particular, inappropriate activation of STAT5 is a common event that leads to increased expression of genes regulating cell cycle progression and survival [3–5]. STAT5 is constitutively active in chronic myelogenous leukemia (CML) [6, 7], acute myelogenous leukemia (AML), acute lymphocytic leukemia (ALL) [3, 8], and Hodgkin lymphoma [9]. STAT5 phosphorylation can be mediated by mutated tyrosine kinases (TKs, such as BCR-ABL1 and JAK2V617F [10, 11]), or autocrine secretion of cytokines that signal through Janus kinase (JAK) [9]. STAT5 plays a crucial role in mediating survival signals emanating from these upstream oncogenic kinases, since disruption of STAT5 abrogate tumorigenesis induced by the oncogenic kinases.

STAT3 is activated in leukemia and lymphoma often through Janus kinases (JAKs). Recently it was found that in anaplastic large cell lymphoma, multiple driver genetic alterations leads to oncogenic STAT3 activation. JAK/STAT3 pathway inhibition consistently impaired lymphoma cell growth in vitro and in vivo [12]. STAT3 also mediates oncogenic addiction to TEL-AML1 in t(12;21) ALL. Consequently, human leukemic cell lines carrying this translocation are highly sensitive to treatment with STAT3 inhibitor [13].

3.2.2 Solid Tumors

STAT activation in solid tumors often occurs through autocrine or paracrine secretion of cytokines and this is also mediated through JAKs. Reflecting how oncogenic pathways often subvert physiologic signaling events, STAT5 plays an important role in normal mammary gland development, and it frequently becomes constitutively activated in breast cancer. The activation of STAT5 in breast cancer may be due to the autocrine, paracrine, or endocrine secretion of prolactin. In the mammary gland, STAT5 is activated late in pregnancy in response to prolactin to promote terminal differentiation and milk production [14–16]. In breast cancer, constitutively activated STAT5 enhances both survival and anchorage-independent growth of human mammary carcinoma cells [17]. Mice that express a constitutively activated form of STAT5 develop mammary carcinomas, whereas mice that lack STAT5A are protected against mammary tumors induced by transforming growth factor α [15, 18, 19].

Using immunohistochemistry to tyrosine phosphorylated STAT3, and similar techniques, it has been found that STAT3 is constitutively activated in an even wider range of solid tumors compared to STAT5, including breast cancer [20], ovarian cancer [21, 22], gastric cancer [23], colorectal cancer [24], lung cancer [25], glioblastoma [26], and pancreatic cancer [27]. Other methods have also revealed a critical role for STAT3 in human cancers. For example, by combining genome-wide RNAi screens with regulatory network analysis, STAT3 has been identified as a critically activated master regulator of HER2(+) breast cancers [28]. In these systems, STAT3 is frequently activated through an IL-6-dependent JAK2-calprotectin axis and inhibition of this axis alone or in combination with HER2 inhibitors reduces tumorigenicity of hormone receptor (−)/HER2(+) breast cancers.

3.3 Critical Role of STATs in the Survival of Cancer Stem-Like Cells

Persistence of cancer stem cells may promote resistance and recurrence of cancer after treatment. Therefore, therapies that target stem and progenitor cells may be particularly important in achieving long-term remissions of cancer. STAT activation has been suggested to play a critical role in cancer stem cell survival in both hematopoietic and solid cancers. Constitutive STAT activation has been implicated in leukemia stem cell self-renewal [29–31]. For example, STAT signaling is enriched in and critical for leukemia stem cell self-renewal in MN1- and HOXA9-co-expressing leukemias, types that harbor a particularly poor prognosis [29]. STAT5 can confer long-term expansion exclusively on human HSCs, by directly modulating Hypoxia-induced factor 2α (HIF2α) expression [31]. In comparing JAK/STAT signaling between leukemia stem cells (LSCs) and normal stem cells from clinical samples, it was found that JAK/STAT signaling is significantly increased in LSCs, particularly from high-risk AML patients. JAK2 inhibition using small molecule inhibitors or RNA interference reduced the growth of AML LSCs while sparing normal stem cells both in vitro and in vivo [32]. Recently it was found that CML stem cell survival is not dependent on the BCR-ABL1 protein kinase, but rather JAK/STAT5 signaling. Thus, while treatment with an ABL tyrosine kinase inhibitor alone may not cure CML patients, dual inhibition of both JAK and BCR-ABL1 may be critical for eradicating primitive quiescent CML stem cells [33]. This observation not only further supports the importance of inhibiting STAT5 in eliminating leukemia stem cells, but also highlights the fact that STAT5 can be activated by multiple aberrant kinases within leukemic stem cells to maintain their survival. Inhibiting STAT5 directly, as the convergence point of multiple upstream oncogenic kinases, may be crucial in achieving a durable therapeutic response.

The critical role of STATs was also found in solid tumor stem-like cells. In glioblastoma, STAT3 was only found to be activated in stem-like cells where it promoted tumorigenicity, but not in more differentiated cells populations [34]. In breast cancer, the JAK2/STAT3 signaling pathway is preferentially active in and required for growth of CD44$^+$CD24$^-$ stem cell-like cancer cells in human tumors [35]. In endometrial cancer, IL-6/JAK1/STAT3 signaling is essential for maintenance of an ALDH^{hi}/CD126$^+$ stem-like component [36]. Furthermore, a small molecule inhibitor targeting STAT3 is effective in inhibiting expression of "stemness" genes and suppresses cancer relapse and metastasis [37]. All of these observations suggest that targeting STATs has the potential to reduce a stem-like cancer cell compartment, which may be the cause of resistance to therapy and tumor recurrence.

3.4   STAT Activation as an Important Mechanism of Resistance to Cancer Therapy

While oncogenic kinase targeted therapy has been extremely successful in the treatment of CML, resistance to targeted therapies develops rapidly in most forms of cancer. One of the important common pathways that mediate this resistance is alternative activation of STATs. It was found that AML cells quickly developed resistance to multi-targeted tyrosine kinase inhibitors through activated JAK2/STAT5 signaling [38]. Even in CML, patients who initially responded well to TKIs could acquire resistance leading to progression of their disease. Indeed, increased activation of STAT5 has been associated with leukemia progression and TKI resistance in

CML [39, 40]. In addition, it has been suggested that an increased level of STAT5 triggers BCR-ABL1 mutation, leading to an increase in inhibitor-resistant BCR-ABL1 mutations [41].

STAT activation has also been found to be an important resistance mechanism in solid tumors. It was found that JAK-mediated STAT5 signaling closely interacts with the PI3K/AKT pathway and mediates resistance to PI3K/AKT inhibition in breast cancer [42]. In melanoma, activation of STAT3 can be induced by MEK or BRAF inhibitors, leading to melanoma cells that are not only resistant to those inhibitors, but also acquire a more invasive phenotype [43, 44]. Thus BRAF inhibitors may need to be combined with STAT3 inhibition to achieve a clinically sustainable response in melanoma [45]. Similarly, in ovarian cancer, resistance to anti-VEGF therapy was found to be mediated through autocrine IL-6/STAT3 signaling [46].

STAT3 activation not only accounts for resistance to targeted therapy, but also plays an important role in resistance to traditional cytotoxic cancer therapies. For example, activated STAT3 can upregulate BCL2 in metastatic breast cancer to promote resistance to chemotherapy [47]. In addition, inhibiting STAT3 activation by blocking IL-6 signaling has been shown to sensitize multiple tumor types to chemotherapy [48]. Tumor permeability is a critical determinant of drug delivery and sensitivity. Using three-dimensional (3D) culture condition, JAK/STAT3 signaling pathway was identified as an essential regulator of tumor permeability barrier function, and STAT3 inhibition increased drug sensitivity. The combination of STAT3 inhibition and 5-FU chemotherapy markedly reduced tumor growth compared to monotherapy. STAT3 activation was also found to be associated with proneural-to-mesenchymal transition observed in gliomas upon radiation therapy [49]. Thus, STAT3 inhibition could be helpful in preventing emergence of therapy-resistant mesenchymal glioma at relapse.

3.5   STAT-Mediated Modulation of the Tumor Microenvironment

STAT3 activation not only directly regulates genes that mediate anti-apoptotic signals and promote malignant cells survival within cells, STAT3 also modulates genes that modify the tumor microenvironment to promote tumor cell survival. For example, not only does activated STAT3 promote angiogenesis, activation of STAT3 also contributes to tumor immune evasion [50]. In STAT3-deficient mice, hyperplastic and early adenoma-like lesions initially formed, but they later completely regressed. This tumor regression correlated with massive immune infiltration into the STAT3-deficient lesions, leading to their elimination [51]. In head and neck squamous cells carcinoma, STAT3 inhibition by siRNA knock-down resulted in enhanced expression and secretion of both pro-inflammatory cytokines and chemokines, and led to the activation of dendritic cells and lymphocytes [52]. STAT3 inhibition was also found to enhance the therapeutic efficacy of immunogenic chemotherapeutic drugs, such as anthracyclines, by stimulating type 1 interferon production by cancer cells

[53]. The important immune checkpoint pathway mediated through programmed death-1 (PD-1) is activated by STAT3 in classic Hodgkin's lymphoma, with JAK-STAT signaling found to promote the induction and increase the abundance of PD-1 ligands expressed on Reed-Sternberg cells [54], which upon binding with PD-1 on tumor infiltrating lymphocytes (TILs), leads to TIL dysfunction.

3.6   Potential Disadvantages of Targeting STAT Transcription Factors in Cancer

Despite the convincing evidence that inappropriate activation of STAT3 and STAT5 can promote oncogenesis, there is evidence showing that in certain cellular context, STAT3 or STAT5 may exert tumor suppressive activities. Identifying and characterizing these cellular contexts is equally essential in designing effective targeted therapies for these proteins. For example, it has been found that mouse models with STAT5-deficiency in hematopoietic cells are permissive for Myc-induced B-cell leukemogenesis [55]. In JAK2V617F-driven myeloproliferative neoplasms in mouse models, deletion of STAT3 enhances myeloid cell expansion and increases the severity of myeloproliferative diseases [56]. In a Pten-deficient prostate cancer mouse model, genetic inactivation of STAT3 or IL-6 signaling accelerates cancer progression leading to metastasis. In addition, loss of STAT3 signaling was found to disrupt the ARF-Mdm2-p53 tumor suppressor axis through bypassing senescence [57].

The role of STAT3 in KRAS-induced malignancy is more complicated, with different mouse models showing distinct roles of STAT3 in KRAS-driven malignancy. In mouse pancreatic cancer models, STAT3 was shown to be essential for pancreatic ductal adenocarcinoma initiation and progression driven by KRAS [58, 59]. On the other hand, in lung adenocarcinoma models also driven by KRAS, two different groups demonstrated that depletion of STAT3 accelerates RAS-induced lung cancer [60–62]. Since the mitochondrial role of STAT3 in supporting KRAS-induced transformation has been well established [63], it is possible that the conflicting effects of STAT3 in KRAS-dependent malignancy may be related to its role as a transcription factor. STAT3 may drive different sets of target genes expression that either support or antagonize KRAS-induced transformation in different cellular contexts.

In breast cancer, both molecular and epidemiological evidence suggests that the co-activation of STAT5 with STAT3 leads to a less aggressive tumor. This may be mediated, at least in part, by modulation of expression of the oncogenic transcriptional regulator BCL6. Whereas expression of this gene is induced by STAT3, it is repressed by STAT5, even in the presence of activated STAT3 [64, 65]. Thus, it remains unclear as to whether inhibition of STAT5 will be of therapeutic value in the large fraction of breast cancers in which both STAT3 and STAT5 are activated.

3.7 Unbiased Approaches to Identify STAT Inhibitors

Based on our understanding of the mechanism of STAT activation in cancer, various strategies to inhibit STAT transcriptional function have been designed. One approach is to use structure-based design, targeting specific STAT domains or critical steps in STAT function [4]. Such approaches include cytokine receptor-directed monoclonal antibodies, tyrosine kinase inhibitors, SH2 domain inhibitors [66], and antisense oligonucleotides or small molecules [67] that target the STAT DNA binding domain [4]. An alternate approach is to use screening strategies to identify compounds that inhibit STAT-based transcription. One way to do this is to use a chemical biology approach in which a cell-based system is developed that allows the quantitative high-throughput measurement of STAT-dependent gene expression. Another screening strategy makes use of a computational approach using databases that catalog the effect of thousands of drugs on gene expression [68] and gene expression signatures that reflect the activation of STATs in human cancers [69] to identify drugs that lead to gene expression signatures that are the opposite of the STAT signature. These unbiased approaches greatly expand the range of potential STAT inhibitors that can be identified. Compounds identified by these strategies also serve as biological probes that provide insight into the physiologic mechanisms of STAT regulation in a cell, and identify new targets for therapeutic inhibition.

3.8 Post-Translational Modifications and STAT Transcriptional Function

While STATs can be activated by cytokine-induced JAK activation, or receptor or non-receptor tyrosine kinases, there are additional subtleties that regulate their transcriptional function. STAT proteins can be post-translationally modified at different locations, in addition to the canonical tyrosine phosphorylation, and several of those modifications have been shown to modulate STAT transcriptional function (Fig. 3.1). For example, STATs can be phosphorylated, acetylated, methylated or ubiquitinated on several amino acid residues. In many tumor types, phosphorylation of both Tyr-705 (Y705) and Ser-727 (S727) is important for STAT3 transcriptional function. Phosphorylation of S727 was believed to occur after Y705 phosphorylation and binding with the target promoter to further augment the transcriptional function of STATs [70]. In certain cancers such as chronic lymphocytic leukemia (CLL), only S727 phosphorylation of STAT3 is observed [71], though this is sufficient to drive target gene expression [72]. In renal cell carcinoma, STAT3 was found to be phosphorylated by glycogen synthase kinase 3α and -β (GSK-3α/β) at T714 and S727, but not Y705, to drive target gene expression [73]. There is also evidence that acetylation of STAT3 enhances the stability and interaction of STAT3 with P300 bromodomain protein to increase transcription [74].

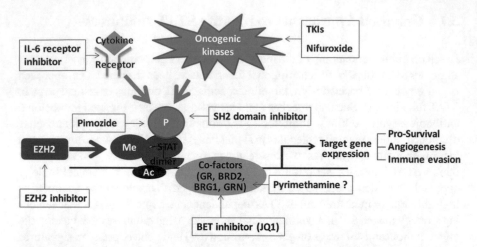

Fig. 3.1 Inappropriate activation of STAT transcription factors drive the expression of critical target genes in cancer, and so STATs represent targets with a potentially high therapeutic index. STATs can become activated constitutively in cancer cells through phosphorylation by mutated oncogenic tyrosine kinases, or through cytokines that are present in the tumor microenvironment through autocrine or paracrine mechanisms, thereby activating JAKs. Upon tyrosine phosphorylation, STATs form active dimers, translocate to the nucleus, bind to DNA, and regulate transcription of target genes that regulate self-renewal ("stemness"), survival, angiogenesis, and immune evasion. The transcriptional function of STATs is modulated by post-translational modifications including phosphorylation, methylation and acetylation. Co-factors that interact with STATs at the genomic level serve as another level of transcriptional regulation. Understanding these mechanisms of regulating STAT function has led to a number of therapeutic opportunities to target these proteins. (*P* phosphorylation, *Me* methylation, *Ac* acetylation)

STAT5 encompass two isoforms, STAT5A and STAT5B. The canonical activation marker for STAT5A is Y694 and for STAT5B is Y699 [75–78]. STAT5A can also be serine phosphorylated at multiple sites such as S726, S780 and S127/128. At least in the case of ERBB4/HER4 activated STAT5A, S779 phosphorylation seemed dispensable for phosphorylation of STAT5A at Y694 and subsequent DNA binding. However S127/S128 was required for ERBB4-induced phosphorylation of Y694 of STAT5A [79]. STAT5B can be serine phosphorylated at S731 and S193 [75, 80]. Furthermore, although Y699 is absolutely required for transcriptional activation of STAT5B, tyrosines 725, 740, and 743 may be involved in a negative regulation of STAT5B-mediated transcription [81].

Recently, key methylation sites that modulate STAT3 transcriptional activity have been identified, though methylation at different sites on STAT3 may exert completely opposite effects on transcriptional activity. For example, following its tyrosine phosphorylation, STAT3 is methylated on K140 by the histone methyl transferase SET9 and demethylated by LSD1. This methylation of K140 is a negative regulatory event [70]. On the other hand, STAT3 can be methylated at different sites by the same enzyme, enhancer of Zeste homolog 2 (EZH2) to activate its transcriptional function. EZH2 is a lysine methyl transferase and EZH2-containing PRC2 catalyzes trimethylation of histone 3 at lysine 27 (H3K27me3) [82].

It has recently been appreciated that EZH2 also methylates non-histone proteins. Two independent studies have demonstrated that EZH2 modulates STAT3 transcriptional activity by methylating distinct sites of STAT3. In glioblastoma stem cells, EZH2 trimethylates STAT3 on K180. Trimethylation at K180 promoted Y705 phosphorylation of STAT3 and activated STAT3 transcriptional activity [34]. It is still unknown how trimethylation at K180 synergize with Y705 phosphorylation of STAT3 in glioblastoma stem cells. In another cellular system in which STAT3 is activated by IL-6, perturbation of EZH2 function did not inhibit Y705 phosphorylation of STAT3, although it significantly reduced STAT3 transcriptional activity. It was found that in this IL-6 dependent system, dimethylation of K49 of STAT3 by EZH2 was crucial for full activation of STAT3 transcriptional activity. Unlike K180 trimethylation that promoted Y705 phosphorylation, dimethylation of K49 had no effect on Y705 phosphorylation. On the contrary, Y705 phosphorylation was required for K49 dimethylation of STAT3 to occur [83]. The mechanism by which K49 modification altered STAT3-dependent gene expression is unclear. It does not appear that K49 methylation affected the binding of STAT3 to its genomic binding site. It has been suggested that K49 methylation of STAT3 promotes the recruitment of co-regulatory factors to genomic target sites to facilitate maximal transcriptional function of STAT3, although these postulated co-regulators have not yet been identified.

3.9   Identification of Clinically-Translatable STAT Inhibitors

Although different modifications can affect STAT3 transcriptional function, it is clear that Y705 phosphorylation is nearly always essential for transcriptional activity. Thus drug screening and structure-based design of STAT inhibitors have mainly focused on inhibition of this phosphorylation event in STAT3. Many inhibitors of STAT tyrosine phosphorylation have been identified that block the STAT3 SH2 domain, which is required for both recruitment to activated kinase-receptor complexes as well as for activating dimerization. In addition, a number of natural products have been described that inhibit STAT3 phosphorylation. While these molecules have encouraging properties in vitro, and some have shown activity in animal models, progress in advancing STAT-targeted small molecules into clinical trials in cancer patients has been slow.

As noted, cell-based screening systems can be used to identify inhibitors of STAT-dependent transcription. This approach can allow the screening of chemical libraries that contain drugs that are already known to be safe in humans, including those that are approved for human use. This approach has identified several notable compounds, two of which function by blocking STAT3 tyrosine phosphorylation, albeit through different mechanisms. Nifuroxazide, an oral antibiotic that is used in many countries to treat colitis and diarrhea in humans, was found to be an inhibitor of STAT3 transcriptional function with an EC 50 of approximately 3 μM [84]. In analyzing its mechanism of action, it was found that nifuroxazide inhibited Y705 phosphorylation of

STAT3 through inhibiting the kinase activity of both TYK2 and JAK2 (but not JAK1). Nifuroxazide was found to induce apoptosis and reduce the viability of multiple myeloma cells that are dependent on activated STAT3 for survival.

Another compound identified through this approach is pimozide, which is clinically used as a neuroleptic for the treatment of Tourette syndrome. This drug was found to decrease STAT5 tyrosine phosphorylation. Interestingly, pimozide inhibits STAT5 phosphorylation irrespective of the upstream kinases that activate STAT5. Indeed, pimozide inhibits STAT5 phosphorylation in CML cells in which STAT5 is activated by the BCR-ABL1 fusion kinase [85], AML cells in which STAT5 is activated by FLT3-ITD [86], and myeloproliferative neoplasms in which STAT5 is activated by the mutated kinase JAK2(V617F) [5]. However, pimozide is not a kinase inhibitor. It does not inhibit JAKs, ABL1 or SRC family members in in vitro kinase assays, nor does it inhibit other signaling pathways downstream of those activated kinases. These findings suggested that pimozide inhibits STAT5 phosphorylation using a completely independent mechanism. The exact mechanism by which pimozide mediates this effect is not known, although it may involve modulation of negative regulators of STAT function. However, this non-kinase dependent STAT5 inhibition by pimozide may provide an important therapeutic opportunity. First, kinase mutation or amplification frequently leads to a reduction or loss of efficacy of kinases inhibitors. Therapies that target STAT5 independent of upstream kinases may still be able to achieve therapeutic efficacy. Indeed, hematopoietic cells with the T315I mutation in BCR-ABL are completely resistant to the BCR-ABL1 kinase inhibitor imatinib, but they are still sensitive to STAT5 inhibition by pimozide [85]. Second, even without BCR-ABL mutation, increased amount of STAT5 have been seen in the accelerated stage of CML and can render CML cells more resistant to imatinib [39]. In this situation, it is conceivable that a drug like pimozide that targets STAT5 without depending on upstream kinase inhibition will be valuable in controlling diseases. In addition, two compounds that inhibit different steps of the same oncogenic pathway may have greater efficacy with a lower chance of the emergence of resistance. Consistent with this idea, combining pimozide with kinase inhibition augmented the therapeutic efficacy of a JAK inhibitor in myeloproliferative diseases [5].

3.10   Therapeutic Modulation of Co-Factors of STATs

As with other transcription factors, STATs recruit co-factors to activate transcription, which can include other transcription factors, as well as chromatin remodeling proteins, among others. Cross talk between STATs and members of the nuclear receptor family has been observed in normal breast tissue and breast cancer [87–92]. Progesterone receptor (PR), androgen receptor (AR), and glucocorticoid receptor

(GR), have all been shown to synergistically interact with STAT5 and enhance STAT5 target gene expression.

BRG1, the ATPase subunit of a chromatin remodeling complex, is another factor that is essential for STAT3 target gene transcription. Genome-wide STAT3 binding in pluripotent embryonic stem cells (ESCs) is dependent on BRG1, since BRG1 is required to establish chromatin accessibility at STAT3 binding targets [93].

To identify STAT3-interacting proteins that contribute to STAT3 tumorigenesis, one can use mass-spectrometry to profile STAT3-interacting proteins. This approach has allowed the identification of granulin (GRN) as a novel STAT3 interacting protein in triple negative breast cancer cells [94]. GRN can act as an autocrine growth factor [95], and it can bind to and alter the subcellular distribution of positive transcription elongation factor (P-TEFb), leading to the repression of the transcription of tumor suppressor genes [96]. In breast cancer cells, GRN enhances STAT3 DNA binding and increases the time-integrated amount of LIF-induced STAT3 phosphorylation in breast cancer cells. Furthermore, silencing GRN neutralizes STAT3-mediated proliferation and migration of breast cancer cells. The correlation between GRN and STAT3 was also observed in primary breast cancer samples, where GRN mRNA levels were positively correlated with STAT3 gene expression signatures and with reduced patient survival.

Many of the co-regulators of STATs that have been identified may be difficult targets for pharmacological intervention. However, one group of key transcriptional co-factors is the BET (bromodomains and extra-terminal domain) family of bromodomain-containing proteins, which includes BRD2, BRD3, BRD4 and BRDT. Nuclear BET-protein interactome studies have indicated that BET proteins are integral components of a large number of nuclear protein complexes [97, 98]. Consistent with a role for BET proteins as key modulators of STAT signaling, it was found that the bromodomain inhibitor JQ1 inhibits STAT5 transcriptional activity. Further RNA interference-based experiments demonstrated that among the three BET bromodomain proteins expressed in hematological malignancies and targeted by JQ1, only BRD2 is necessary for STAT5 transcriptional function [99]. BRD2 likely participates in the STAT5 transcriptional complex, and acts as a critical co-activator for STAT5 function. The recruitment of STAT5 to its genomic binding sites is not dependent on BRD2, but rather maximal transcriptional initiation of these target genes requires BRD2. Interestingly, although JQ1 significantly reduces the transcriptional function of STAT5, it had essentially no effects on STAT3-dependent gene expression. Given the structural similarity between STAT5 and STAT3, further genomic and structural studies are necessary to elucidate the mechanism of this selectivity. The therapeutic implication of targeting STAT5 by dual BET bromodomain inhibition (JQ1) and tyrosine kinase inhibition (TKIs) was investigated in a clinically aggressive disease, acute T lymphocytic leukemia. Strong synergy in the induction of apoptosis was found in T-ALL cells when JQ1 was combined with TKIs [99]. Over-expression of a constitutively activated STAT5 rescued cell death induced by the combination of JQ1 and TKIs, supporting the notion that the synergistic effect is, at least partially, mediated through STAT5 inhibition. These findings also reaffirm the important role of STAT5 activation in the pathogenesis of T-ALL.

3.11 Limitations of Transcription-Based Drug Discovery for STATs Inhibitors

While most approaches to developing STAT inhibitors are based on inhibition of its transcriptional function, there are some limitations on relying on this approach. Although most of the known oncogenic properties of STATs are attributed to their roles as transcriptional factors, there is evidence that cytoplasmic [77] or mitochondrial STATs [63] can play important roles in malignant cell transformation and survival. It is conceivable that compounds that target these aspects of STAT function may not be discovered from transcription-based drug discovery methods. On the other hand, modifications of STATs that regulate their transcriptional function could also influence their cytoplasmic or mitochondrial localization.

Another potential caveat in transcription-based drug discovery is that STAT activation in these assays is generally induced by exogenous cytokine stimulation. Cytokine-induced STAT activation is transient, generally returning to baseline in 60–90 min. This differs from the continual activation seen in most tumor systems. In addition, the magnitude of the phosphorylation of STATs induced by cytokines, and the induction of transcription, is considerably greater in cytokine-induced systems than that seen with constitutive activation. Thus it is possible that compounds or genetic perturbations that modulate STAT transcriptional activity in a cytokine-induced system may not have the same activity in the setting of constitutively activated STATs as seen in cancer. Finally, it is clear that there are differences in STAT driven gene expression and STAT function that is dependent on the cellular context. Thus, compounds identified in a given system may not have uniform effects in other cells or tissues. Even within a given tumor type, unique aspects related to epigenetic states or the presence or absence of co-regulatory proteins may affect the activity of pharmacological modulators of STAT function. Nonetheless, the large amount of encouraging data generated in pre-clinical systems has generated a great interest in testing the approach of targeting STATs in human cancer.

3.12 Clinical Trials of STAT3 Inhibitors

Despite the large number of papers on developing and testing STAT inhibitors in model systems, relatively few true STAT inhibitors, i.e., compounds designed to specifically inhibit STAT function, have been introduced into clinical trials. This reflects a number of factors, including a relative lack of enthusiasm for targeting transcription factors among many in the field of cancer drug development, due to the pharmacologic challenges in inhibiting these proteins. Thus, for STAT inhibitors being introduced into clinical use, it is essential that appropriate pharmacodynamic markers be followed, to ensure that the target is, in fact, being inhibited. While this should be true for all targeted drug development efforts, it is particularly important for such a novel target as an inhibitor of an oncogenic transcription factor.

Particularly in a Phase 1 trial in heavily pre-treated cancer patients, the chance of a large clinical response may be limited. In order to learn as much as possible from every patient who volunteers to participate in such a trial, it is important to first ask the question of whether the designated target is being inhibited. For a compound that blocks the activating tyrosine phosphorylation of STAT3, it can be relatively easy to monitor tyrosine phosphorylation by immunocytochemistry, immunofluo-rescence, or immunoblots. Where malignant cells and tissue can easily be obtained, as in hematological cancers or superficial lesions, this can be relatively straightfor-ward. For other tumor types, it might be necessary to perform biopsies to obtain the necessary material. To minimize morbidity in patients with advanced cancer, one can also consider approaches such as examining circulating tumor cells to assess functional STAT activation.

For inhibitors that do not alter STAT3 phosphorylation, but inhibit the transcrip-tional response, it can be even more challenging to measure inhibition of STAT func-tion. In those cases, one can evaluate the mRNA levels of STAT3 target gene signatures. Again, it may be necessary to perform relatively invasive biopsies to obtain adequate tissue, but the use of circulating tumor cells may make this more feasible.

Two clinical trials of true STAT3 inhibitors are particularly illustrative. The first, built on pioneering work from the laboratory of Jennifer Grandis, highlighted sev-eral key points [100]. The first is to use an inhibitor that has been tested extensively and rigorously in pre-clinical systems to ensure on target activity. While much work in developing STAT3 inhibitors is focused on inhibitors of the SH2 domain, these investigators used an approach based on blocking DNA binding of activated STAT3 dimers. They used a short double-stranded oligonucleotide that contained a canoni-cal STAT3 binding site. They then were able to show that when this molecule was introduced into cancer cells with activated STAT3, it titrated the active STAT3 dimers away from the endogenous genomic sites to this "decoy". After validating this approach in cell culture and animal studies, the investigators were then ready to test this approach in human cancer patients. The next key issue, in which physician investigators or collaborators are essential, was to determine the appropriate tumor type in which to test this strategy. These scientists chose squamous cell carcinoma of the head and neck, a disease in which constitutive STAT3 is common, and which is often accessible to direct visualization and injection. They performed a so-called "Phase 0" clinical trial (#NCT00696176), in which patients who were going to have their tumor resected had a single intratumoral injection of either the STAT3 decoy or saline control. No toxicity was noted from this therapy. When the tumor was resected 4–6 h later, assessment of expression of STAT3 regulated cyclin D1 and Bcl-xl were lower in the tumors treated with the STAT3 decoy than in the tumors treated with saline. Although this work is at an early stage, and these genes are regu-lated by a number of transcription factors, it represented a significant advance in actually translating STAT3 inhibitors from the laboratory to the clinic.

In contrast to this macromolecular approach to STAT3 inhibition, the first small molecule inhibitor of STAT3 to enter a clinical trial was based on a drug, pyrimeth-amine, that was identified from a chemical library screen for STAT3 inhibition. Pyrimethamine is an anti-microbial drug that is used clinically to treat malaria and toxoplasmosis. Pyrimethamine inhibits the transcriptional function of STAT3, but not that of other STAT family members or unrelated transcription factors like NF-kB [101, 102]. Furthermore, pyrimethamine exerts this effect at low micromolar concentrations, which are known to be readily achieved in human patients, and can safely be sustained for months on end. While pyrimethamine was very desirable from the standpoint of efficacy, specificity, and safety, it had one disadvantage. At the lower range of concentrations at which it inhibits STAT3 transcriptional function, it does not significantly reduce phosphorylation of STAT3. Thus, it seems that this drug acts through a relatively novel mechanism, likely involving disruption of co-activator complexes. However, this property of pyrimethamine would alter the way its activity would have to be monitored in a patient.

In considering a clinical trial with this drug, again it was important to focus on a cancer that was known to be dependent on activated STAT3 in a large majority of patients, to forestall the need to either test tumors prior to study entry or to enroll a large enough cohort so that an adequate number of patients with activated STAT3 were included. In addition, it was necessary to focus on a cancer in which it was easy to obtain sufficient tumor cells to perform pharmacodynamic evaluation of whether STAT3 function was definitively being inhibited. Since the phosphorylation of STAT3 was not affected, this analysis would have to rely on measurements of STAT3-dependent gene expression. The cancer chosen for this trial was chronic lymphocytic leukemia (CLL), and its essentially equivalent counterpart of small lymphocytic lymphoma (SLL). From a logistic standpoint, CLL has the advantage that most patients have a very large number of circulating malignant cells, so that assessment of pharmacodynamic endpoints can easily be achieved with a simple blood draw. CLL is characterized by essentially uniform phosphorylation of STAT3 in leukemic cells [71]. However, although the STAT3 is in the nucleus and transcriptionally active, it is phosphorylated on S727 rather than Y705. Nonetheless, since pyrimethamine could block the transcriptional function of STAT3 in CLL, and could decrease viability of CLL cells in vitro, this disease was chosen for a phase I/II clinical trial (#NCT01066663).

In this study, which is currently ongoing, patients are treated in cohorts of increasing daily doses of oral pyrimethamine. Trough concentrations of pyrimethamine are obtained in both the plasma and the white blood cell fraction (which contains the leukemic cells), so that effects on gene expression can be correlated with drug exposure. Not only are changes in STAT3 target genes determined from the cells taken immediately from the patient, but parallel in vitro experiments are performed on cells obtained from the patient prior to entry on the trial, to determine whether changes in gene expression and survival of the cells treated *ex vivo* with pyrimethamine match the clinical response.

Should this study show evidence of on-target effects, the integrated pharmacokinetic and pharmacodynamic data can then be used to guide trials in other diseases commonly driven by activated STAT3. If STAT3 inhibition is not occurring, then consideration needs to be given as to whether adequate drug concentrations and exposures over a 24 h time period are being achieved. For example, increased dose levels may need to be considered. If gene expression analyses show that STAT3 is adequately being inhibited, yet there is little clinical benefit, then one could consider combining a STAT3 inhibitor with another modality, including some of the conventional or novel targeted agents in use to treat this disease. For example, by decreasing expression of pro-survival genes like BCL-2 or BCL-xL, a STAT3 inhibitor like pyrimethamine might sensitize CLL cells to conventional cytotoxic drugs like fludarabine and cyclophosphamide, as well as novel kinase inhibitors like ibrutinib or idelalisib.

3.13   Conclusion

Although drug development in oncology had been dominated since its inception by cytotoxic drugs that non-specifically damage DNA or microtubules, or inhibited metabolic pathways, the field is now shifting to a new, more rational approach. Targeted molecular therapies first showed dramatic efficacy when specific kinases, activated by mutation, could be specifically inhibited. However, the targets are now broadening so-that non-mutated kinases that are oncogenic dependencies have become appealing targets. Finally, non-kinase targets, like the pro-survival protein BCL-2, are becoming tractable to pharmacologic intervention. One of the next frontiers in targeted molecular therapy for cancer is oncogenic transcription factors. While usually not directly mutated, these proteins are key convergence points from oncogenic signaling pathways. Since normal cells are generally tolerant of their inhibition, while cancer cells may be completely dependent on their function, transcription factors like STAT3 or STAT5 represent important targets with the potential of having a very high therapeutic index. While somewhat challenging from a medicinal chemistry standpoint, these high value targets can be inhibited using a number of creative strategies, and clinical trials of STAT inhibitors are currently under way. In the coming years, we will gain a better appreciation of the feasibility and potential of targeting STATs and other oncogenic transcription factors for the rational molecular therapy of cancer.

References

1. Darnell JE Jr (1997) STATs and gene regulation. Science 277:1630–1635
2. Frank DA (2003) STAT signaling in cancer: insights into pathogenesis and treatment strategies. Cancer Treat Res 115:267–291
3. Lin TS, Mahajan S, Frank DA (2000) STAT signaling in the pathogenesis and treatment of leukemias. Oncogene 19:2496–2504
4. Benekli M, Baumann H, Wetzler M (2009) Targeting signal transducer and activator of transcription signaling pathway in leukemias. J Clin Oncol 27:4422–4432
5. Bar-Natan M, Nelson EA, Walker SR et al (2012) Dual inhibition of Jak2 and STAT5 enhances killing of myeloproliferative neoplasia cells. Leukemia 26:1407–1410

6. Frank DA, Varticovski L (1996) BCR/abl leads to the constitutive activation of Stat proteins, and shares an epitope with tyrosine phosphorylated Stats. Leukemia 10:1724–1730
7. Carlesso N, Frank DA, Griffin JD (1996) Tyrosyl phosphorylation and DNA-binding activity of STAT proteins in hematopoietic cell lines transformed by Bcr/Abl. J Exp Med 183:811–820
8. Sternberg DW, Gilliland DG (2004) The role of signal transducer and activator of transcription factors in leukemogenesis. J Clin Oncol 22:361–371
9. Scheeren FA, Diehl SA, Smit LA et al (2008) IL-21 is expressed in Hodgkin lymphoma and activates STAT5: evidence that activated STAT5 is required for Hodgkin lymphomagenesis. Blood 111(9):4706–4715
10. Hoelbl A, Kovacic B, Kerenyi MA et al (2006) Clarifying the role of Stat5 in lymphoid development and Abelson-induced transformation. Blood 107:4898–4906
11. Walz C, Medrzycki M, Bunting ST et al (2012) Essential role for Stat5a/b in myeloproliferative neoplasms induced by BCR-ABL1 and Jak2V617F in mice. Blood 119:3550–3560
12. Crescenzo R, Abate F, Lasorsa E et al (2015) Convergent mutations and kinase fusions lead to oncogenic STAT3 activation in anaplastic large cell lymphoma. Cancer Cell 27:516–532
13. Mangolini M, De Boer J, Walf-Vorderwulbecke V et al (2013) STAT3 mediates oncogenic addiction to TEL-AML1 in t(12;21) acute lymphoblastic leukemia. Blood 122:542–549
14. Cui Y, Riedlinger G, Miyoshi K et al (2004) Inactivation of Stat5 in mouse mammary epithelium during pregnancy reveals distinct functions in cell proliferation, survival, and differentiation. Mol Cell Biol 24:8037–8047
15. Iavnilovitch E, Groner B, Barash I (2002) Overexpression and forced activation of stat5 in mammary gland of transgenic mice promotes cellular proliferation, enhances differentiation, and delays postlactational apoptosis. Mol Cancer Res 1:32–47
16. Liu X, Robinson GW, Gouilleux F, Groner B, Hennighausen L (1995) Cloning and expression of Stat5 and an additional homologue (Stat5b) involved in prolactin signal transduction in mouse mammary tissue. Proc Natl Acad Sci U S A 92:8831–8835
17. Tang JZ, Zuo ZH, Kong XJ et al (2010) Signal transducer and activator of transcription (STAT)-5A and STAT5B differentially regulate human mammary carcinoma cell behavior. Endocrinology 151:43–55
18. Ren S, Cai HR, Li M, Furth PA (2002) Loss of Stat5a delays mammary cancer progression in a mouse model. Oncogene 21:4335–4339
19. Iavnilovitch E, Cardiff RD, Groner B, Barash I (2004) Deregulation of Stat5 expression and activation causes mammary tumors in transgenic mice. Int J Cancer 112:607–619
20. Walker SR, Nelson EA, Yeh JE et al (2009) Reciprocal effects of STAT5 and STAT3 in breast cancer. Mol Cancer Res 7:966–976
21. Walker SR, Chaudhury M, Nelson EA, Frank DA (2010) Microtubule-targeted chemotherapeutic agents inhibit signal transducer and activator of transcription 3 (STAT3) signaling. Mol Pharmacol 78:903–908
22. Burke WM, Jin X, Lin HJ et al (2001) Inhibition of constitutively active Stat3 suppresses growth of human ovarian and breast cancer cells. Oncogene 20:7925–7934
23. Putoczki TL, Thiem S, Loving A et al (2013) Interleukin-11 is the dominant IL-6 family cytokine during gastrointestinal tumorigenesis and can be targeted therapeutically. Cancer Cell 24:257–271
24. Rokavec M, Oner MG, Li H et al (2014) IL-6R/STAT3/miR-34a feedback loop promotes EMT-mediated colorectal cancer invasion and metastasis. J Clin Invest 124:1853–1867
25. Errico A (2015) Lung cancer: driver-mutation-dependent stratification: learning from STAT3. Nat Rev Clin Oncol 12:251
26. Fan QW, Cheng CK, Gustafson WC et al (2013) EGFR phosphorylates tumor-derived EGFRvIII driving STAT3/5 and progression in glioblastoma. Cancer Cell 24:438–449
27. Baumgart S, Chen NM, Siveke JT et al (2014) Inflammation-induced NFATc1-STAT3 transcription complex promotes pancreatic cancer initiation by KrasG12D. Cancer Discov 4:688–701
28. Rodriguez-Barrueco R, Yu J, Saucedo-Cuevas LP et al (2015) Inhibition of the autocrine IL-6-JAK2-STAT3-calprotectin axis as targeted therapy for HR-/HER2+ breast cancers. Genes Dev 29:1631–1648

29. Heuser M, Sly LM, Argiropoulos B et al (2009) Modeling the functional heterogeneity of leukemia stem cells: role of STAT5 in leukemia stem cell self-renewal. Blood 114:3983–3993
30. Yoshimoto G, Miyamoto T, Jabbarzadeh-Tabrizi S et al (2009) FLT3-ITD up-regulates MCL-1 to promote survival of stem cells in acute myeloid leukemia via FLT3-ITD-specific STAT5 activation. Blood 114:5034–5043
31. Fatrai S, Wierenga AT, Daenen SM, Vellenga E, Schuringa JJ (2011) Identification of HIF2alpha as an important STAT5 target gene in human hematopoietic stem cells. Blood 117:3320–3330
32. Cook AM, Li L, Hoy Y et al (2014) Role of altered growth factor receptor-mediated JAK2 signaling in growth and maintenance of human acute myeloid leukemia stem cells. Blood 123:2826–2837
33. Gallipoli P, Cook A, Rhodes S et al (2014) JAK2/STAT5 inhibition by nilotinib with ruxolitinib contributes to the elimination of CML CD34+ cells in vitro and in vivo. Blood 124:1492–1501
34. Kim E, Kim M, Woo DH et al (2013) Phosphorylation of EZH2 activates STAT3 signaling via STAT3 methylation and promotes tumorigenicity of glioblastoma stem-like cells. Cancer Cell 23:839–852
35. Marotta LL, Almendro V, Marusyk A et al (2011) The JAK2/STAT3 signaling pathway is required for growth of CD44(+)CD24(–) stem cell-like breast cancer cells in human tumors. J Clin Invest 121:2723–2735
36. van der Zee M, Sacchetti A, Cansoy M et al (2015) IL6/JAK1/STAT3 Signaling blockade in endometrial cancer affects the ALDHhi/CD126+ stem-like component and reduces tumor burden. Cancer Res 75:3608–3622
37. Li Y, Guo G, Li L et al (2015) Suppression of cancer relapse and metastasis by inhibiting cancer stemness. Proc Natl Acad Sci U S A 112:1839–1844
38. Nishioka C, Ikezoe T, Yang J, Yokoyama A (2009) Multitargeted tyrosine kinase inhibitor stimulates expression of IL-6 and activates JAK2/STAT5 signaling in acute myelogenous leukemia cells. Leukemia 23:2304–2308
39. Warsch W, Kollmann K, Ecklehart E et al (2011) High STAT5 levels mediate imatinib resistance and indicate disease progression in chronic myeloid leukemia. Blood 117:3409–3420
40. Nishioka C, Ikezoe T, Yang J, Yokoyama A (2010) Long-term exposure of leukemia cells to multi-targeted tyrosine kinase inhibitor induces activations of AKT, ERK and STAT5 signaling via epigenetic silencing of the PTEN gene. Leukemia 24:1631–1640
41. Warsch W, Grunschober E, Berger A et al (2012) STAT5 triggers BCR-ABL1 mutation by mediating ROS production in chronic myeloid leukaemia. Oncotarget 3:1669–1687
42. Britschgi A, Andraos R, Brinkhaus H et al (2012) JAK2/STAT5 inhibition circumvents resistance to PI3K/mTOR blockade: a rationale for cotargeting these pathways in metastatic breast cancer. Cancer Cell 22:796–811
43. Vultur A, Villanueva J, Krepler C et al (2014) MEK inhibition affects STAT3 signaling and invasion in human melanoma cell lines. Oncogene 33:1850–1861
44. Liu F, Cao J, Wu J et al (2013) Stat3-targeted therapies overcome the acquired resistance to vemurafenib in melanomas. J Invest Dermatol 133:2041–2049
45. Girotti MR, Pedersen M, Sanchez-Laorden B et al (2013) Inhibiting EGF receptor or SRC family kinase signaling overcomes BRAF inhibitor resistance in melanoma. Cancer Discov 3:158–167
46. Eichten A, Su J, Adler A et al (2016) Resistance to anti-VEGF therapy mediated by autocrine IL-6/STAT3 signaling and overcome by IL-6 blockade. Cancer Res 76(8):2327–2339
47. Real PJ, Sierra A, De Juan A et al (2002) Resistance to chemotherapy via Stat3-dependent overexpression of Bcl-2 in metastatic breast cancer cells. Oncogene 21:7611–7618
48. Zhong H, Davis A, Ouzounova M et al (2016) A novel IL6 antibody sensitizes multiple tumor types to chemotherapy including trastuzumab-resistant tumors. Cancer Res 76:480–490
49. Lau J, Ilkhandizadeh S, Wang S et al (2015) STAT3 blockade inhibits radiation-induced malignant progression in glioma. Cancer Res 75:4302–4311

50. Wang T, Niu G, Kortylewski M et al (2004) Regulation of the innate and adaptive immune responses by Stat-3 signaling in tumor cells. Nat Med 10:48–54
51. Jones LM, Broz ML, Ranger JJ et al (2016) Stat3 establishes an immunosuppressive microenvironment during the early stages of breast carcinogenesis to promote tumor growth and metastasis. Cancer Res 76:1416–1428
52. Albesiano E, Davis M, See AP et al (2010) Immunologic consequences of signal transducers and activators of transcription 3 activation in human squamous cell carcinoma. Cancer Res 70:6467–6476
53. Yang H, Yamazaki T, Pietrocola F et al (2015) STAT3 inhibition enhances the therapeutic efficacy of immunogenic chemotherapy by stimulating type 1 interferon production by cancer cells. Cancer Res 75:3812–3822
54. Green MR, Monti S, Rodig SJ et al (2010) Integrative analysis reveals selective 9p24.1 amplification, increased PD-1 ligand expression, and further induction via JAK2 in nodular sclerosing Hodgkin lymphoma and primary mediastinal large B-cell lymphoma. Blood 116:3268–3277
55. Wang Z, Medrzycki M, Bunting ST, Bunting KD (2015) Stat5-deficient hematopoiesis is permissive for Myc-induced B-cell leukemogenesis. Oncotarget 6:28961–28972
56. Yan D, Jobe F, Hutchison RE, Mohi G (2015) Deletion of Stat3 enhances myeloid cell expansion and increases the severity of myeloproliferative neoplasms in Jak2V617F knock-in mice. Leukemia 29:2050–2061
57. Pencik J, Schlederer M, Gruber W et al (2015) STAT3 regulated ARF expression suppresses prostate cancer metastasis. Nat Commun 6:7736
58. Fukuda A, Wang SC, Morris JPT et al (2011) Stat3 and MMP7 contribute to pancreatic ductal adenocarcinoma initiation and progression. Cancer Cell 19:441–455
59. Lesina M, Kurkowski MU, Ludes K et al (2011) Stat3/Socs3 activation by IL-6 transsignaling promotes progression of pancreatic intraepithelial neoplasia and development of pancreatic cancer. Cancer Cell 19:456–469
60. Zhou J, Qu Z, Yan S et al (2015) Differential roles of STAT3 in the initiation and growth of lung cancer. Oncogene 34:3804–3814
61. Qu Z, Sun F, Zhou J et al (2015) Interleukin-6 prevents the initiation but enhances the progression of lung cancer. Cancer Res 75:3209–3215
62. Grabner B, Schramek D, Mueller KM et al (2015) Disruption of STAT3 signalling promotes KRAS-induced lung tumorigenesis. Nat Commun 6:6285
63. Gough DJ, Corlett A, Schlessinger K et al (2009) Mitochondrial STAT3 supports Ras-dependent oncogenic transformation. Science 324:1713–1716
64. Walker SR, Nelson EA, Frank DA (2007) STAT5 represses BCL6 expression by binding to a regulatory region frequently mutated in lymphomas. Oncogene 26:224–233
65. Walker SR, Nelson EA, Yeh JE et al (2013) STAT5 outcompetes STAT3 to regulate the expression of the oncogenic transcriptional modulator BCL6. Mol Cell Biol 33:2879–2890
66. Yue P, Lopez-Tapia F, Paladino D et al (2016) Hydroxamic acid and benzoic acid-based Stat3 inhibitors suppress human glioma and breast cancer phenotypes in vitro and in vivo. Cancer Res 76:652–663
67. Huang W, Dong Z, Chen Y et al (2016) Small-molecule inhibitors targeting the DNA-binding domain of STAT3 suppress tumor growth, metastasis and STAT3 target gene expression in vivo. Oncogene 35:783–792
68. Lamb J, Crawford ED, Peck D et al (2006) The Connectivity Map: using gene-expression signatures to connect small molecules, genes, and disease. Science 313:1929–1935
69. Alvarez JV, Febbo PG, Ramaswamy S et al (2005) Identification of a genetic signature of activated signal transducer and activator of transcription 3 in human tumors. Cancer Res 65:5054–5062
70. Yang J, Huang J, Dasgupta M et al (2010) Reversible methylation of promoter-bound STAT3 by histone-modifying enzymes. Proc Natl Acad Sci U S A 107:21499–21504
71. Frank DA, Mahajan S, Ritz J (1997) B lymphocytes from patients with chronic lymphocytic leukemia contain signal transducer and activator of transcription (STAT) 1 and STAT3 constitutively phosphorylated on serine residues. J Clin Invest 100:3140–3148

72. Hazan-Halevy I, Harris D, Liu Z et al (2010) STAT3 is constitutively phosphorylated on serine 727 residues, binds DNA, and activates transcription in CLL cells. Blood 115:2852–2863
73. Waitkus MS, Chandrasekharan UM, Willard B et al (2014) Signal integration and gene induction by a functionally distinct STAT3 phosphoform. Mol Cell Biol 34:1800–1811
74. Hou T, Ray S, Lee C, Brasier AR (2008) The STAT3 NH2-terminal domain stabilizes enhanceosome assembly by interacting with the p300 bromodomain. J Biol Chem 283: 30725–30734
75. Mitra A, Ross JA, Rodriguez G et al (2012) Signal transducer and activator of transcription 5b (Stat5b) serine 193 is a novel cytokine-induced phospho-regulatory site that is constitutively activated in primary hematopoietic malignancies. J Biol Chem 287:16596–16608
76. Berger A, Hoelbl-Kovacic A, Bougeais J et al (2014) PAK-dependent STAT5 serine phosphorylation is required for BCR-ABL-induced leukemogenesis. Leukemia 28:629–641
77. Friedbichler K, Kerenyi MA, Kovacic B et al (2010) Stat5a serine 725 and 779 phosphorylation is a prerequisite for hematopoietic transformation. Blood 116:1548–1558
78. Gouilleux F, Wakao H, Mundt M, Groner B (1994) Prolactin induces phosphorylation of Tyr694 of Stat5 (MGF), a prerequisite for DNA binding and induction of transcription. EMBO J 13:4361–4369
79. Clark DE, Williams CC, Duplessis TT et al (2005) ERBB4/HER4 potentiates STAT5A transcriptional activity by regulating novel STAT5A serine phosphorylation events. J Biol Chem 280:24175–24180
80. Weaver AM, Silva CM (2007) S731 in the transactivation domain modulates STAT5b activity. Biochem Biophys Res Commun 362:1026–1030
81. Kloth MT, Catling AD, Silva CM (2002) Novel activation of STAT5b in response to epidermal growth factor. J Biol Chem 277:8693–8701
82. Cao R, Wang L, Wang H et al (2002) Role of histone H3 lysine 27 methylation in Polycomb-group silencing. Science 298:1039–1043
83. Dasgupta M, Dermawan JK, Willard B, Stark GR (2015) STAT3-driven transcription depends upon the dimethylation of K49 by EZH2. Proc Natl Acad Sci U S A 112:3985–3990
84. Nelson EA, Walker SR, Kepich A et al (2008) Nifuroxazide inhibits survival of multiple myeloma cells by directly inhibiting STAT3. Blood 112:5095–5102
85. Nelson EA, Walker SR, Weisberg E et al (2011) The STAT5 inhibitor pimozide decreases survival of chronic myelogenous leukemia cells resistant to kinase inhibitors. Blood 117:3421–3429
86. Nelson EA, Walker SR, Xiang M et al (2012) The STAT5 inhibitor pimozide displays efficacy in models of acute myelogenous leukemia driven by FLT3 mutations. Genes Cancer 3:503–511
87. Cerliani JP, Guillardoy T, Giulianelli S et al (2011) Interaction between FGFR-2, STAT5, and progesterone receptors in breast cancer. Cancer Res 71:3720–3731
88. Bertucci PY, Quaglino A, Pozzi AG, Kordon EC, Pecci A (2010) Glucocorticoid-induced impairment of mammary gland involution is associated with STAT5 and STAT3 signaling modulation. Endocrinology 151:5730–5740
89. Subtil-Rodriguez A, Millan-Arino L, Quiles I et al (2008) Progesterone induction of the 11beta-hydroxysteroid dehydrogenase type 2 promoter in breast cancer cells involves coordinated recruitment of STAT5A and progesterone receptor to a distal enhancer and polymerase tracking. Mol Cell Biol 28:3830–3849
90. Carsol JL, Gingras S, Simard J (2002) Synergistic action of prolactin (PRL) and androgen on PRL-inducible protein gene expression in human breast cancer cells: a unique model for functional cooperation between signal transducer and activator of transcription-5 and androgen receptor. Mol Endocrinol 16:1696–1710
91. Richer JK, Lange CA, Manning NG et al (1998) Convergence of progesterone with growth factor and cytokine signaling in breast cancer. Progesterone receptors regulate signal transducers and activators of transcription expression and activity. J Biol Chem 273:31317–31326
92. Wyszomierski SL, Yeh J, Rosen JM (1999) Glucocorticoid receptor/signal transducer and activator of transcription 5 (STAT5) interactions enhance STAT5 activation by prolonging STAT5 DNA binding and tyrosine phosphorylation. Mol Endocrinol 13:330–343

93. Ho L, Miller EL, Ronan JL et al (2011) esBAF facilitates pluripotency by conditioning the genome for LIF/STAT3 signalling and by regulating polycomb function. Nat Cell Biol 13:903–913

94. Yeh JE, Kreimer S, Walker SR et al (2015) Granulin, a novel STAT3-interacting protein, enhances STAT3 transcriptional function and correlates with poorer prognosis in breast cancer. Genes Cancer 6:153–168

95. Lu R, Serrero G (2001) Mediation of estrogen mitogenic effect in human breast cancer MCF-7 cells by PC-cell-derived growth factor (PCDGF/granulin precursor). Proc Natl Acad Sci U S A 98:142–147

96. Hoque M, Young TM, Lee CG et al (2003) The growth factor granulin interacts with cyclin T1 and modulates P-TEFb-dependent transcription. Mol Cell Biol 23:1688–1702

97. Dawson MA, Prinjha RK, Dittmann A et al (2011) Inhibition of BET recruitment to chromatin as an effective treatment for MLL-fusion leukaemia. Nature 478:529–533

98. Dawson MA, Kouzarides T, Huntly BJ (2012) Targeting epigenetic readers in cancer. N Engl J Med 367:647–657

99. Liu S, Walker SR, Nelson EA et al (2014) Targeting STAT5 in hematologic malignancies through inhibition of the bromodomain and extra-terminal (BET) bromodomain protein BRD2. Mol Cancer Ther 13:1194–1205

100. Sen M, Grandis JR (2012) Nucleic acid-based approaches to STAT inhibition. JAKSTAT 1:285–291

101. Takakura A, Nelson EA, Haque N et al (2011) Pyrimethamine inhibits adult polycystic kidney disease by modulating STAT signaling pathways. Hum Mol Genet 20:4143–4154

102. Nelson EA, Sharma SV, Settleman J, Frank DA (2011) A chemical biology approach to developing STAT inhibitors: molecular strategies for accelerating clinical translation. Oncotarget 2:518–524

Chapter 4
Historical Development of STAT3 Inhibitors and Early Results in Clinical Trials

Chao-Lan Yu, Richard Jove, and James Turkson

Abstract Since the initial reports of constitutive STAT3 activation in cells transformed by viral oncoproteins, the critical role of STAT3 signaling in human cancers has been firmly established. Detailed understanding of how STAT3 activity is tightly regulated by the balance between activating and inhibitory circuits provides important insights of how STAT3 becomes deregulated in cancer cells. A large number of STAT3 inhibitors have been developed. The predominant emphasis of the early rational drug discovery strategies was on disrupting phospho-tyrosine (pY) interactions with the Src-homology 2 (SH2) domain due to its requirement for STAT3:STAT3 dimerization and STAT3 function. Following the first reported direct STAT3 inhibitor peptide, PpYLKTK and its derivatives and peptidomimetics, several other peptides, peptide mimetics, and small molecules have been developed. However, their slow clinical development is in a large part due to the significant challenges of targeting transcription factors by disrupting protein:protein interactions. Two other major strategies to directly target STAT3 signaling are the decoy oligodeoxynucleotide (ODN) and antisense oligonucleotide (ASO) approaches, which have their own challenges for clinical development relating to their physicochemcial properties. Moreover, a large variety of natural products have been found to inhibit STAT3

C.-L. Yu
Department of Biomedical Sciences, College of Medicine, Chang Gung University,
259 Wenhua 1st Road, Taoyuan City 33302, Taiwan, ROC

Division of Hematology, Chang Gung Memorial Hospital,
Taoyuan City, Linkou, Taiwan
e-mail: clyu@mail.cgu.edu.tw

R. Jove
Cell Therapy Institute, Nova Southeastern University, 3301 College Avenue,
Fort Lauderdale, FL 33314, USA
e-mail: rjove@nova.edu

J. Turkson (✉)
Cancer Biology and Natural Products and Experimental Therapeutics Programs,
University of Hawaii Cancer Center, 701 Ilalo Street, Honolulu, HI 96813, USA
e-mail: jturkson@cc.hawaii.edu

© Springer International Publishing Switzerland 2016
A.C. Ward (ed.), *STAT Inhibitors in Cancer*, Cancer Drug
Discovery and Development, DOI 10.1007/978-3-319-42949-6_4

signaling pathways and tumor growth, although their precise mechanisms of action are often unclear. Tyrosine kinase inhibitors (TKIs), which impact STAT3 signaling indirectly through their inibitory effects on tyrosine phosphorylation, are the most advanced in clinical trials to date. Several TKIs are at various stages of clincal evaluation for safety and efficacy.

Keywords STAT3 • Solid tumors • Blood cancers • Protein tyrosine kinases • Protein tyrosine phosphatases • Cytokine signaling • Growth factor receptors • Mitochondria • Metabolism • Drug discovery • Small molecule inhibitors • Tyrosine kinase inhibitors • Decoy oligonucleotides • Natural products • Anticancer agents

4.1 Introduction

4.1.1 STAT3 Activation in Human Cancers

STAT proteins were initially identified in the context of cellular responses to interferon (IFN) and other cytokines [1]. There are seven STAT family members in mammalian cells: STAT1, STAT2, STAT3, STAT4, STAT5A, STAT5B and STAT6. They are latent cytoplasmic transcription factors and share highly conserved structural and functional domains. Upon ligand stimulation, STAT proteins are recruited to tyrosine-phosphorylated receptors, and are subsequently phosphorylated by receptor-associated Janus kinases (JAK) on the highly conserved tyrosine residues (Fig. 4.1). Tyrosine-phosphorylated STAT proteins dimerize, translocate to the nucleus, and regulate target gene expression by binding to distinct *cis*-acting elements in promoter regions. STAT3 was first discovered as a transcription factor, acute phase response factor (APRF), binding to an enhancer element in the promoter region of acute-phase genes in hepatocytes after stimulation with interleukin-6 (IL-6) [2]. Subsequent studies showed that STAT3 can be activated by other cytokines and growth factors, such as epidermal growth factor (EGF) [3]. STAT3 plays a critical role in tumor progression by regulating many target genes involved in cell proliferation, differentiation, apoptosis, metastasis, angiogenesis, metabolism, inflammation and immune evasion.

Uncontrolled cell proliferation and resistance to apoptosis are major cancer hallmarks [4]. This strongly implicates a critical role of STAT3 in carcinogenesis. The first line of evidence was reported in 1995 demonstrating constitutive STAT3 activation in cells transformed by the viral Src oncoprotein [5] and by HTLV-1 [6]. In the past 20 years, overexpression and/or abnormal activation of STAT3 has been reported in a wide variety of human solid tumors, including breast, colon, gastric, lung, ovarian, endometrial, cervical, pancreatic, brain, renal, head and neck, skin, and prostate [7, 8]. Constant STAT3 activation is also common in blood malignancies, including lymphomas, leukemias and multiple myeloma.

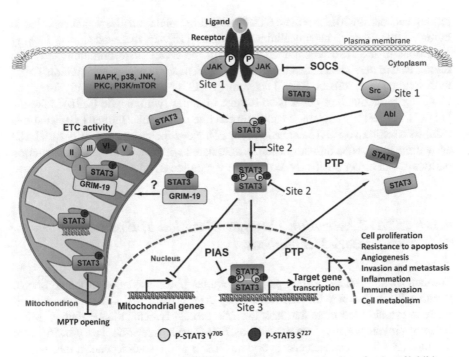

Fig. 4.1 Canonical and non-canonical STAT3 signal transduction and the sites of action of inhibitory modalities. STAT3 activity is tightly regulated in cells largely through phosphorylation and dephosphorylation of the highly conserved Y705 and S727 residues. Ligand-induced activation of receptor and non-receptor protein tyrosine kinases (such as JAK, Src and Abl) leads to Y705 phosphorylation, dimerization, nuclear translocation, and activation of many target genes associated with cancer hallmarks. Phosphorylation of S727 by a number of protein serine/threonine kinases can further enhance STAT3 activity. To prepare cells for the next round of ligand stimulation, the JAK-STAT3 pathway can be downregulated by multiple mechanisms, including suppressor of cytokine signaling (SOCS), protein tyrosine phosphatase (PTP), and protein inhibitor of activated STAT (PIAS). In addition to its canonical activity in the nucleus, STAT3 phosphorylated on S727 also translocates to mitochondria through a less defined mechanism. Mitochondrial STAT3 contributes to mitochondrial respiration as a complex with GRIM-19, a component of the electron transport chain (ETC). Mitochondrial STAT3 may also protect cells from apoptosis by inhibiting the opening of mitochondrial permeability transition pore (MPTP). Interestingly, consistent with the reported role of STAT3 in inhibiting nucleus-encoded mitochondrial genes, STAT3 may also bind to the circular mitochondrial genome and inhibit mitochondrion-encoded ETC components. Coordinated nuclear and mitochondrial actions of STAT3 on two distinct sets of mitochondrial genes may aid in metabolic reprogramming in cancer cells. The sites of action for tyrosine kinase inhibitors (Site 1), SH2 domain-binding, dimerization inhibitors (Site 2) and oligonucleotide-based modalities or DNA-binding inhibitors (Site 3) are shown

4.1.2   STAT3 as an Oncogene

Soon after the initial report of STAT3 activation in transformed cells, the role of STAT3 as an oncogene was confirmed by direct transformation of mouse fibroblasts with a constitutively-active mutant form of STAT3 [9]. Unlike many oncogenes, however, STAT3 mutations leading to its persistent activation are rarely identified in human cancers. In 2011, somatic STAT3 activating mutations were first reported in human inflammatory hepatocellular adenomas [10]. In these adenomas lacking mutations in the IL-6 receptor, mutations in the STAT3 Src homology 2 (SH2) region lead to persistent activation of STAT3 independent of IL-6 stimulation. Other than solid tumors, somatic STAT3 activating mutations were subsequently identified in a large percentage of patients with large granular lymphocytic (LGL) leukemia [11, 12]. Interestingly, a mouse leukemic cell line that mimics human LGL leukemia exhibits constitutive STAT3 activation [13, 14]. Nevertheless, the majority of STAT3 activation observed in human cancers is associated with aberrant signal transduction pathways that either positively or negatively regulate STAT3 activity.

4.1.3   STAT3 Activation Through Elevation of Positive Regulatory Mechanisms

The canonical STAT3 signaling pathway requires phosphorylation of the conserved tyrosine 705, adjacent to the SH2 domain, by the upstream JAK kinases upon recruitment to cytokine receptors that lack intrinsic protein tyrosine kinase activity. Many receptor protein tyrosine kinases, such as EGFR and platelet-derived growth factor receptor (PDGFR), can also phosphorylate STAT3 in a ligand-dependent manner [8]. Moreover, other non-receptor tyrosine kinases, such as Src and Abl family kinases, can phosphorylate STAT3 either in the context of receptor complexes or directly. Constitutive activation of these upstream kinases either by overexpression or as a result of mutations has been reported in many cancer types [15, 16]. In addition to tyrosine 705, STAT3 has a conserved serine 727 near the carboxy-terminal transactivation domain. Phosphorylation of serine 727 also contributes to maximal STAT3 activation in certain cell types and ligand stimulation contexts. Numerous pathways, such as mitogen-activated protein kinase (MAPK), p38, c-Jun N-terminal kinase (JNK), protein kinase C and PI3K/mTOR, are involved in STAT3 serine 727 phosphorylation [17]. STAT3 serine phosphorylation represents an important mechanism in fine-tuning STAT3 activity and in the crosstalk among different signaling pathways.

A third mechanism of STAT3 activation is acetylation on lysine 685 by histone acetyltransferase [18]. STAT3 acetylation enhances dimer stability and subsequent DNA-binding and target gene expression. Compared to STAT3 tyrosine phosphorylation, however, STAT3 serine phosphorylation and acetylation in human cancers are much less well defined.

4.1.4   STAT3 Activation Through Inhibition of Negative Regulatory Mechanisms

Like other STAT family members, STAT3 activation is both rapid and transient in response to ligand stimulation. The transient nature of STAT3 activation under physiological conditions is controlled by multiple negative regulatory mechanisms

(Fig. 4.1). Inhibition of one or more of these mechanisms can lead to constitutive STAT3 activation in human cancers.

Suppressor of cytokine signaling (SOCS) is the key negative feedback regulator in STAT3 signaling. Active STAT proteins induce the expression of SOCS family genes, which in turn downregulate further STAT signaling by inhibiting the upstream JAK kinase activity or by blocking STAT recruitment to the receptor complex. Among eight SOCS family members, SOCS3 exhibits more specific inhibitory effects toward STAT3. Other than JAK, SOCS can also inhibit many oncogenic protein tyrosine kinases capable of activating STAT3. Consistent with its role as a tumor suppressor, SOCS expression and/or activity have been shown to be inhibited in human cancers. Epigenetic silencing of SOCS genes by promoter hyper-methylation is the most common mechanism reported in human cancers [19].

Protein tyrosine phosphatases (PTP) inhibit STAT3 and its upstream activating kinases by removing phosphates from their key regulatory tyrosine residues. Cytosolic and membrane-associated phosphatases, such as SH2-containing phosphatase-1 (SHP-1), SHP-2, CD45, PTEN, PTPRD, PTPRT and protein tyrosine phosphatase 1B (PTP1B), can inhibit JAK and/or STAT3 [20–23]. Nuclear phosphatases, such as T-cell PTP, also can dephosphorylate and inhibit STAT3 [24, 25]. Many PTPs are known as tumor suppressors and inhibited by mutations or epigenetic silencing in human cancers [26]. Protein inhibitor of activated STAT (PIAS) represents another group of proteins that inhibit nuclear STAT proteins. Among four PIAS family members, PIAS3 specifically interacts with phosphorylated STAT3 to inhibit STAT3 DNA-binding and transactivation abilities [27]. Reduced PIAS3 expression has also been reported in human cancers that exhibit high levels of STAT3 activation, such as glioblastoma and lung cancer [28, 29].

4.1.5   STAT3 Target Gene Expression in Human Cancers

Genome-wide analysis of STAT3 target genes has identified numerous genes tightly associated with all aspects of cancer hallmarks [30, 31]. The gene expression patterns also overlap between cancer and wound healing processes [32]. They include genes important in cell proliferation (such as c-Myc, c-Fos, c-Jun, Cyclin D1, p21WAF1/CIP1), resistance to apoptosis (such as Bcl-xL, Bcl-2, Mcl-1, Survivin), angiogenesis (such as VEGF, bFGF, HGF), invasion and metastasis (such as MMPs, Vimentin, ICAM-1), inflammation (such as COX-2), immune evasion (such as IL-10, IL-23), and cell metabolism (such as HIF-1α). Depending on the cell types and context of genes, STAT3 can also repress distinct target gene expression. For example, STAT3 downregulates the expression of several mitochondrial electron transport chain (ETC) components encoded in the nuclear genome [33]. Reduced ETC protein expression can lead to decreased mitochondrial respiration and promote aerobic glycolysis, commonly known as the "Warburg effect" in cancer cells.

4.1.6   Mitochondrial STAT3 and Oncogenesis

Most of the earlier reports on STAT3 activation in human cancer focus on STAT3-mediated upregulation of nuclear target genes that contribute to different aspects of the tumorigenic process. However, it has become increasingly evident that STAT3 exhibits additional functions outside the nuclear compartment (Fig. 4.1). Mitochondrial STAT3 represents one of the most intriguing non-canonical STAT3 activities. It was first reported that STAT3 interacts with GRIM-19, a component of ETC Complex I embedded in the mitochondrial inner membrane [34]. Mitochondrial localization of STAT3 requires phosphorylation of the conserved serine 727 and not tyrosine 705. As a resident protein, mitochondrial STAT3 participates in mitochondrial respiration through oxidative phosphorylation to generate ATP [35]. Subsequent studies revealed the role of mitochondrial STAT3 in Ras-dependent cellular transformation [36] and as a potential therapeutic target for pancreatic cancer [37]. Nevertheless, it remains unclear how mitochondrial STAT3 contributes to the metabolic shift away from mitochondrial respiration observed in many cancer cells.

In addition to energy production, mitochondrial STAT3 may contribute to tumor growth through other mechanisms. In breast cancer cells, mitochondrial STAT3 has been proposed to have a role in regulating reactive oxygen species (ROS) levels that drive cancer cell growth and differentiation [38]. Mitochondrial STAT3 also interacts with cyclophilin D (CypD) to regulate the mitochondrial permeability transition pore (MPTP) [39]. Inhibition of MPTP opening can protect cells from apoptosis and may be advantageous for cancer cell survival [40]. The mitochondrion also has multiple copies of its own circular DNA encoding 13 essential ETC components and its own translational machinery. Most of the earlier reports demonstrated mitochondrial STAT3 functions independent of STAT3 binding to mitochondrial DNA. However, in keratinocytes, STAT3 binding to mitochondrial DNA is associated with reduced levels of mitochondrial-encoded transcripts [41]. Similarly, STAT5 also has been shown to translocate into mitochondria and bind mitochondrial DNA in both cytokine-stimulated cells and in leukemic cells [42]. In contrast to STAT3, STAT5 translocation into mitochondria correlates with phosphorylation of the conserved tyrosine residue. STAT5 is another STAT family member widely implicated in human cancer. Regulation of mitochondrial genome through direct binding of STAT3 and STAT5 may serve as another key mechanism in metabolic reprogramming in human cancer and represents an attractive target in cancer therapy.

4.2   STAT Inhibitory Modalities

4.2.1   Peptides and Peptidomimetic Approaches to Target
STAT3 Signaling

The design of peptide inhibitors of STAT3 preceded all the other strategies, and included the first generation of native pTyr peptides, PpYLKTK, PpYL, and ApYL and their modified forms and peptidomimetics, including ISS-610

[43–46]. These were all developed via a semi-rational, structure-based design approach to target the pTyr-SH2 domain interaction. Accordingly, these modalities disrupt STAT3:STAT3 dimerization (Fig. 4.1, site 2), with biochemical and cellular activities ranging from 35 μM to 1 mM, and they have preferential affinity for STAT3 over STAT1 and relatively minimal impact on STAT5 activity. A modified version of the phospho-peptide, PpYLKTK, which is appended at the carboxy-terminus with a membrane-translocation sequence (mts, AAVLLPVLLAAP) composed of hydrophobic amino acids to aid cell membrane permeability, demonstrated intracellular inhibitory activity against STAT3 signaling and STAT3-dependent tumor processes *in vitro* [44]. However, the PpYLKTK-mts peptide had to be used at concentrations up to 1 mM for measurable intracellular effects.

Other phospho-peptide inhibitors have the primary structure, pYNNQ, where N represents any amino acid, and were derived from the leukemia inhibitory factory (LIF), interleukin 10 receptor (IL-10R), epidermal growth factor receptor (EGFR), granulocyte colony-stimulating factor receptor (GCSF), or glycoprotein 130 (gp130) [47, 48]. These and their peptidomimetic analogs such as Ac-pYLPQTV-NH$_2$ reportedly inhibited STAT3 activity, with an IC$_{50}$ of 150 nM [48, 49]. Moreover, a 28-mer peptide derived from the STAT3 SH2 domain, SPI (amino acid sequence, NH$_2$-FISKERERAILSTKPPGTFLLRFSESS-COOH), was functionally active at 25–50 μM [50]. Additional peptidomimetic modalities that also target the STAT3 SH2 domain and the pTyr-SH2 domain interaction include CJ-1383 [51] and the phosphatase-stable, cell-permeable phosphopeptide mimetic prodrug, PM-73G [52].

Besides the inhibition of both constitutive and ligand-induced STAT3 phosphorylation, DNA-binding, and transcriptional activities, studies of these modalities showed suppressive effects against tumor cell viability. They caused induction of apoptosis *in vitro* of human breast, pancreatic, prostate and non-small cell lung cancer, and other human tumor and mouse transformed cells harboring aberrantly-active STAT3, with varying activities [3, 43, 44, 46–51, 53–57]. Studies further showed S3I-M2001 [46] and PM-73G [57] are active and efficacious *in vivo* against the growth of human breast tumor xenografts in mice. The authors of the studies of PM-73G reported no observed changes in the expression of Cyclin D1, Bcl-2 or Survivin, which are known STAT3-regulated genes, and no evidence of apoptosis induction in response to the lowest concentration that inhibited STAT3 activity [52]. Moreover, the inhibition of cell proliferation occurred at 50-fold higher concentrations [52]. Therefore, STAT3-independent effects likely contribute to the biological responses to PM-73G at higher concentrations. Notwithstanding, the large body of data support the viewpoint that inhibition of STAT3 activity leads to tumor cell growth suppression and apoptosis. Despite the prolific research into peptide inhibitors of STAT3, metabolic instability, poor cell permeability, and other peptide-associated liabilities have precluded their clinical development as therapeutics.

4.2.2   Small Molecules that Target STAT3 Signaling

The development of peptide inhibitors of STAT3 gave way to small molecules as therapeutic approaches. These initiatives were established largely through the use of computational modeling, docking studies, and the virtual screening of chemical libraries. Like the peptides, this strategy is focused on targeting the pTyr-SH2 domain interaction, and most of the small molecule STAT3 inhibitors disrupt STAT3:STAT3 dimerization (Fig. 4.1, site 2). Among them are STA-21 (NSC628869), which was identified from the screening of the National Cancer Institute (NCI) chemical library, and its structural analog, LLL-3, and a catechol (1,2-dihydroxybenzene) compound [58]. These compounds inhibit STAT3 dimerization, DNA-binding activity and/or transcriptional function in tumor cells at 20–106 µM. The more membrane permeable compound, LLL-3, suppressed intracranial glioblastoma tumors [59]. An oxazole-based small molecule, S3I-M2001 emerged from the optimization of the lead peptidomimetic inhibitor, ISS-610 [43], and it showed improved activity *in vitro* and efficacy *in vivo* against human breast cancer [46].

Separately, the STAT3 SH2 domain-focused structure-based, virtual docking and screening of the NCI chemical library discovered S3I-201 (NSC74859) as a disruptor of STAT3 dimerization and activation, with potency of 86±33 µM, and a strong *in vivo* antitumor efficacy against human breast tumor xenografts [60]. Subsequent medicinal chemistry and lead optimization efforts have generated several derivatives, including S3I-201.1066, S3I-1757, BP-1-102, SH4-54 and SH5-07 [61–64]. These analogs show improved STAT3-inhibitory potencies of 35, 13.5, 6.8, 4.7 and 3.9 µM, respectively, and inhibited DNA-binding and transcriptional activities, tumor cell growth, malignant transformation, survival, migration and invasiveness *in vitro* of solid and hematological tumor cells harboring aberrantly-active STAT3. In particular, BP-1-102, SH4-54 and SH5-07 inhibited growth of human breast, non-small cell lung cancer, and glioblastoma xenografts in mice, and all are fairly orally-bioavailable [62, 64].

Other compounds similarly discovered through virtual ligand screening are Cpd30 (4-(5-((3-ethyl-4-oxo-2-thioxo-1,3-thiazolidin-5-ylidene)methyl)-2-furyl) benzoic acid) and its related compound, Cpd188 4-(((3-((carboxymethyl)thio)-4-hydroxy-1-naphthyl)amino)sulfonyl)benzoic acid [65], Stattic [66], STX-0119 [67, 68], and HJC0123 [69], which interfere with the SH2 domain function. These compounds inhibited constitutive and/or ligand (IL-6)-induced STAT3 activation and induced apoptosis *in vitro* in tumor models harboring abnormal STAT3 activity, including breast, pancreatic, head and neck squamous cell carcinoma (HNSCC), and lymphoma cells. *In vivo*, these compounds inhibited growth of tumor xenografts of the same cancer cells. In combination studies, Cpd188 and docetaxel suppressed tumor growth in a chemotherapy-resistant human breast cancer model [65].

The niclosamide-derived agent, HJC0152 [70], compound 6 [71], WP1066 [72], LLL-3 [59, 73], LLL12 [74], ML116 [75, 76], and OPB-31121 [77–83] are other small molecule STAT3 signaling inhibitors that induced anti-tumor responses *in vitro* and *in vivo* with varying potencies against diverse tumor models harboring constitutively active STAT3. Other inhibitors are inS3-54 and inS3-54A18 [84], XZH-5 and its derivatives [85–87], LY5 (5,8-dioxo-6-(pyridin-3-ylamino)-5,8-dihydronaphthalene-1-sulfonamide) [88], compound 1 [89], compound 9 and compound 16w [90], HJC0416 [91], HO-3867 [92, 93], compound 23 [94], and platinum (IV) complexes, such as IS3 295 [95], CPA-7 and CPA-1 [96], which potentially target the pTyr:SH2 domain interaction and/or the STAT3 DNA-binding domain (Fig. 4.1, sites 2 and 3). These inhibitors induced biological responses in diverse human tumor models *in vitro* and antitumor effects *in vivo*.

Except for OPB-31121, none of the aforementioned agents have advanced to clinical trials in part due to low potency and other pharmacological weaknesses. Further, for many of these inhibitors, the exact mechanisms of inhibition of STAT3 activation are not as clearly defined. Surprisingly, despite that OPB-31121 has gone through clinical trials, its mode of inhibition of STAT3 signaling is not entirely clear. Reports suggest it modulates STAT3 signaling at the level of the receptor by inducing the down regulation of the IL-6 receptor/gp130 and further that it inhibits JAK activity [80], which would suggest it functions by way of a gp130/JAK TK inhibitor. It is also surprising that the structure of OPB-31121 is not in the public domain to enable its synthesis for mechanistic studies. Given these issues, it is therefore unclear if the antitumor responses of OPB-31121 are due to the combination of effects on STAT3, STAT5, JAKs and other potential targets that are as yet undetermined. Another compound that has gone through clinical trials as a STAT3 inhibitor is OPB-51602 [97], which similarly lacks pre-clinical studies on its mechanism(s) of inhibition of STAT3 and has no structural information. The outcome of the clinical trials of both OPB-31121 and OPB-51602 are discussed later in the chapter.

4.2.3 Oligonucleotide Decoy Approach to Inhibit STAT3 Activity

Decoy oligodeoxynucleotide (ODN) modalities compete with endogenous promoter sequences for the binding of target transcription factors and consequently suppress gene expression [98, 99]. Specific ODN sequences have been evaluated for inhibitory effects against STAT3 DNA-biniding and transcriptional activities (Fig. 4.1, site 3) [99]. The intra-tumoral administration of the ODN 5′-CATTTCCCGTAAATC-3′, a modified version of high-affinity *sis*-inducible element (hSIE) of the *c-fos* promoter, downregulated STAT3 target gene expression and decreased tumor growth *in vivo* in glioblastoma xenograft models [98]. The ODN-induced inhibition of STAT3 function sensitized resistant HNSCC and bladder cancer cells to cetuximab and erlotinib [100]. The biological effects of the ODN agents appear to be STAT1-independent, despite that conceptually the ODN agents are expected to interfere with STAT1 transcriptional activity [101]. More stable cyclic versions of the decoy, 5′-CATTTCCCGTAAATC-3′ that are resistant to serum nucleases have also been developed, tested, and found to downregulate STAT3 target gene expression and to induce the loss of viability in HNSCC and bladder cancer models [100]. A hairpin ODN version with a modified consensus sequence containing two STAT3-binding sites and that discriminates between STAT1 and STAT3 was shown to be effective against SW480 colon cancer cells [99]. Studies thus far show great promise for the clinical development of the STAT3 ODN decoy approach. This strategy has already progressed to clinical trials, which will be further discussed later in the chapter.

4.2.4 Antisense Oligonucleotides as Inhibitors of STAT3 Functions

Oligonucleotide sequences complementary to the specific STAT3 messenger RNA (mRNA) have also been evaluated as modalities to inhibit STAT3 expression and functions [102]. Antisense oligonucleotide (ASO) agents have been tested for their ability to target STAT3 signaling and for efficacy against STAT3-dependent tumor models, including HCC [103], melanoma [102], breast [102], and prostate [104] cancer models. The antisense agent, ISIS 481464 was developed as a phosphorothioate-modified chimeric sequence to target the human STAT3 mRNA for therapeutic application [105]. Its evaluation in tumor models *in vivo* showed responses that included the downregulation of both the STAT3 mRNA and protein levels and the inhibition of cell proliferation. The application of ISIS 481464 at 10 mg/kg/week in monkeys led to the suppression of the STAT3 protein level, and the agent was well tolerated up to 30 mg/kg/week dose, with no signs of toxicity or any treatment-related deaths [105]. This approach is also further along in its development, including testing clinical studies, which will be discussed later in the chapter.

4.2.5 Natural Products that Inhibit STAT3 Signaling

There are reports of natural products and their inhibitory effects against the JAK/STAT3 signaling pathway. For many of these, the modes of inhibition of STAT3 activity are rather unclear, with the possibility that the inhibition of STAT3 signaling may be indirect. Also, it is likely that additional targets are modulated that contribute to the overall responses for these compounds, and the challenge is defining the contribution of the STAT3 inhibition to the overall antitumor responses.

Curcumin [106, 107], a phenolic compound derived from the perennial herb *Curcuma longa* and a series of derivatives, including FLLL32 [108, 109], HO-3867 [93, 110], LLL12 [109, 111–113], and FLLL62 [114], were all reported to suppress the JAK/STAT signaling at micromolar concentrations. These compounds decreased STAT3 recruitment to the receptor, phospho-STAT3 and total STAT3 levels, interfered with STAT3 dimerization, and promoted the induction of STAT3 ubiquitination and proteasomal degradation [108, 112]. Suppression of IL-6 production by interleukin-1β (IL-1β)-stimulated myeloid-derived suppressor cells in gastric cancer xenografts was also observed following curcumin treatment [107]. The associated biological responses include cycle arrest, loss of cell viability, decreased colony formation, migration and invasion behaviors, sensitization of resistant ovarian cancer cells to cisplatin, induction of apoptosis *in vitro*, the inhibition of tumor vasculature development, and the suppression of tumor growth *in vivo* in human tumors [93, 109, 110, 112, 113]. The latter include glioblastoma, osteosarcoma, small cell lung, breast and ovarian cancers, and BRCA1-mutated ovarian cancer models. BBMD3 derived from bis-benzylsioquinoline alkaloid berbamine (BBM) from *Berberis amurensis* inhibited pJAK2, pSrc, and pSTAT3 in melanoma cells and induced loss of cell viability, with a potency of 2.9 μM [115]. BBMD3 is likely functiioning as a JAK inhibitor, because it directly inhibited the auto-phosphorylation of the mutant JAK2^{V617F} in *in vitro* kinase assay [115].

The bis-indole alkaloid, indirubin from a mixture of Danggui Longhui Wan plants used in the traditional Chinese medicine, and its derivatives inhibited vascular endothelial growth factor receptor (VEGFR)-mediated JAK/STAT3 activation and angiogenesis in both chick embryo chorio-allantoic membrane and mice corneal micropocket assays [116]. Moreover, IRD E804 and MLS-2488, which are also derivatives of indirubin, similarly inhibited c-Src activity *in vitro* at 0.43 μM, and suppressed pJAK, pSTAT3, pAkt, and STAT3 DNA binding activity, downregulated Mcl-1 and Survivin expression, and induced apoptosis in human breast cancer cells [117, 118]. The more water-soluble IRD, E738, strongly inhibited the kinase activities of JAK1 (IC$_{50}$ of 10.4 nM), JAK2 (74.1 nM), Tyk2 (0.7 nM), and Src (IC$_{50}$ of 10.7 nM), and downregulated pSrc and pSTAT3 levels, and STAT3 transcriptional activity in pancreatic cancer cells at 1–2 μM [119].

Resveratrol (3, 5, 4'-trihydroxystilbene), found in red grapes and other plants, its analogs, piceatannol (3, 3', 4, 4'-transtrihydroxystilbene) and LYR71, caffeic acid, a phenolic acid present in fruits, wine and coffee and its synthetic derivative, CAPDE and its analog, and WP1193 were reported to inhibit constitutive and/or ligand-induced STAT3 activation [120–123]. These compounds inhibit multiple myeloma, leukemia, melanoma, renal carcinoma, glioma, pancreatic, prostate cancer, and other tumor cells at moderate to high micromolar concentrations [120–125]. It is unclear how these agents modulate pSTAT3 and STAT3 signaling. The responses further include decreased expression of matrix metalloproteinase (MMP)-9, Bcl-2, Bcl-xL, and other anti-apoptotic proteins, induction of apoptosis, and sensitization to chemotherapy or radiation in the models of lung carcinoma, multiple myeloma, prostate cancer, pancreatic cancer, and glioblastoma multiforme patient-derived CD133-positive cells *in vitro*. Treatment with resveratrol also prolonged the survival of leukemia-bearing mice, in parallel with decreased pSTAT3 levels in liver tissue lysates [121]. Moreover, caffeic acid and CAPDE both inhibited tumor growth and angiogenesis in renal cancer mouse xenografts, which was associated with decreased active STAT3 and HIF1α and VEGF expression, while WP1193 blocked murine melanoma and human glioma tumor growth *in vivo* [126–128].

Capsaicin (trans-8-methyl-*N*-vanillyl-6-nonenamide, 100 μM) from hot red and chili peppers, cryptotanshinone from the *Salvia miltiorrhiza* Bunge (Danshen), celastrol, a triterpene derived from the Chinese medicinal plant, *Tripterygium wilfordii*, and avicin D, a triterpenoid saponin that is present in the cactus plant *Acacia victoriae*, were all reported to inhibit both constitutive or inducible STAT3 phosphorylation, activation, and/or STAT3 nuclear translocation [129–133]. The exact mechanisms by which these natural products modulate STAT3 activation remain poorly understood, with some evidence that capsaicin promotes gp130 depletion and cryptotanshinne may bind to the STAT3 SH2 domain [129, 130]. These natural products further promote decreased expression of Cyclin D1, Survivin, Bcl-xL, and/or Bcl-2 expression, known STAT3-regulated genes, inhibit cell proliferation, induce apoptosis, and enhance sensitivity to chemotherapy *in vitro* and *in vivo* [130, 131, 133]. These studies were performed in models of multiple myeloma, prostate cancer, HCC, and cutaneous T-cell lymphoma (CTCL), and CD4+ T-cells isolated from patients with Sézary Syndrome [133].

Other natural products, including withaferin A (triterpenoid derived found in *Withania somnifera*), betulinic acid (pentacyclic triterpene isolated from the bark of the plant *Zizyphus mauritiana*), ursolic acid (3β-hydroxy-urs-12-en-28-oic-acid; pentacyclic triterpenoid, a dietary component found in many fruits), and oleanolic acid (from *Ganoderma lucidum* other other plants) and its more potent derivative, CDDO-Me, inhibited constitutive and ligand-induced STAT3 activation, nuclear translocation, and DNA binding activity in tumor cells [56, 134–141]. These effects were observed in breast cancer, renal carcinoma, multiple myeloma, prostate cancer, multidrug-resistant (MDR) ovarian cancer, and osteosarcoma cells. Except for the activity of CDDO-Me at 0.1 nM [138], these natural products are moderately active. The mechanisms of inhibition of STAT3 activation are also unclear and suggested to include decreased STAT3 and JAK2 protein levels, blockade of JAK1, JAK2, and c-Src activities, modulation of EGFR, and the induction of the SHP-1 protein Tyr phosphatase [56, 136, 137, 141]. Treatment with these natural products further caused decreased cyclin D1, Bcl-2, survivin, Mcl-1 and VEGF expression [56], sensitization to apoptosis induced in response to bortezomib and thalidomide in multiple myeloma cells [136], and the inhibition of tumor growth *in vivo* in an aggressive ER⁻ (negative) breast cancer model [141]. More recent studies identified a group of hirsutinolides that inhibited STAT3 phosphorylation and DNA-binding activity by mechanisms that involve the direct interference with the DNA-binding domain. These effects contributed to decreased cell viability, cell growth, and colony formation, cell cycle arrest, and tumor growth inhibition in glioblastoma model *in vitro* and *in vivo* [142].

Cucurbitacin agents (from Cucurbitaceae, Cruciferae and other plant families) also modulated the JAK/STAT3 pathway. These include cucurbitacin I (JSI-124) that inhibited JAK/STAT3 signaling, with a potency of 500 nM, cucurbitacin B that inhibited STAT3 signaling in combination with cisplatin, and cucurbitacin E that blocked VEGFR2-induced JAK2/STAT3 activation in human umbilical vein endothelial cells (HUVEC) [143–145]. These natural products also promoted the loss of cell viability, cell growth inhibition, and apoptosis of human and mouse tumors harboring aberrantly-active STAT3, and suppressed both angiogenesis and tumor growth *in vitro* and *in vivo* [145]. These findings were reported in models of laryngeal squamous carcinoma, medulloblastoma, thyroid, prostate, pancreatic, or bladder cancer [144, 146–149]. Additional responses included inhibition of cell proliferation and enhanced radiation-sensitivity of CD133-positive cancer stem cells (CSC) from non-small cell lung cancer patients [150].

Diosgenin (plant steroidal saponin), emodin (from the root and rhizome of *Rhenum palmatum*), and thymoquinone (from the volatile oil of black seed, *Nigella sativa*), all inhibited both constitutive and inducible STAT3 signaling with potencies of 8.5–10 μM [151–154]. The mechanisms of action remain unclear and likely involve the suppression of STAT3 nuclear translocation, inhibition of Tyr kinases, including Src and JAK2 activation, and/or the induction of protein Tyr phosphatases, including SH-PTP2 [151, 153, 154]. These resulted in the downregulation of the expression of STAT3 target genes, loss of cell viability, decreased cell proliferation, and chemosensitization in tumor models, including HCC and multiple myeloma. Similarly, honokiol (from the bark of *Magnolia officialis*) and evodiamine (an alkaloid isolated from *Evodia rutaecarpa*) weakly to moderately inhibited STAT3 activation in HNSCC, HCC, and gastric cancer cells by poorly understood mechanisms that likely involve JAK and EGFR suppression, and SHP-1 phosphatase induction [155–158]. These natural products also induced antitumor response *in vivo* in a HCC xenograft model.

Carbazole (the active compound of coal tar) and its *N*-alkyl derivatives, and the clinically used drug, sanguarine (a benzophenantridine alkaloid extracted primarily from the bloodroot plant), inhibited constitutive STAT3 and/or IL-6 stimulated STAT3 activation and DNA-binding activity in embryonic kidney or human monocytic leukemia cells via mechanisms that are presently unclear [159–161]. These changes likely contribute to the suppression of cell proliferation, migration and invasion of prostate tumor cells. γ-Tocotrienol (a member of the vitamin E superfamily), acetyl-11-keto-β-boswellic acid (AKBA) (the active compound isolated from the Indian *Boswellia serrate* plant), 3,3′-diindolmethane (DIM; an indole compound found in cruciferous vegetables), and brevilin A (isolated from *Litsea glutinosa*) inhibited constitutive or inducible JAK/STAT signaling [162–165]. Again, the mechanisms of action are not fully understood and are likely to involve inhibition of the JAK JH1 (Janus homology 1) domain and other tyrosine kinases and the induction of SHP-1 phosphatase activity in HCC, multiple myeloma, prostate and/or breast cancer cells [162, 163, 166]. These effects led to decreased expression of Cyclin D1, Bcl-2, Mcl-1 and VEGF, inhibition of cell proliferation, and induction of apoptosis *in vitro*, antitumor effects *in vivo*, and enhanced cisplatin sensitivity in an ovarian cancer model [163–166].

4.2.6   Tyrosine Kinase Inhibitors of STAT3 Signaling

Tyrosine kinases have long been attractive targets for therapeutic development due to their importance in many cellular processes and human diseases. It is feasible that the modulation of STAT3 function could be part of the underlying mechanisms for the therapeutic responses to TKIs, in so long as STAT signaling is dysregulated downstream of the Tyr kinase (Fig. 4.1, site 1). Several Tyr kinase modulators have been approved for the treatment of different types of cancers. Most of these are small molecule kinase inhibitors or antibody-based therapeutics that compete for binding to the cell surface receptors. The discussion of TK modulators in this volume will focus on JAK inhibitors.

JAK inhibitors are becoming more prominent in clinical application, and there are presently JAK inhibitors undergoing clinical trials against a variety of diseases. Notable ones include tofacitinib (CP690,550), which abrogated anti-CD3-induced IFN-γ, IL-4 and IL-17 production in CD4+ T cells isolated from the peripheral blood of healthy volunteers and was efficacious in rheumatoid arthritis [167]. CP690,550 inhibited STAT3 and the activation of other STATs in cultured anti-CD3-stimulated T cells [167]. Also, ruxolitinib inhibits JAK1 ($IC_{50} = 3.3$ nM) and JAK2 ($IC_{50} = 2.8$ nM), blocks both STAT3 and STAT5 activation in a human erythroleukemia cell line (HEL) expressing JAK2^{V617F}, and inhibits STAT3 activity, soft-agar growth, and tumor growth *in vivo* in a NSCLC model [168, 169]. AZD1480 inhibits JAK1 ($IC_{50} = 1.3$ nM) and JAK2 ($IC_{50} = 0.4$ nM) [170]. This drug preferentially blocks STAT3 activation over other STATs in prostate, ovarian, and breast cancers, glioma, and human and murine kidney carcinoma, and myeloid-derived suppressor cells in a murine renal carcinoma model *in vitro* [171–173], and induces antitumor effects in the prostate and ovarian tumor models *in vivo* [171]. Despite its potent activity against JAKs, AZD1480 inhibited cell proliferation of Hodgkin lymphoma cells harboring activated JAK only at higher concentration (5 µM) [170], suggesting additional mechanisms contribute to the anti-proliferative effects. Atiprimod (SK&F 106615) suppressed pJAK2 and JAK2 protein levels, blocked STAT3 and STAT5 phosphorylation, and induced antiproliferative and pro-apoptotic effects in model lines of K562, multiple myeloma, or essential thrombocythemia harboring an active JAK2 mutation [174–176]. Auranofin, which is currently undergoing Phase II clinical trials, also inhibited JAK1 activity in *in vitro* kinase assays, and it further blocked IL6-induced JAK1 and STAT3 activation, suppressed Mcl-1 expression, and induced Caspase 3 activation in multiple myeloma cells [177, 178]. Nevertheless, the exact mechanism of action remains to be defined. It is noteworthy that treatment with TKIs may not always lead to a suppressive response on STAT3 signaling, likely due to compensatory mechanisms from the non-targeted tyrosine kinases.

4.3   Early Results from Clinical Studies of JAK/STAT3 Inhibitors

With the exception of Tyr kinase modulators, inhibitors of STAT3 signaling are currently unavailable for clinical application. Multiple reasons account for this, including physicochemical liabilities of reported inhibitors that impact their pharmacological properties. The last several years have seen a few cases of clinical trials of modalities that directly modulate STAT3 signaling. The compound, OPB-31121, is the only small molecule STAT3 inhibitor to go through clinical trials (Phases I and II) and it inhibits STAT3 signaling by as yet undefined mechanisms [77, 82, 83]. Separate Phase I trials have been conducted against advanced solid tumors, including gastric and colo-rectal cancers (#NCT00955812) and hepatocellular carcinoma (#NCT01406574). The common adverse events were gastrointestinal (grade 1–2 nausea; grade 1–3 vomiting; grade 1–3 diarrhea), fatigue (grade 1–2), malaise, anorexia, and peripheral sensory neuropathy, which were reported to occur at 300 mg dose and higher. Two of the reports indicated that the observed pharmacokinetics did not demonstrate dose-proportionality, the plasma concentrations were several hundreds to 4000-fold lower than the target concentrations from pre-clinical studies, and further that the agent demonstrated a high inter-subject variability [77, 82]. Despite these, there were reports of cases of patients showing stable disease and/or tumor shrinkage (one colon cancer and one rectal cancer), while other patients showed disease progression.

Two other reports focused on another small molecule identified as a STAT3 inhibitor, OPB-51602, which was evaluated in two separate Phase I clinical trials in relapsed/refractory NSCLC or hematological tumors at much lower administered doses [81, 97]. The most common treatment-related toxicities included nausea, vomiting, diarrhea, fatigue, anorexia, and peripheral sensory neuropathy. Dose limiting toxicities included grade 3 hyponatremia, grade 3 dehydration, grade 3 lactic acidosis and increased blood lactic acid levels, and grade 1–2 peripheral neuropathy. Evidence of inhibition of pSTAT3 was observed in peripheral blood mononuclear cells [97], and there were partial responses in two of the NSCLC patients [97], while no clear therapeutic response was observed in the case of the hematological malignancies, except for a durable stable disease observed in two patients with acute myeloid leukemia and one with multiple myeloma [81].

A Phase 0 clinical trial (#NCT00696176) of the ODN decoy was pursued for the safety of a single dose of intratumoral injection in HNSCC patients and for pharmacodynamic monitoring [98], which showed suppressive effects on the STAT3-regulated gene expreession and minimal toxicity [179]. A Phase I/Ib clinical trial (#NCT01839604) for patients with advanced/metastatic HCC to evaluate the safety, tolerability, pharmacokinetics and preliminary anti-tumor activity of STAT3 antisense oligonucleotide, AZD9150 (ISIS-STAT3Rx), has been completed, although the results are yet to be publicly disclosed. A recent published report alluded to an initial clinical study that showed a single-agent antitumor activity of AZD9150 in patients with highly treatment-refractory lymphoma and NSCLC in a Phase 1 dose-escalation study. Another clinical study (#NCT01563302) is ongoing, which is intended to provide more data on the clinical and therapeutic significance of the inhibition of STAT3 function in cancer patients and on the efficacy of the ASO approach [180].

The potential to safely modulate aberrant STAT3 signaling in human cancers can also be evaluated by way of TKIs, and there are many TKIs in clinical application against human cancers. These include a Phase II study in chronic myelogenous leukemia (CLL) patients (#NCT01441882) of dasatinib based on the *in vitro* evidence of cytotoxic effects against primary CLL cells, and a Phase I/II trial (#NCT00124657) of erlotinib in combination with radiation therapy in young patients who are newly diagnosed with glioma to determine the dose-limiting toxicity. It is envisioned that the effects on STAT3 signaling would contribute to the overall responses in these studies, in so long as aberrantly-active STAT3 is prevalent in these tumors as a consequence of the hyperactive Tyr kinase target. Other studies that could be relevant to STAT3 signaling is the evaluation of curcumin on pancreatic cancer in a Phase II trial (#NCT00094445), the studies of the tolerability and pharmacodynamic properties of resveratrol in colorectal cancer patients (#NCT00433576), and the Phase II/III study (#NCT01391689) of the effectiveness of DIM in breast cancer, based on pre-clinical studies that these natural products modulate STAT3 signaling in addition to other mechanisms.

A phase II study will also evaluate the pharmacodynamic effects of the TKI, AZD0530 on c-Src, STAT3, STAT5 activation in metastatic HNSCC patients (#NCT00513435). In addition, a Phase I clinical trial (#NCT01431664) of the multi-kinase inhibitor, AT9283, in young patients with relapsed or refractory acute leukemia, will determine the MTD, the pharmacokinetic profile, and the effects on pSTAT5 *ex vivo* and *in vivo*. Furthermore, an observational clinical study (#NCT01633346) will determine the activation status of STAT3 and other STATs in leukocytes isolated from rheumatoid arthritis patients treated with tocilizumab, a humanized anti IL-6 receptor monoclonal antibody. There also is a Phase II clinical trial (#NCT01712659) to examine the safety and effectiveness of the JAK inhibitor, AZD1480, in adult T-cell leukemia patients. Finally, the reponses to auranofin, currently undergoing Phase II clinical trials in chronic lymphocytic leukemia (CLL) and ovarian and lung cancers (#NCT01419691, #NCT01747798, #NCT01737502), may potentially involve the role of STAT3. The clinical benefits and potential toxicities of targeting constitutively-active STAT3 signaling in human diseases remain to be fully characterized in these ongoing clinical trials.

4.4   Conclusion

In normal cellular physiology, STAT3 activation is very tightly controlled by a multitude of complex signal transduction pathways emanating primarily from cytokine and growth factor receptors on the cell surface. These normal signaling pathways control STAT3 activity through precise positive and negative regulatory circuits, often involving crosstalk among different signal transduction networks. Positive regulation of STAT3 is mediated largely by protein kinases, especially tyrosine and serine kinases induced by cytokines and growth factors. Negative STAT3 regulation involves protein tyrosine phosphatases as well as other proteins that inhibit STAT3 phosphorylation or DNA-binding and gene regulation.

Disruption of this delicate balance in normal STAT3 signaling contributes to cancer by inducing persistent STAT3 activation. The constitutive activation of STAT3 results in continuous expression of STAT3 target genes involved in cell proliferation, differentiation, apoptosis, metastasis, angiogenesis, metabolism, inflammation and immune evasion [181]. The resulting permanent change in gene expression programs contributes to the malignant phenotype. Deregulation of any of the above STAT3 positive and negative regulators, through a variety of different mechanisms, is the most common cause of STAT3 activation in cancer. Mutation of the STAT3 gene itself can be oncogenic, although this is a less common mechanism of STAT3 activation in cancer. Thus, the positive and negative regulators of STAT3 are the most promising molecular targets for cancer therapy.

Numerous inhibitors of STAT3 activity have been developed, although a viable clinical candidate has yet to be demonstrated. These inhibitors include small-molecule drugs, natural products, and gene therapy approaches. Given the wide diversity of fundamental cellular processes regulated by STAT3 signaling, the challenge will be to develop inhibitors of this pathway that do not have toxic side effects in normal cellular physiology. The solution to this challenge may be that tumor cells are more dependent on STAT3 signaling, and therefore could be more sensitive than normal cells to STAT3 inhibitors. Furthermore, normal cells may be able to utilize alternative signaling pathways that are not available to tumor cells, thereby circumventing the toxic effects of STAT3 inhibitors. Another possible approach to limit potential toxicity is local application of STAT3 inhibitors rather than systemic administration. Because STAT3 is activated in a plethora of human cancers, such STAT3 inhibitors may have broad applicability in cancer therapy, most likely in combination with other cancer treatments.

References

1. Darnell JE Jr, Kerr IM, Stark GR (1994) Jak-STAT pathways and transcriptional activation in response to IFNs and other extracellular signaling proteins. Science 264:1415–1421
2. Akira S, Nishio Y, Inoue M et al (1994) Molecular cloning of APRF, a novel IFN-stimulated gene factor 3 p91-related transcription factor involved in the gp130-mediated signaling pathway. Cell 77:63–71
3. Turkson J, Jove R (2000) STAT proteins: novel molecular targets for cancer drug discovery. Oncogene 19:6613–6626
4. Hanahan D, Weinberg RA (2011) Hallmarks of cancer: the next generation. Cell Death Differ 144:646–674
5. Yu C-L, Meyer DJ, Campbell GS et al (1995) Enhanced DNA-binding activity of a Stat3-related protein in cells transformed by the Src oncoprotein. Science 269:81–83
6. Migone TS, Lin JX, Cereseto A et al (1995) Constitutively activated Jak-STAT pathway in T cells transformed with HTLV-I. Science 269:79–81
7. Levy DE, Lee CK (2002) What does Stat3 do? J Clin Invest 109:1143–1148
8. Yu H, Jove R (2004) The STATS of cancer—new molecular targets come of age. Nat Rev Cancer 4:97–105
9. Bromberg JF, Wrzeszczynska MH, Devgan G et al (1999) *Stat3* as an oncogene. Cell 98:295–303
10. Pilati C, Amessou M, Bihl MP et al (2011) Somatic mutations activating STAT3 in human inflammatory hepatocellular adenomas. J Exp Med 208:1359–1366
11. Koskela HL, Eldfors S, Ellonen P et al (2012) Somatic STAT3 mutations in large granular lymphocytic leukemia. N Engl J Med 366:1905–1913
12. Jerez A, Clemente MJ, Makishima H et al (2012) STAT3 mutations unify the pathogenesis of chronic lymphoproliferative disorders of NK cells and T-cell large granular lymphocyte leukemia. Blood 120:3048–3057

13. Chueh F-Y, Cronk RJ, Alsuwaidan AN et al (2014) Mouse LSTRA leukemia as a model of human natural killer T cell and highly aggressive lymphoid malignancies. Leuk Lymphoma 55:706–708

14. Yu C-L, Jove R, Burakoff SJ (1997) Constitutive activation of the Janus kinase-STAT pathway in T lymphoma overexpressing the Lck protein tyrosine kinase. J Immunol 159:5206–5210

15. Jechlinger M, Sommer A, Moriggl R et al (2006) Autocrine PDGFR signaling promotes mammary cancer metastasis. J Clin Invest 116:1561–1570

16. Yue P, Zhang X, Paladino D et al (2012) Hyperactive EGF receptor, Jaks and Stat3 signaling promote enhanced colony-forming ability, motility and migration of cisplatin-resistant ovarian cancer cells. Oncogene 31:2309–2322

17. Decker T, Kovarik P (2000) Serine phosphorylation of STATs. Oncogene 19:2628–2637

18. Yuan ZL, Guan YJ, Chatterjee D et al (2005) Stat3 dimerization regulated by reversible acetylation of a single lysine residue. Science 307:269–273

19. He B, You L, Uematsu K et al (2003) SOCS-3 is frequently silenced by hypermethylation and suppresses cell growth in human lung cancer. Proc Natl Acad Sci U S A 100:14133–14138

20. Veeriah S, Brennan C, Meng S et al (2009) The tyrosine phosphatase PTPRD is a tumor suppressor that is frequently inactivated and mutated in glioblastoma and other human cancers. Proc Natl Acad Sci U S A 106:9435–9440

21. Zhang X, Guo A, Yu J et al (2007) Identification of STAT3 as a substrate of receptor protein tyrosine phosphatase. Proc Natl Acad Sci U S A 104:4060–4064

22. Sun S, Steinberg BM (2002) PTEN is a negative regulator of STAT3 activation in human papillomavirus-infected cells. J Gen Virol 83:1651–1658

23. Irie-Sasaki J, Sasaki T, Matsumoto W et al (2001) CD45 is a JAK phosphatase and negatively regulates cytokine receptor signalling. Nature 409:349–354

24. Fukushima A, Loh K, Galic S et al (2010) T-cell protein tyrosine phosphatase attenuates STAT3 and insulin signaling in the liver to regulate gluconeogenesis. Diabetes 59:1906–1914

25. Ren F, Geng Y, Minami T et al (2015) Nuclear termination of STAT3 signaling through SIPAR (STAT3-interacting protein as a repressor)-dependent recruitment of T cell tyrosine phosphatase TC-PTP. FEBS Lett 589:1890–1896

26. Östman A, Hellberg C, Böhmer FD (2006) Protein-tyrosine phosphatases and cancer. Nat Rev Cancer 6:307–320

27. Chung CD, Liao J, Liu B et al (1997) Specific inhibition of Stat3 signal transduction by PIAS3. Science 278:1803–1805

28. Brantley EC, Nabors LB, Gillespie GY et al (2008) Loss of protein inhibitors of activated STAT-3 expression in glioblastoma multiforme tumors: implications for STAT-3 activation and gene expression. Clin Cancer Res 14:4694–4704

29. Abbas R, McColl KS, Kresak A et al (2015) PIAS3 expression in squamous cell lung cancer is low and predicts overall survival. Cancer Med 4:325–332

30. Alvarez JV, Febbo PG, Ramaswamy S et al (2005) Identification of a genetic signature of activated signal transducer and activator of transcription 3 in human tumors. Cancer Res 65:5054–5062

31. Carpenter RL, Lo H-W (2014) STAT3 target genes relevant to human cancers. Cancers (Basel) 6:897–925

32. Dauer DJ, Ferraro B, Song L et al (2005) Stat3 regulates genes common to both wound healing and cancer. Oncogene 24:3397–3408

33. Demaria M, Giorgi C, Lebiedzinska M et al (2010) A STAT3-mediated metabolic switch is involved in tumour transformation and STAT3 addiction. Aging (Albany NY) 2:823–842

34. Wegrzyn J, Potla R, Chwae Y-J et al (2009) Function of mitochondrial Stat3 in cellular respiration. Science 323:793–797

35. Meier JA, Larner AC (2014) Toward a new STATe: the role of STATs in mitochondrial function. Semin Immunol 26:20–28

36. Gough DJ, Corlett A, Schlessinger K et al (2009) Mitochondrial STAT3 supports Ras-dependent oncogenic transformation. Science 324:1713–1716

37. Mackenzie GG, Huang L, Alston N et al (2013) Targeting mitochondrial STAT3 with the novel phospho-valproic acid (MDC-1112) inhibits pancreatic cancer growth in mice. PLoS One 8:e61532
38. Ralph SJ, Rodriguez-Enriquez S, Neuzil J et al (2010) The causes of cancer revisited: "mitochondrial malignancy" and ROS-induced oncogenic transformation—why mitochondria are targets for cancer therapy. Mol Aspects Med 31:145–170
39. Boengler K, Hilfiker-Kleiner D, Heusch G (2010) Inhibition of permeability transition pore opening by mitochondrial STAT3 and its role in myocardial ischemia/reperfusion. Basic Res Cardiol 105:771–785
40. Mantel C, Messina-Graham S, Moh A et al (2012) Mouse hematopoietic cell-targeted STAT3 deletion: stem/progenitor cell defects, mitochondrial dysfunction, ROS overproduction, and a rapid aging-like phenotype. Blood 120:2589–2599
41. Macias E, Rao D, Carbajal S et al (2014) Stat3 binds to mtDNA and regulates mitochondrial gene expression in keratinocytes. J Invest Dermatol 134:1971–1980
42. Chueh F-Y, Leong K-F, Yu C-L (2010) Mitochondrial translocation of signal transducer and activator of transcription 5 (STAT5) in leukemic T cells and cytokine-stimulated cells. Biochem Biophys Res Commun 402:778–783
43. Turkson J, Kim JS, Zhang S et al (2004) Novel peptidomimetic inhibitors of signal transducer and activator of transcription 3 dimerization and biological activity. Mol Cancer Ther 3:261–269
44. Turkson J, Ryan D, Kim JS et al (2001) Phosphotyrosyl peptides block Stat3-mediated DNA binding activity, gene regulation, and cell transformation. J Biol Chem 276:45443–45455
45. Turkson J (2004) STAT proteins as novel targets for cancer drug discovery. Expert Opin Ther Targets 8:409–422
46. Siddiquee KA, Gunning PT, Glenn M et al (2007) An oxazole-based small-molecule Stat3 inhibitor modulates Stat3 stability and processing and induces antitumor cell effects. ACS Chem Biol 2:787–798
47. Ren Z, Cabell LA, Schaefer TS et al (2003) Identification of a high-affinity phosphopeptide inhibitor of Stat3. Bioorg Med Chem Lett 13:633–636
48. McMurray JS (2008) Structural basis for the binding of high affinity phosphopeptides to Stat3. Biopolymers 90:69–79
49. Coleman DRI, Ren Z, Mandal PK et al (2005) Investigation of the binding determinants of phosphopeptides targeted to the Src homology 2 domain of the Signal transducer and activator of transcription 3. Development of a high-affinity peptide inhibitor. J Med Chem 48:6661–6670
50. Zhao W, Jaganathan S, Turkson J (2010) A cell-permeable Stat3 SH2 domain mimetic inhibits Stat3 activation and induces antitumor cell effects in vitro. J Biol Chem 285:35855–35865
51. Chen J, Bai L, Bernard D et al (2010) Structure-based design of conformationally constrained, cell-permeable STAT3 inhibitors. ACS Med Chem Lett 1:85–89
52. Mandal PK, Gao F, Lu Z et al (2011) Potent and selective phosphopeptide mimetic prodrugs targeted to the Src homology 2 (SH2) domain of signal transducer and activator of transcription 3. J Med Chem 54:3549–3563
53. Gunning PT, Katt WP, Glenn M et al (2007) Isoform selective inhibition of STAT1 or STAT3 homo-dimerization via peptidomimetic probes: structural recognition of STAT SH2 domains. Bioorg Med Chem Lett 17:1875–1878
54. Gunning PT, Glenn MP, Siddiquee KA et al (2008) Targeting protein–protein interactions: suppression of Stat3 dimerization with rationally designed small-molecule, nonpeptidic SH2 domain binders. Chembiochem 9:2800–2803
55. Mandal PK, Liao WS, McMurray JS (2009) Synthesis of phosphatase-stable, cell-permeable peptidomimetic prodrugs that target the SH2 domain of Stat3. Org Lett 11:3394–3397
56. Pathak AK, Bhutani M, Nair AS et al (2007) Ursolic acid inhibits STAT3 activation pathway leading to suppression of proliferation and chemosensitization of human multiple myeloma cells. Mol Cancer Res 5:943–955

57. Auzenne EJ, Klostergaard J, Mandal PK et al (2012) A phosphopeptide mimetic prodrug targeting the SH2 domain of Stat3 inhibits tumor growth and angiogenesis. J Exp Ther Oncol 10:155–162

58. Song H, Wang R, Wang S (2005) A low-molecular-weight compound discovered through virtual database screening inhibits Stat3 function in breast cancer cells. Proc Natl Acad Sci U S A 102:4700–4705

59. Fuh B, Sobo M, Cen L et al (2009) LLL-3 inhibits STAT3 activity, suppresses glioblastoma cell growth and prolongs survival in a mouse glioblastoma model. Br J Cancer 100:106–112

60. Siddiquee K, Zhang S, Guida WC et al (2007) Selective chemical probe inhibitor of Stat3, identified through structure-based virtual screening, induces antitumor activity. Proc Natl Acad Sci U S A 104:7391–7396

61. Zhang X, Yue P, Fletcher S et al (2010) A novel small-molecule disrupts Stat3 SH2 domain-phosphotyrosine interactions and Stat3-dependent tumor processes. Biochem Pharmacol 79:1398–1409

62. Zhang X, Yue P, Page BD et al (2012) Orally bioavailable small-molecule inhibitor of transcription factor Stat3 regresses human breast and lung cancer xenografts. Proc Natl Acad Sci U S A 109:9623–9628

63. Zhang X, Sun Y, Pireddu R et al (2013) A novel inhibitor of STAT3 homodimerization selectively suppresses STAT3 activity and malignant transformation. Cancer Res 73:1922–1933

64. Yue P, Lopez-Tapia F, Paladino D et al (2015) Hydroxamic acid and benzoic acid-based Stat3 inhibitors suppress human glioma and breast cancer phenotypes in vitro and in vivo. Cancer Res 58:7734–7748

65. Dave B, Landis MD, Tweardy DJ et al (2012) Selective small molecule Stat3 inhibitor reduces breast cancer tumor-initiating cells and improves recurrence free survival in a human-xenograft model. PLoS One 7:e30207

66. Schust J, Sperl B, Hollis A et al (2006) Stattic: a small-molecule inhibitor of STAT3 activation and dimerization. Chem Biol 13:1235–1242

67. Ashizawa T, Miyata H, Ishii H et al (2011) Antitumor activity of a novel small molecule STAT3 inhibitor against a human lymphoma cell line with high STAT3 activation. Int J Oncol 38:1245–1252

68. Matsuno K, Masuda Y, Uehara Y et al (2010) Identification of a new series of STAT3 inhibitors by virtual screening. ACS Med Chem Lett 1:371–375

69. Chen H, Yang Z, Ding C et al (2013) Fragment-based drug design and identification of HJC0123, a novel orally bioavailable STAT3 inhibitor for cancer therapy. Eur J Med Chem 62:498–507

70. Chen H, Yang Z, Ding C et al (2013) Discovery of O-alkylamino tethered niclosamide derivatives as potent and orally bioavailable anticancer agents. ACS Med Chem Lett 4:180–185

71. Zhang M, Zhu W, Ding N et al (2013) Identification and characterization of small molecule inhibitors of signal transducer and activator of transcription 3 (STAT3) signaling pathway by virtual screening. Bioorg Med Chem Lett 23:2225–2229

72. Horiguchi A, Asano T, Kuroda K et al (2010) Stat3 inhibitor WP1066 as a novel therapeutic agent for renal cell carcinoma. Br J Cancer 102:1592–1599

73. Mencalha AL, Du Rocher B, Salles D et al (2010) LLL-3, a STAT3 inhibitor, represses BCR-ABL-positive cell proliferation, activates apoptosis and improves the effects of Imatinib mesylate. Cancer Chemother Pharmacol 65:1039–1046

74. Lin L, Hutzen B, Li PK et al (2010) A novel small molecule, LLL12, inhibits STAT3 phosphorylation and activities and exhibits potent growth-suppressive activity in human cancer cells. Neoplasia 12:39–50

75. Assi HH, Paran C, VanderVeen N et al (2014) Preclinical characterization of signal transducer and activator of transcription 3 small molecule inhibitors for primary and metastatic brain cancer therapy. J Pharmacol Exp Ther 349:458–469

76. Madoux F, Koenig M, Sessions H et al (2009–2010) Modulators of STAT transcription factors for the targeted therapy of cancer (STAT3 inhibitors). Probe Reports from the NIH

Molecular Libraries Program [Internet]. National Center for Biotechnology Information (US), Bethesda, MD; 2009–2010, 28 Aug (updated 2011 Mar 25)
77. Bendell JC, Hong DS, Burris HA 3rd et al (2014) Phase 1, open-label, dose-escalation, and pharmacokinetic study of STAT3 inhibitor OPB-31121 in subjects with advanced solid tumors. Cancer Chemother Pharmacol 74:125–130
78. Brambilla L, Genini D, Laurini E et al (2015) Hitting the right spot: mechanism of action of OPB-31121, a novel and potent inhibitor of the signal transducer and activator of transcription 3 (STAT3). Mol Oncol 9:1194–1206
79. Hayakawa F, Sugimoto K, Harada Y et al (2013) A novel STAT inhibitor, OPB-31121, has a significant antitumor effect on leukemia with STAT-addictive oncokinases. Blood Cancer J 3, e166
80. Kim MJ, Nam HJ, Kim HP et al (2013) OPB-31121, a novel small molecular inhibitor, disrupts the JAK2/STAT3 pathway and exhibits an antitumor activity in gastric cancer cells. Cancer Lett 335:145–152
81. Ogura M, Uchida T, Terui Y et al (2015) Phase I study of OPB-51602, an oral inhibitor of signal transducer and activator of transcription 3, in patients with relapsed/refractory hematological malignancies. Cancer Sci 106:896–901
82. Oh DY, Lee SH, Han SW et al (2015) Phase I study of OPB-31121, an oral STAT3 inhibitor, in patients with advanced solid tumors. Cancer Res Treat 47:607–615
83. Okusaka T, Ueno H, Ikeda M et al (2015) Phase 1 and pharmacological trial of OPB-31121, a signal transducer and activator of transcription-3 inhibitor, in patients with advanced hepatocellular carcinoma. Hepatol Res 45:1283–1291
84. Huang W, Dong Z, Chen Y et al (2016) Small-molecule inhibitors targeting the DNA-binding domain of STAT3 suppress tumor growth, metastasis and STAT3 target gene expression in vivo. Oncogene 35:783–792
85. Daka P, Liu A, Karunaratne C et al (2015) Design, synthesis and evaluation of XZH-5 analogues as STAT3 inhibitors. Bioorg Med Chem 23:1348–1355
86. Liu A, Liu Y, Jin Z et al (2012) XZH-5 inhibits STAT3 phosphorylation and enhances the cytotoxicity of chemotherapeutic drugs in human breast and pancreatic cancer cells. PLoS One 7(10):e46624
87. Liu A, Liu Y, Xu Z et al (2011) Novel small molecule, XZH-5, inhibits constitutive and interleukin-6-induced STAT3 phosphorylation in human rhabdomyosarcoma cells. Cancer Sci 102:1381–1387
88. Yu W, Xiao H, Lin J et al (2013) Discovery of novel STAT3 small molecule inhibitors via in silico site-directed fragment-based drug design. J Med Chem 56:4402–4412
89. Leung KH, Liu LJ, Lin S et al (2015) Discovery of a small-molecule inhibitor of STAT3 by ligand-based pharmacophore screening. Methods 71:38–43
90. Zhang M, Zhu W, Li Y (2013) Discovery of novel inhibitors of signal transducer and activator of transcription 3 (STAT3) signaling pathway by virtual screening. Eur J Med Chem 62:301–310
91. Chen H, Yang Z, Ding C et al (2014) Discovery of potent anticancer agent HJC0416, an orally bioavailable small molecule inhibitor of signal transducer and activator of transcription 3 (STAT3). Eur J Med Chem 82:195–203
92. Rath KS, Naidu SK, Lata P et al (2014) HO-3867, a safe STAT3 inhibitor, is selectively cytotoxic to ovarian cancer. Cancer Res 74:2316–2327
93. Selvendiran K, Ahmed S, Dayton A et al (2011) HO-3867, a curcumin analog, sensitizes cisplatin-resistant ovarian carcinoma, leading to therapeutic synergy through STAT3 inhibition. Cancer Biol Ther 12:837–845
94. Pallandre JR, Borg C, Rognan D et al (2015) Novel aminotetrazole derivatives as selective STAT3 non-peptide inhibitors. Eur J Med Chem 103:163–174
95. Turkson J, Zhang S, Mora LB et al (2005) A novel platinum compound inhibits constitutive Stat3 signaling and induces cell cycle arrest and apoptosis of malignant cells. J Biol Chem 280:32979–32988

96. Turkson J, Zhang S, Palmer J et al (2004) Inhibition of constitutive signal transducer and activator of transcription 3 activation by novel platinum complexes with potent anti-tumor activity. Mol Cancer Ther 3:1533–1542
97. Wong AL, Soo RA, Tan DS et al (2015) Phase I and biomarker study of OPB-51602, a novel signal transducer and activator of transcription (STAT) 3 inhibitor, in patients with refractory solid malignancies. Ann Oncol 26:998–1005
98. Sen M, Tosca PJ, Zwayer C et al (2009) Lack of toxicity of a STAT3 decoy oligonucleotide. Cancer Chemother Pharmacol 63:983–995
99. Souissi I, Ladam P, Cognet JA et al (2012) A STAT3-inhibitory hairpin decoy oligodeoxy-nucleotide discriminates between STAT1 and STAT3 and induces death in a human colon carcinoma cell line. Mol Cancer 11:12
100. Sen M, Joyce S, Panahandeh M et al (2012) Targeting Stat3 abrogates EGFR inhibitor resistance in cancer. Clin Cancer Res 18:4986–4996
101. Lui VW, Boehm AL, Koppikar P et al (2007) Antiproliferative mechanisms of a transcription factor decoy targeting signal transducer and activator of transcription (STAT) 3: the role of STAT1. Mol Pharmacol 71:1435–1443
102. Niu G, Wright KL, Huang M et al (2002) Constitutive Stat3 activity up-regulates VEGF expression and tumor angiogenesis. Oncogene 21:2000–2008
103. Li WC, Ye SL, Sun RX et al (2006) Inhibition of growth and metastasis of human hepatocellular carcinoma by antisense oligonucleotide targeting signal transducer and activator of transcription 3. Clin Cancer Res 12:7140–7148
104. Barton BE, Murphy TF, Shu P et al (2004) Novel single-stranded oligonucleotides that inhibit signal transducer and activator of transcription 3 induce apoptosis in vitro and in vivo in prostate cancer cell lines. Mol Cancer Ther 3:1183–1191
105. Burel SA, Han SR, Lee HS et al (2013) Preclinical evaluation of the toxicological effects of a novel constrained ethyl modified antisense compound targeting signal transducer and activator of transcription 3 in mice and cynomolgus monkeys. Nucleic Acid Ther 23:213–227
106. Yang CL, Liu YY, Ma YG et al (2012) Curcumin blocks small cell lung cancer cells migration, invasion, angiogenesis, cell cycle and neoplasia through Janus kinase-STAT3 signalling pathway. PLoS One 7:e37960
107. Tu SP, Jin H, Shi JD et al (2012) Curcumin induces the differentiation of myeloid-derived suppressor cells and inhibits their interaction with cancer cells and related tumor growth. Cancer Prev Res (Phila) 5:205–215
108. Fossey SL, Bear MD, Lin J et al (2011) The novel curcumin analog FLLL32 decreases STAT3 DNA binding activity and expression, and induces apoptosis in osteosarcoma cell lines. BMC Cancer 11:112
109. Onimoe GI, Liu A, Lin L et al (2012) Small molecules, LLL12 and FLLL32, inhibit STAT3 and exhibit potent growth suppressive activity in osteosarcoma cells and tumor growth in mice. Invest New Drugs 30:916–926
110. Tierney BJ, McCann GA, Cohn DE et al (2012) HO-3867, a STAT3 inhibitor induces apoptosis by inactivation of STAT3 activity in BRCA1-mutated ovarian cancer cells. Cancer Biol Ther 13:766–775
111. Lin L, Hutzen B, Zuo M et al (2010) Novel STAT3 phosphorylation inhibitors exhibit potent growth-suppressive activity in pancreatic and breast cancer cells. Cancer Res 70:2445–2454
112. Bid HK, Oswald D, Li C et al (2012) Anti-angiogenic activity of a small molecule STAT3 inhibitor LLL12. PLoS One 7:e35513
113. Lin L, Deangelis S, Foust E et al (2010) A novel small molecule inhibits STAT3 phosphorylation and DNA binding activity and exhibits potent growth suppressive activity in human cancer cells. Mol Cancer 9:217
114. Bill MA, Nicholas C, Mace TA et al (2012) Structurally modified curcumin analogs inhibit STAT3 phosphorylation and promote apoptosis of human renal cell carcinoma and melanoma cell lines. PLoS One 7:e40724
115. Nam S, Xie J, Perkins A et al (2012) Novel synthetic derivatives of the natural product berbamine inhibit Jak2/Stat3 signaling and induce apoptosis of human melanoma cells. Mol Oncol 6:484–493

116. Zhang X, Song Y, Wu Y et al (2011) Indirubin inhibits tumor growth by antitumor angiogenesis via blocking VEGFR2-mediated JAK/STAT3 signaling in endothelial cell. Int J Cancer 129:2502–2511
117. Nam S, Buettner R, Turkson J et al (2005) Indirubin derivatives inhibit Stat3 signaling and induce apoptosis in human cancer cells. Proc Natl Acad Sci U S A 102:5998–6003
118. Liu L, Kritsanida M, Magiatis P et al (2012) A novel 7-bromoindirubin with potent anticancer activity suppresses survival of human melanoma cells associated with inhibition of STAT3 and Akt signaling. Cancer Biol Ther 13:1255–1261
119. Nam S, Wen W, Schroeder A et al (2012) Dual inhibition of Janus and Src family kinases by novel indirubin derivative blocks constitutively-activated Stat3 signaling associated with apoptosis of human pancreatic cancer cells. Mol Oncol 7:369–378
120. Shakibaei M, Harikumar KB, Aggarwal BB (2009) Resveratrol addiction: to die or not to die. Mol Nutr Food Res 53:115–128
121. Li T, Wang W, Chen H et al (2010) Evaluation of anti-leukemia effect of resveratrol by modulating STAT3 signaling. Int Immunopharmacol 10:18–25
122. Kim JE, Kim HS, Shin YJ et al (2008) LYR71, a derivative of trimeric resveratrol, inhibits tumorigenesis by blocking STAT3-mediated matrix metalloproteinase 9 expression. Exp Mol Med 40:514–522
123. Yang YP, Chang YL, Huang PI et al (2012) Resveratrol suppresses tumorigenicity and enhances radiosensitivity in primary glioblastoma tumor initiating cells by inhibiting the STAT3 axis. J Cell Physiol 227:976–993
124. Gupta SC, Kannappan R, Reuter S et al (2011) Chemosensitization of tumors by resveratrol. Ann N Y Acad Sci 1215:150–160
125. Santandreu FM, Valle A, Oliver J et al (2011) Resveratrol potentiates the cytotoxic oxidative stress induced by chemotherapy in human colon cancer cells. Cell Physiol Biochem 28:219–228
126. Lin CL, Chen RF, Chen JY et al (2012) Protective effect of caffeic acid on paclitaxel induced anti-proliferation and apoptosis of lung cancer cells involves NF-kappaB pathway. Int J Mol Sci 13:6236–6645
127. Kong LY, Gelbard A, Wei J et al (2010) Inhibition of p-STAT3 enhances IFN-alpha efficacy against metastatic melanoma in a murine model. Clin Cancer Res 16:2550–2561
128. Sai K, Wang S, Balasubramaniyan V et al (2012) Induction of cell-cycle arrest and apoptosis in glioblastoma stem-like cells by WP1193, a novel small molecule inhibitor of the JAK2/STAT3 pathway. J Neurooncol 107:487–501
129. Lee HK, Seo IA, Shin YK et al (2009) Capsaicin inhibits the IL-6/STAT3 pathway by depleting intracellular gp130 pools through endoplasmic reticulum stress. Biochem Biophys Res Commun 382:445–450
130. Shin DS, Kim HN, Shin KD et al (2009) Cryptotanshinone inhibits constitutive signal transducer and activator of transcription 3 function through blocking the dimerization in DU145 prostate cancer cells. Cancer Res 69:193–202
131. Kannaiyan R, Hay HS, Rajendran P et al (2011) Celastrol inhibits proliferation and induces chemosensitization through down-regulation of NF-kappaB and STAT3 regulated gene products in multiple myeloma cells. Br J Pharmacol 164:1506–1521
132. Rajendran P, Li F, Shanmugam MK et al (2012) Celastrol suppresses growth and induces apoptosis of human hepatocellular carcinoma through the modulation of STAT3/JAK2 signaling cascade in vitro and in vivo. Cancer Prev Res (Phila) 5:631–643
133. Zhang C, Li B, Gaikwad AS et al (2008) Avicin D selectively induces apoptosis and down-regulates p-STAT-3, bcl-2, and survivin in cutaneous T-cell lymphoma cells. J Invest Dermatol 128:2728–2735
134. Lee J, Hahm ER, Singh SV (2010) Withaferin A inhibits activation of signal transducer and activator of transcription 3 in human breast cancer cells. Carcinogenesis 31:1991–1998
135. Um HJ, Min KJ, Kim DE et al (2012) Withaferin A inhibits JAK/STAT3 signaling and induces apoptosis of human renal carcinoma Caki cells. Biochem Biophys Res Commun 427:24–29

136. Pandey MK, Sung B, Aggarwal BB (2010) Betulinic acid suppresses STAT3 activation pathway through induction of protein tyrosine phosphatase SHP-1 in human multiple myeloma cells. Int J Cancer 127:282–292

137. Shanmugam MK, Rajendran P, Li F et al (2011) Ursolic acid inhibits multiple cell survival pathways leading to suppression of growth of prostate cancer xenograft in nude mice. J Mol Med (Berl) 89:713–727

138. Honda T, Rounds BV, Bore L et al (2000) Synthetic oleanane and ursane triterpenoids with modified rings A and C: a series of highly active inhibitors of nitric oxide production in mouse macrophages. J Med Chem 43:4233–4246

139. Duan Z, Ames RY, Ryan M et al (2009) CDDO-Me, a synthetic triterpenoid, inhibits expression of IL-6 and Stat3 phosphorylation in multi-drug resistant ovarian cancer cells. Cancer Chemother Pharmacol 63:681–689

140. Ryu K, Susa M, Choy E et al (2010) Oleanane triterpenoid CDDO-Me induces apoptosis in multidrug resistant osteosarcoma cells through inhibition of Stat3 pathway. BMC Cancer 10:187

141. Tran K, Risingsong R, Royce D et al (2012) The synthetic triterpenoid CDDO-methyl ester delays estrogen receptor-negative mammary carcinogenesis in polyoma middle T mice. Cancer Prev Res (Phila) 5:726–734

142. Miklossy G, Youn UJ, Yue P et al (2015) Hirsutinolide series inhibit Stat3 activity, modulate GCN1, MAP1B, Hsp105, G6PD, Vimentin, and importin α-2 expression, and induce antitumor effects against human glioma. J Med Chem 58:7734–7748

143. Blaskovich MA, Sun J, Cantor A et al (2003) Discovery of JSI-124 (cucurbitacin I), a selective Janus kinase/signal transducer and activator of transcription 3 signaling pathway inhibitor with potent antitumor activity against human and murine cancer cells in mice. Cancer Res 63:1270–1279

144. Liu T, Peng H, Zhang M et al (2010) Cucurbitacin B, a small molecule inhibitor of the Stat3 signaling pathway, enhances the chemosensitivity of laryngeal squamous cell carcinoma cells to cisplatin. Eur J Pharmacol 641:15–22

145. Dong Y, Lu B, Zhang X et al (2010) Cucurbitacin E, a tetracyclic triterpenes compound from Chinese medicine, inhibits tumor angiogenesis through VEGFR2-mediated Jak2-STAT3 signaling pathway. Carcinogenesis 31:2097–2104

146. Chang CJ, Chiang CH, Song WS et al (2012) Inhibition of phosphorylated STAT3 by cucurbitacin I enhances chemoradiosensitivity in medulloblastoma-derived cancer stem cells. Childs Nerv Syst 28:363–373

147. Tseng LM, Huang PI, Chen YR et al (2012) Targeting signal transducer and activator of transcription 3 pathway by cucurbitacin I diminishes self-renewing and radiochemoresistant abilities in thyroid cancer-derived CD133+ cells. J Pharmacol Exp Ther 341:410–423

148. Sun C, Zhang M, Shan X et al (2010) Inhibitory effect of cucurbitacin E on pancreatic cancer cells growth via STAT3 signaling. J Cancer Res Clin Oncol 136:603–610

149. Huang WW, Yang JS, Lin MW et al (2012) Cucurbitacin E induces G(2)/M phase arrest through STAT3/p53/p21 signaling and provokes apoptosis via Fas/CD95 and mitochondria-dependent pathways in human bladder cancer T24 cells. Evid Based Complement Alternat Med 2012:952762

150. Hsu HS, Huang PI, Chang YL et al (2011) Cucurbitacin I inhibits tumorigenic ability and enhances radiochemosensitivity in nonsmall cell lung cancer-derived CD133-positive cells. Cancer 117:2970–2985

151. Li F, Fernandez PP, Rajendran P (2010) Diosgenin, a steroidal saponin, inhibits STAT3 signaling pathway leading to suppression of proliferation and chemosensitization of human hepatocellular carcinoma cells. Cancer Lett 292:197–207

152. Muthukumaran G, Kotenko S, Donnelly R (1997) Chimeric erythropoietin-interferon gamma receptors reveal differences in functional architecture of intracellular domains for signal transduction. J Biol Chem 272:4993–4999

153. Badr G, Mohany M, Abu-Tarboush F (2011) Thymoquinone decreases F-actin polymerization and the proliferation of human multiple myeloma cells by suppressing STAT3 phosphorylation and Bcl2/Bcl-XL expression. Lipids Health Dis 10:236

154. Li F, Rajendran P, Sethi G (2010) Thymoquinone inhibits proliferation, induces apoptosis and chemosensitizes human multiple myeloma cells through suppression of signal transducer and activator of transcription 3 activation pathway. Br J Pharmacol 161:541–554
155. Leeman-Neill RJ, Cai Q, Joyce SC et al (2010) Honokiol inhibits epidermal growth factor receptor signaling and enhances the antitumor effects of epidermal growth factor receptor inhibitors. Clin Cancer Res 16:2571–2579
156. Rajendran P, Li F, Shanmugam MK et al (2012) Honokiol inhibits signal transducer and activator of transcription-3 signaling, proliferation, and survival of hepatocellular carcinoma cells via the protein tyrosine phosphatase SHP-1. J Cell Physiol 227:2184–2195
157. Liu SH, Wang KB, Lan KH et al (2012) Calpain/SHP-1 Interaction by Honokiol Dampening Peritoneal Dissemination of Gastric Cancer in nu/nu Mice. PLoS One 7:e43711
158. Yang J, Cai X, Lu W et al (2012) Evodiamine inhibits STAT3 signaling by inducing phosphatase shatterproof 1 in hepatocellular carcinoma cells. Cancer Lett 328:243–251
159. Arbiser JL, Govindarajan B, Battle TE et al (2006) Carbazole is a naturally occurring inhibitor of angiogenesis and inflammation isolated from antipsoriatic coal tar. J Invest Dermatol 126:1396–1402
160. Saturnino C, Palladino C, Napoli M et al (2013) Synthesis and biological evaluation of new N-alkylcarbazole derivatives as STAT3 inhibitors: preliminary study. Eur J Med Chem 60:112–119
161. Sun M, Liu C, Nadiminty N et al (2012) Inhibition of Stat3 activation by sanguinarine suppresses prostate cancer cell growth and invasion. Prostate 72:82–89
162. Kannappan R, Yadav VR, Aggarwal BB (2010) gamma-Tocotrienol but not gamma-tocopherol blocks STAT3 cell signaling pathway through induction of protein-tyrosine phosphatase SHP-1 and sensitizes tumor cells to chemotherapeutic agents. J Biol Chem 285:33520–33528
163. Rajendran P, Li F, Manu KA et al (2011) gamma-Tocotrienol is a novel inhibitor of constitutive and inducible STAT3 signalling pathway in human hepatocellular carcinoma: potential role as an antiproliferative, pro-apoptotic and chemosensitizing agent. Br J Pharmacol 163:283–298
164. Kandala PK, Srivastava SK (2012) Regulation of Janus-activated kinase-2 (JAK2) by diindolylmethane in ovarian cancer in vitro and in vivo. Drug Discov Ther 6:94–101
165. Kandala PK, Srivastava SK (2012) Diindolylmethane suppresses ovarian cancer growth and potentiates the effect of cisplatin in tumor mouse model by targeting signal transducer and activator of transcription 3 (STAT3). BMC Med 10:9
166. Kunnumakkara AB, Nair AS, Sung B (2009) Boswellic acid blocks signal transducers and activators of transcription 3 signaling, proliferation, and survival of multiple myeloma via the protein tyrosine phosphatase SHP-1. Mol Cancer Res 7:118–128
167. Migita K, Miyashita T, Izumi Y et al (2011) Inhibitory effects of the JAK inhibitor CP690,550 on human CD4(+) T lymphocyte cytokine production. BMC Immunol 12:51
168. Quintas-Cardama A, Vaddi K, Liu P et al (2010) Preclinical characterization of the selective JAK1/2 inhibitor INCB018424: therapeutic implications for the treatment of myeloproliferative neoplasms. Blood 115:3109–3117
169. Looyenga BD, Hutchings D, Cherni I et al (2012) STAT3 is activated by JAK2 independent of key oncogenic driver mutations in non-small cell lung carcinoma. PLoS One 7:e30820
170. Derenzini E, Lemoine M, Buglio D et al (2011) The JAK inhibitor AZD1480 regulates proliferation and immunity in Hodgkin lymphoma. Blood Cancer J 1:e46
171. Hedvat M, Huszar D, Herrmann A et al (2009) The JAK2 inhibitor AZD1480 potently blocks Stat3 signaling and oncogenesis in solid tumors. Cancer Cell 16:487–497
172. McFarland BC, Ma JY, Langford CP et al (2011) Therapeutic potential of AZD1480 for the treatment of human glioblastoma. Mol Cancer Ther 10:2384–2393
173. Xin H, Herrmann A, Reckamp K et al (2011) Antiangiogenic and antimetastatic activity of JAK inhibitor AZD1480. Cancer Res 71:6601–6610

174. Faderl S, Ferrajoli A, Harris D et al (2007) Atiprimod blocks phosphorylation of JAK-STAT and inhibits proliferation of acute myeloid leukemia (AML) cells. Leuk Res 31:91–95
175. Amit-Vazina M, Shishodia S, Harris D et al (2005) Atiprimod blocks STAT3 phosphorylation and induces apoptosis in multiple myeloma cells. Br J Cancer 93:70–80
176. Quintas-Cardama A, Manshouri T, Estrov Z et al (2011) Preclinical characterization of atiprimod, a novel JAK2 AND JAK3 inhibitor. Invest New Drugs 29:818–826
177. Kim NH, Lee MY, Park SJ et al (2007) Auranofin blocks interleukin-6 signalling by inhibiting phosphorylation of JAK1 and STAT3. Immunology 122:607–614
178. Nakaya A, Sagawa M, Muto A et al (2011) The gold compound auranofin induces apoptosis of human multiple myeloma cells through both down-regulation of STAT3 and inhibition of NF-kappaB activity. Leuk Res 35:243–249
179. Sen M, Thomas SM, Kim S et al (2012) First-in-human trial of a STAT3 decoy oligonucleotide in head and neck tumors: implications for cancer therapy. Cancer Discov 2:694–705
180. Hong D, Kurzrock R, Kim Y et al (2015) AZD9150, a next-generation antisense oligonucle-otide inhibitor of STAT3 with early evidence of clinical activity in lymphoma and lung cancer. Sci Transl Med 7:314ra185
181. Yu H, Lee H, Hermann A et al (2014) Revisiting STAT3 signaling in cancer: new and unex-pected biological functions. Nat Rev Cancer 14:736–746

Chapter 5
STAT3 Inhibitors in Cancer: A Comprehensive Update

Uddalak Bharadwaj, Moses M. Kasembeli, and David J. Tweardy

Abstract STAT3 is an important signaling molecule that modulates a wide range of genes by relaying extracellular signals from the plasma membrane to the nucleus in response to peptide hormone binding. It is known to play a prominent role in the initiation and progression of cancer, as it is constitutively activated in 25–100 % of more than 25 different malignancies and has been implicated in nearly all the hallmarks of cancer. In addition, STAT3 contributes to development and maintenance of cancer stem cells, as well as to cancer immune evasion and resistance to chemotherapy and radiotherapy, making it an even more attractive target for cancer therapy. In this chapter, we give an overview of strategies involved in targeting STAT3 and discuss recent advances in the development of STAT3 modulating agents.

Keywords Cancer • Oncogene • Kinase • Inhibitor • Signaling • Phosphorylation • High throughput screen • Transcriptional activation • Therapeutic • Dysregulated • SH2 • Peptidomimetics • Aptamer • Decoy • Drug design • Nuclear • Allosteric • Interference • Rational • Clinic • Clinical trial • STAT3 • Resistance

5.1 Introduction

Signal transducer and activator of transcription 3 (STAT3) is a member of a family of seven proteins that are known to play important roles in growth factor and cytokine signaling [1]. Canonical signal transduction by STAT3 is initiated by the recruitment

U. Bharadwaj • M.M. Kasembeli
Department of Infectious Disease, Infection Control and Employee Health,
The University of Texas MD Anderson Cancer Center, Houston, TX, USA
e-mail: Ubharadwaj@mdanderson.org; MMKasembeli@mdanderson.org

D.J. Tweardy (✉)
Department of Infectious Disease, Infection Control and Employee Health,
The University of Texas MD Anderson Cancer Center, Houston, TX, USA

Department of Molecular and Cellular Oncology, The University of Texas
MD Anderson Cancer Center, Houston, TX, USA
e-mail: DJTweardy@mdanderson.org

© Springer International Publishing Switzerland 2016   95
A.C. Ward (ed.), *STAT Inhibitors in Cancer*, Cancer Drug
Discovery and Development, DOI 10.1007/978-3-319-42949-6_5

of STAT3 to ligand activated membrane receptor complexes leading to a key phosphorylation event on Y705, which in turn induces a configuration change leading to tail-to-tail dimerization mediated by reciprocal SH2/pY705-peptide ligand interactions [2, 3]. The active dimer accumulates in the nucleus, where it binds to promoters and transcriptionally regulates a large number of target genes encoding proteins involved in cell survival, cell cycle progression, homeostasis, and inflammation.

Under normal physiological conditions the phosphorylation status of STAT3 in the cell is closely tied to receptor activation in response to extracellular stimuli, such that the intensity and duration of the intended signal is tightly regulated. Regulation of STAT3 is achieved by a number of elements that either act through negative feedback control on the phosphorylation of STAT3 or deactivation by dedicated nuclear phosphatases. Pathological conditions may arise in those instances where anomalies in the STAT3 signaling cascade lead to constitutive activation [1]. Hyperphosphorylation of STAT3 has been shown to occur through a variety of mechanisms, including, unregulated autocrine and paracrine secretion of cytokines and growth hormones [4], expression of intrinsically activated tyrosine kinases or receptors [5], or reduced levels of endogenous negative regulators of STAT3 signaling such as SOCS3, PIAS3, nuclear phosphatases [6, 7].

5.2 STAT3, The Oncogene

Dysregulated activation of STAT3 has been linked to the etiology and molecular pathogenesis of many diseases, most prominently cancer [4, 8], where the STAT3 signaling pathway has been implicated in nearly all features of cancer biology [7], including anti-apoptosis [9], cell transformation [8], growth and proliferation [2], angiogenesis [10], metastasis [11], and cancer stem cell maintenance [12]. Accordingly, over-expression or constitutive activation of STAT3 frequently occurs in a large number of both solid and hematological tumors (Table 5.1).

In addition to its established role in cell transformation and tumorigenesis, STAT3 oncogenic signaling has been implicated in immune regulatory mechanisms of multiple tumors [13]. For example, several studies showed that persistent activation of STAT3 leads to the suppression of anti-tumor immunity by promoting Treg recruitment within the tumor microenvironment, while negatively regulating antitumor Th1-mediated immune response [14, 15]. In addition, recent findings also revealed that STAT3 plays a crucial role in tumor immune resistance, as constitutive STAT3 activation has been shown to drive the expression of PD-L1, an immune checkpoint ligand that mediates immune inhibition within the tumor microenvironment [16]. Overall, it appears that STAT3 plays an important role in anti-tumor immune response by up regulating immune inhibitors while at the same time suppressing tumor immune activators.

From a therapeutic perspective, another significant aspect of STAT3 signaling that also merits attention is its role in chemotherapy resistance. Despite initial clinical responses to both targeted and cytotoxic cancer drugs, relapses are frequent and drug resistance remains a major obstacle in curing cancer [17, 18]. Because STAT3

Table 5.1 Constitutively activated STAT3 in various cancers

Tumor type	STAT3 activity in tumor tissue	STAT3 and clinicopathological features
Acute myelogenous leukemia (AML)	33 % pY-STAT3+ve compared to bone marrow cells from normal donors [95]	NA
Chronic myelogenous leukemia (CML)	48.5 % CML patients pY-STAT3+ve compared to 36.8 controls (P=0.033) [316]	pY-STAT3 higher in advanced phase CML patients than in chronic phase patients (22.77±4.41 % vs. 11.47±3.14 %), P=0.003 [316]
T cell large granular lymphocytic (T-LGL) leukemia	100 % of T-LGL pY-STAT3+ve [317] ~40 % of T-LGL patients harbor mutations in *STAT3* gene and/or STAT3 pathway related genes and harbor increased pY-STAT3 activity [318]	NA
Chronic lymphocytic leukemia (CLL)	100 % of CLL patients PBMC constitutive pS-STAT3+ve in contrast to none among normal PBMC or CD5+ B cells isolated from tonsil [319, 320]	NA
Lymphoma	87 % of Hodgkins Lymphoma (HL), 45 % of B-cell NHL, 73 % of T-cell NHL stained pY-STAT3+ve [321] 100 % lymphoma pY-STAT3+ve, most intense staining in marginal sinus [210]	61 % ALCL tumors constitutive STAT3 activation (84 % of ALK+, 47 % of ALK−). ALK correlates with STAT3 activation (P<0.0001). ALK− group: lack of STAT3 activation correlated with a favorable 5-year overall survival (P=0.0076) [322]
Sézary syndrome (SS), type of cutaneous T-cell lymphoma (CTCL)	100 % of SS pY-STAT3+ve compared to CD4+ T-cells from healthy controls [323]	NA
NPM-ALK+ve anaplastic large cell lymphoma (ALCL)	95 % NPM-ALK+ ALCL tumors nuclear STAT3+ve, vs. surrounding non- neoplastic lymphocytes. ALK-ve cases primarily cytoplasmic STAT3 [324]	Survivin associate to nuclear pY-STAT3 (P=0.007). ALK+ve group: 5-year failure-free survival (FFS): 34 % in survivin+ve vs 100 % in survivin-ve (p=0.009). ALK-ve group: 5-year FFS: 46 % in survivin+ve vs. 89 % in survivin-ve (p=0.03) [325]
Diffuse large B-cell lymphoma (DLBCL)	Strong pY-STAT3 (32.4 %) and nuclear STAT3 (25.7 %), more frequent in non-germinal center B cell-like (non-GCB) DLBCL than in GCB [326]	High nuclear STAT3 correlated with poor overall survival (OS, p=0.005), and is an independent prognostic factor for DLBCL [326]. Detectable pY-STAT3 associated with improved 5-year EFS (93% vs. 47 %, p=0.006) [327]

(continued)

Table 5.1 (continued)

Tumor type	STAT3 activity in tumor tissue	STAT3 and clinicopathological features
Non-germinal center B-cell–like (GCB-DLBCL) including activated B-cell–like (ABC-DLBCL)	61 % non-GCB-DLBCL positive for pY-STAT3 [328]	pY-STAT3 associated with shorter survival in patients (n=185) treated with RCHOP (rituximab, cyclophosphamide, doxorubicin, vincristine, and prednisone) [329] pY-STAT3 associated with worse event free survival [329]
Breast cancer	46 % expressed high to moderate levels (3, 2+) of nuclear pY-STAT3, 23 % low levels (+1), and 31 % no detectable pY-STAT3 [330]	pY-STAT3 higher in invasive carcinoma (52 %) than in non-neoplastic tissue (27.8 %, $p<0.001$), pY-STAT3 lower in patients showing complete pathologic response, suggesting that higher levels of activated STAT3 made tumors less responsive to the treatment [331]
Lung cancer (non-small-cell)	(64.6 %) pY-STAT3+ve, in carcinoma tissue vs. 37.5 % in normal tissue (p=0.001) [332]	78.8 % lymph node metastasis+ve patients pY-STAT3+ve (p=0.009) [332]. High STAT3/pY-STAT3 strong predictor of poor prognosis [333]
Endometrial cancer	64.9 % pY-STAT3+ve (Scores 2 and 3) compared to normal endometrial tissues [334]	High pY-STAT3 (Scores 2 and 3) detected in 11.8 % of grade I, 25.8 % of grade II, and 27.3 % of grade III patients [334]
Cervical cancer	10.8 % grade II and 10.5 % grade III patients pY-STAT3+ve [334]	56.8 % patients+ve for pY-STAT3 which also correlated with lymph node metastasis, lymph vascular space invasion, and large tumor diameter (>4 cm). pY-STAT3+ve indicative of a poor OS (p=0.006) and DFS (p=0.010) [335]
Clear cell renal cell carcinoma (ccRCC)	76.3 % RCC tissues were nuclear pY-STAT3+ve [336]	High CD44 correlates with high pY-STAT3 (r=0.4013, p=0.0004), high tumor grade (p<0.001), large tumor size (p=0.009) and advanced T stage (p=0.004). CD44-high/pY-STAT3-high had poor survival vs. CD44-low/pY-STAT3-low (p=0.024) [336]
Hepatocellular carcinoma (HCC)	100 % HCC nuclear pY-STAT3+ve, intense, moderate and weak staining in 28.5, 28.5 and 43 %, vs. weak nuclear pY-STAT3 in 40 % of normal liver. Intense/moderate STAT3 in 89 % of HCC vs. normal liver samples [337]	49.3 % HCC, vs. 5.8 % of adjacent non-tumor liver (p<0.001)+ve for pY-STAT3 which correlated with intratumour MVD (p=0.002) and was a predictor of OS (p=0.036) [338]

Cancer type		
Cholangiocarcinoma (CCA)	44 % of CCA tissues STAT3 positive [339]	STAT3 and STAT5b associated with non-papillary, poorly differentiated CCA ($p=0.032$ and $p=0.001$); STAT3 associated with shorter survival ($p<0.001$) [339]
Colorectal cancer	62 % pY-STAT3+ve; 18 % high expression (pY-STAT3 high), 34 % low-level expression (pY-STAT3-low) [340]	pY-STAT3 associated to higher colorectal cancer-specific mortality [log-rank p=0.0020; univariate HR (pY-STAT3-high vs. pY-STAT3-ve): 1.85, 95 % confidence interval (CI) 1.30–2.63, ptrend=0.0005; multivariate HR: 1.61, 95 % CI (1.11–2.34), ptrend=0.015) [340]
Ovarian carcinoma (OC)	74 % nuclear pY-STAT3+ve [341]	pY-STAT3 increased in aggressive, high-grade vs. low-grade, indolent carcinomas ($p<0.005$) [342]
Pancreatic adenocarcinoma (PAC)	70.4 % PAC pY-STAT3+ve compared to none in normal pancreas [343]	pY-STAT3, a risk factor for prognosis, correlated to tumor size, TNM staging and lymphatic metastasis [343]
Head and neck squamous cell carcinoma (HNSCC)	75 % HNSCC tumors increased pY-STAT3+vity vs. normal mucosa [344]	pY-STAT3 levels correlated to presence of lymph node metastasis ($p<0.0001$) [345] in HNSCC and decreased survival in oral and tongue tumors [346, 347]
Glioblastoma (GBM)	55.6 % astrocytomas (AA) and 56.4 %, GBMs were pY-STAT3+ve [348]; 50 % of AA and 51 % of GBM pY-STAT3+ve [226, 346, 348–351]	40 % of Gliomas pY-STAT3+ve with 27 %, 29 %, 57 % and 66 %+vity in Grade I, II, III and IV gliomas, respectively [350]
Extramammary Paget disease (EMPD)	91.6 % Paget cells pY-STAT3+ve [351]	Strong nuclear pY-STAT3 staining in invasive EMPD [351]
Papillary thyroid cancer (PTC)	56.7 % of PTC vs. 10.9 % of adjacent normal thyroid tissues were pY-STAT3+ve [352]	Nuclear pY-STAT3 positively correlated with presence of ETE and LNM, and higher TNM stage ($p<0.05$) [352]

signaling drives gene expression promoting cell growth and resistance to apoptosis, persistent activation of STAT3 is thought to confer resistance to drug mediated apoptosis [19]. Numerous studies show that hyper-activated STAT3 signaling plays a significant role in chemotherapy resistance. Accordingly, the inhibition of activated STAT3 signaling appeared to sensitize resistant tumor cells to the cytotoxic agents [20]. STAT3 is also emerging as a major contributor to adaptive resistance to targeted drug therapy. Notably, it has been demonstrated that STAT3 activation via a positive feedback mechanism underpins frequently observed drug resistance in many oncogene addicted tumor cells. Similarly, inhibition of STAT3 reversed drug resistance to RTK targeting. Taken together, these findings support targeting STAT3 to overcome resistance to cancer therapy [17, 21].

There is an overwhelming amount of clinical and preclinical data in solid and hematological cancers supporting STAT3 as a pharmacological target, which has prompted substantial efforts to develop STAT3 inhibitors. Currently, there are a number of STAT3 inhibitors in clinical trials and many more in active development, as will be discussed later in this chapter. Here we provide an update on efforts to develop inhibitors of STAT3 to treat various cancers and will discuss the strategies involved in targeting STAT3 and the advantages and pitfalls of each approach.

5.3   Strategies for STAT3 Inhibition

The STAT3 signaling cascade provides many opportunities to manipulate its activity, because each step in the activation process can serve as a potential target. In order to pharmacologically modulate STAT3 activity, it is important to understand how each step contributes to the transcriptional function of STAT3, as this information forms a basis for target identification and design of specific inhibitors (Fig. 5.1).

5.3.1   *Structure and Biochemical Properties of STAT3*

The initial steps in STAT3 activation are triggered by tyrosine phosphorylation events that drive key protein-protein interactions, which are necessary for signal transduction from the plasma membrane to the nucleus [22]. STAT signaling initiated by peptide hormones generally occurs through 3 types of receptors—receptor kinases, receptor-linked kinases, or G–coupled receptors [23, 24]. Peptide ligand binding stimulates cytoplasmic receptor-associated kinase activity leading to phosphorylation of receptors at key tyrosine residues. Phosphorylated tyrosine residues on the receptors act as anchors that recruit STAT3 proteins via their SH2 domains [25]. STAT3 is phosphorylated at Y705 and subsequently dimerizes in a tail-tail conformation.

Migration from the cytoplasm into the nucleus is required for STATs to transduce signals and regulate gene expression in response to extracellular stimuli. It has been noted that once dimerized in a tail-to-tail configuration, STATs rapidly accumulate

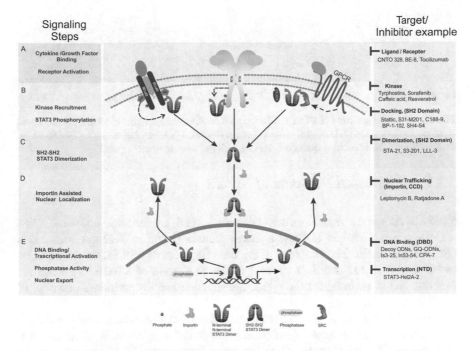

Fig. 5.1 Strategies for targeting STAT3 signaling. STAT3 signaling cascade is triggered by phosphorylation. (**a**) Upstream events including ligand binding, receptor activation or kinase activity can be blocked to prevent STAT3 phosphorylation. (**b**) Blocking STAT3 recruitment onto receptors inhibits phosphorylation of STAT3 at Y705 and consequently SH2-SH2 dimerization. (**c**) Inhibitors that disrupt the SH2-SH2 dimer block the transcriptional activity of STAT3. (**d**) Nuclear localization can be blocked by targeting importins or importin binding sites on STAT3. (**e**) The DNA binding domain can be targeted to inhibit STAT3 DNA binding, consequently transcriptional activity

in the nucleus. Though initially thought to be dependent on tail-to-tail dimerization of STAT3, subsequent studies now suggest that STAT3 is constitutively shuttled between the cytoplasm and nucleus independent of phosphorylation [26]. Studies show that rather than a passive process dependent on diffusion, nuclear translocation of STAT3 is an active process. Indeed, the nuclear import and export of STAT3 as well as other STATs is facilitated by a group of proteins belonging to the karyopherin-B family called importins [27]. Available data shows that importin $\alpha3$, $\alpha5$, $\alpha6$, and $\alpha7$ are involved in the nuclear translocation of STAT3. Importin $\alpha3$ and $\alpha6$ are linked to translocation of unphosphorylated STAT3 while $\alpha5$ and $\alpha7$ are required for pY-STAT3 nuclear import [28]. All importins involved in STAT3 trafficking appear to utilize a NLS located within the coiled-coiled domain of STAT3 [29, 30]. Once localized in the nucleus, STAT3 binds to specific DNA elements via its DNA binding domain (DBD), whereby it engages the transcriptional machinery by recruiting a number of coactivators and chromatin remodelers, such as cAMP response element binding protein/p300 (CBP/p300) complex and steroid receptor coactivator 1 [31, 32].

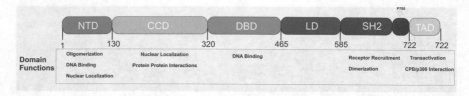

Fig. 5.2 Domains structure of STAT3. STAT3 has 6 domains with specific biochemical functions. NH2-terminal domain (NTD), coil coiled domain (CCD), DNA binding domain (DBD), linker domain (LD), SRC homology domain (SH2), and transactivation domain (TAD)

5.3.2 Functional Domains of STAT3

STAT3 is composed of an N-terminal domain (NTD), a coiled-coil domain (CCD), a DNA-binding domain (DBD), a linker domain (LD), an SH2 domain, and a C-terminal domain. The structure of the core fragment of STAT3, which includes the CCD, DBD, LD and SH2 showed that each domain of STAT3 has a distinct function and is essential for the signal transduction and transcriptional activity of STAT3 (Fig. 5.2).

STAT3 has no enzymatic activity that would make it amenable to small-molecule intervention; rather, its mode of action depends on protein-protein interactions (PPI) and protein-DNA interactions. Thus, strategies for targeting STAT3 mainly rely on the ability to disrupt these interactions. Although the prevailing dogma is that PPI interfaces generally lack special topological features amenable to small molecule inhibition, STAT3, nonetheless, has proven to be a compelling protein to target using small molecules. The available X-ray crystallographic data of both the monomer and dimerized STAT3 bound to DNA have been instrumental in revealing physical chemical properties of phosphotyrosyl (pY) peptide binding, as well as DNA recognition that have laid the foundation for the development of many STAT3 inhibitors by rational design.

5.3.3 Inhibitors Acting Upstream of STAT3 Activation

There is a strong correlation between the phosphorylation status of STAT3 at Y705 with tumor initiation and progression (Table 5.1), yet the reason for dysregulated STAT3 signaling is only rarely due to mutations in the signaling molecule itself. Although the reason for abnormal STAT3 signaling in cancer is not fully understood, most instances of hyper-phosphorylated STAT3 observed in cancer are mediated by receptor tyrosine kinases (RTK), for example EGFR, or non-receptor tyrosine kinases, such as JAK and SRC, more specifically, by unchecked intrinsic tyrosine kinase activity of RTK, over expression of RTK, or persistent stimulation of RTK or tyrosine kinase-associated receptors by cytokines and growth factors [33–35]. As such, intense efforts have focused on inhibiting events upstream of STAT3 that drive STAT3 phosphorylation [36, 37].

There are several therapeutic strategies used to block upstream activation of STAT3, One involves targeting the tyrosine kinase enzymatic activity of specific receptors or associated kinases using small molecule inhibitors of RTKs, JAK2 and SRC kinases. Another strategy involves disruption of protein-protein interactions necessary for receptor mediated signal transmission across the plasma membrane. The later strategy has been achieved in several ways including blocking cytokine binding to the extracellular portions of the receptors, and disruption of receptor oligomerization. These strategies primarily involve blocking cytokine or growth factor activation of cognate receptors with the use of monoclonal antibody-based inhibitors that target either the ligand or critical sites on extracellular portion of receptors. Another strategy in this category involves the use of an aptamer, a short peptide portion derived from a random peptide library integrated into the thioredoxin scaffold protein, which specifically binds to the intracellular domain of the EGF receptor blocking the recruitment of substrate to the receptor [38].

All the above approaches have shown success in targeting STAT3 activation leading to induction of cancer cell death (Table 5.2) and have demonstrated significant clinical efficacy. However, acquired resistance against tyrosine kinase inhibitors remains a significant challenge [21, 39]. Besides, there have been inhibitors (e.g. OPB-31121) that showed very low nanomolar level IC_{50}s in pre-clinical settings, but eventually failed to show efficacy in clinical trials. Moreover, due to the pleiotropic nature of cytokines such as IL-6 there are always concerns of potential toxicity due to off-target effects [40, 41]. Recent studies now provide a rationale for direct targeting of STAT3 by itself or in combination with other therapeutic approaches for combating drug resistance in cancer treatment [21, 42].

5.3.4   Inhibitors Targeting the STAT3 SH2 Domain

The SH2 domain presents a defined and well-characterized targeting site with suitable topological features amenable to small molecule intervention and has proven to be tractable for small molecule inhibition of STAT3. Additionally, the SH2 domain of STATs have a dual function where they act as receptor recruitment modules as well as dimerization domains necessary for high-affinity STAT DNA-binding. The SH2 domain has become the favored target for platforms geared towards rational design, as well as in vitro and cell based screens for several reasons, including: (i) the pY-peptide binding site provides a suitable druggable site for in silico docking screens, (ii) pY705 phosphorylation is a convenient surrogate for STAT3 activation making it amenable to very robust cell based high-throughput screening (HTS) assays, and (iii) the SH2 domain binds short cognate pY-peptide ligands and, thus, provides a platform for competitive inhibition bind assays such as SPR and fluorescence polarization that have routinely been used to directly screen for competitive inhibitors of pY-peptide binding. The greatest effort at designing STAT3 inhibitors has been directed at the SH2 domain, as summarized below (Table 5.3).

Table 5.2 STAT3 upstream inhibitors in development

Inhibitors	Type	Description	Blocks	IC50 STAT3 inhibition (assay)	IC50 cell growth inhibition, cells	Pre-clinical animal models	Ref
PD153035	SM	EGFR TK inhibitor	pY, DM, NT, DB, GT	~100 nM, EGF-stimulated pSTAT3 MDA-MB-468	0.2–2.5 µM, HER2/Neu+ve cancer cells	80 mg/kg, IP, A431 xenografts	[353–355]
Oleanolic Acid	SM	JAK2, SRC, EGFR, STAT3 inhibitor	pY, DM, NT, DB, GT	~20^E µM, constitutive pSTAT3, U373	~20^E µM, U373	NA	[356, 357]
Brevilin A	SM	JAK inhibitor	pY, DM, NT, DB, GT	10.6 µM, constitutive pSTAT3 A549R	>20 µM, A549R	NA	[358]
Tofacitinib (CP-690,550)	SM	JAK3 inhibitor, inhibits pSTAT1/3/4/5/6	pY, DM, NT, DB, GT	0.07 µM, constitutive pSTAT3, JAK2V617F/FDCP-EpoR	0.07 µM, JAK2V617F-transduced FDCP-EpoR	NA	[359–363]
Sorafenib	SM	JAK2/STAT3 inhibitor	pY, DM, NT, DB, GT	<3 µM, constitutive pSTAT3, U87	1–2 µM glioblastoma cells	100 mg/kg, IP, U87-Luc xenografts	[364]
AZD1480	SM	JAK1/2 inhibitor, inhibits pSTAT1/3/5/6	pY, DM, NT, DB, GT	0.35 µM, nuclear translocation	0.36–5.37 µM, Ewing sarcoma cells	30–50 mg/kg, OG, DU145, MDA-MB-468, MDAH2774 xenografts	[41, 269, 272, 365–370]
Atiprimod	SM	JAK2/3 inhibitor, inhibits pSTAT3/5	pY, DM, NT, DB, GT	~4–8^E µM, constitutive pSTAT3, U266-B1	0.5–1.5 µM, HEPG2	50 mg/kg/2d, IV, OPMI xenografts	[371–375]
Auranofin	SM	JAK1/STAT3 inhibitor	pY, DM, NT, DB, GT	<1^E µM, IL6-stimulated pSTAT3, HepG2	0.05 µM, U266	7 mg/kg/d, IP, IM-resistant Bcr-Abl-T315I xenografts	[376–379]
Sanguinarine	SM	JAK2, Src, STAT3 inhibitor	pY, DM, NT, DB, GT	~1–2^E µM, IL6-stimulated pSTAT3, DU145	1.3/1.6 µM, A17, MDA-MB-231	2.5/5 mg/kg/2d, 7d, IG, GTL-16 xenografts	[380–382]
Cucurbitacin I (JSI-124)	SM	JAK2/STAT3 inhibitor	pY, DM, NT, DB, GT	7.5/0.5 µM, constitutive pSTAT3 MD-MB-468, A549	2.9–10.5 µM, cells from CLL patients	1 mg/kg/d, 15d, IP, HRas/3 T3/A549/MDA-MB-468/Calu-1 xenografts	[383, 384]

Cucurbitacins B	SM	JAK2/STAT3 inhibitor	pY, DM, NT, DB, GT	Low nM–high μM, constitutive pSTAT3, PANC-1, K-562	~0.5 nM, leukemia, HCC, breast cancer cells	1 mg/kg, IP, Panc-1 xenografts	[385–392]
Cucurbitacin E	SM	JAK2/STAT3 inhibitor	pY, DM, NT, DB, GT	1.4 μM, constitutive pSTAT3, MD-MB-468	~10 nM, HUVEC, PC3)	3 mg/kg, IL, PC3 xenografts	[393–395]
Celastrol	SM	JAK2, SRC, STAT3 inhibitor	pY, DM, NT, DB, GT	~2.5^E μM, constitutive pSTAT3, C3A	1.1–3 μM, H1650/H1975/H2228	1–2 mg/kg, IP, PLC/PRF5 cells	[396–398]
Emodin	SM	JAK2/STAT3 inhibitor	pY, DM, NT, DB, GT	25–50^E μM, constitutive pSTAT3, HepG2	35.8–46 μM, FaDu/HSC-3	20–50 mg/kg, IP, HCCLM3_Luc2	[399]
Dasatinib	SM	SRC/ABL/KITSTAT3 inhibitor	DM, NT, DB, GT	Does not block pSTAT3	8 nM, MTT CME -1, cells / 13 nM, MTT SYO-1 cells	10 mg/kg, IP, SYO-1 xenografts	[400, 401]
Caffeic Acid (CA)	SM	JAK2, SRC, STAT3 inhibitor	pY, DM, NT, DB, GT	CA: 70–100 μM	~50^E μM, Huh-7	5 mg/kg, IP, Caki-I xenografts	[402–404]
CADPE				CADPE 15–30 μM, hypoxia-induced pSTAT3, Caki-1			
AG490	SM	JAK3	pY, DM, NT, DB, GT	50–100 μM, constitutive pSTAT3, renal/colon cancer cells	40 μM HT29, cells / 50 μM Caki-1 cells	5 mg/kg, IC, EGFRvIII cell intracranial xenografts	[405, 406]
WP1066	SM	JAK2/STAT3 inhibitor	pY, DM, NT, DB, GT	1–2^E μM, constitutive pSTAT3, HEL	2.5 μM Caki-1 cells / 2.3 μM, HEL cells	40 mg/kg, OG, Caki-1, GL26 xenografts	[151, 288, 407]
TG101209	SM	JAK2/STAT3 inhibitor	pY, DM, NT, DB, GT	~2–5^E μM, constitutive pSTAT3, HEL	2–5 μM myeloma cells	100 mg/kg, PO, Ba/F3 V617F-GFP xenografts	[408, 409]
FLL32	SM	JAK2, STAT3 inhibitor, binds to STAT3 SH2 domain	pY, DM, NT, DB, GT	2.5–5 μM, corstitutive pSTAT3, MDA-MB-231, PANC-1	0.11–0.64 μM Pancreatic / 0.14–0.60 μM Breast cancer cells	50 mg/kg, IP MDA-MB-231 xenografts	[410, 411]

(continued)

Table 5.2 (continued)

106 U. Bharadwaj et al.

Inhibitors	Type	Description	Blocks	IC50 STAT3 inhibition (assay)	IC50 cell growth inhibition, cells	Pre-clinical animal models	Ref
Avicin D	SM	JAK1/2/3 and STAT3 inhibitor, acts through SHP1 upregulation too	pY, DM, NT, DB, GT	~1^E μM, pSTAT3, U266 cells	5^E μM, U266 cells, 0.32 μM, Jurkut cells	NA	[412, 413]
E738	SM	SRC and JAK inhibitor	pY, DM, NT, DB, GT	1–5 μM, constitutive pSTAT3, PaCa cells	0.68–2.2 μM, pancreatic cancer cell	NA	[414]
MLS-2384	SM	SRC and JAK inhibitor	pY, DM, NT, DB, GT	1–2.5 μM, constitutive pSTAT3, DU145, MDA-MB-468, A2058, A549	2 μM, DU145, MDA-MB-468, A2058, A549	25 mg/kg, PO, melanoma	[415]
CYT387 (Momelotinib)	SM	JAK2 Inhibitor	pY, DM, NT, DB, GT	NA	1.5 μM, Ba/F3-JAK2V617F, HEL cells	15 mg/kg, PO, HEY cell xenografts	[416, 417]
Ergosterol peroxide (EP)	SM	JAK, SRC, STAT3 inhibitor	pY, DM, NT, DB, GT	8–12.5 μM, constitutive pSTAT3, U266, SCC4, DU145. MDA-MB-231	NA	100 mg/kg, IP, U266 cells xenografts	[418]
PP2	SM	SRC inhibitor/STAT3		μM, LIF-activated pSTAT3	0.2–3 μM, melanoma cell		[419, 420]
Ponatinib	SM	FGFR4 inhibitor	pY, DM, NT, DB, GT	0.2–0.8 μM, constitutive pSTAT3, RH4/RH5/RH41	0.2–0.9 μM, rhabdomyosarcoma	30 mg/kg, PO, RMS722 xenograft	[421]
Benzyl isothiocyanate	SM	Inhibits SRC recruitment and hence STAT3	pY, DM, NT, DB, GT	5–10 μM, constitutive pSTAT3, PaCa cells	8–10 μM, PANC-1, BxPC3	12 μM, PO, BxPC3 xenografts	[308, 422]
CNTO-328 (Siltuximab)	Ab	MAb to IL6 JAK/STAT inhibitor	pY, DM, NT, DB, GT	0.06–0.6 μM, IL6-activated pSTAT3 HKOV3	No effect on viability, H1650 cells	10 mg/kg, 36d, IP, H1650 xenografts, NSCLC PDX	[423, 424]

Toclizimab	Ab	MAb to IL-6R JAK/STAT inhibitor	pY, DM, NT, DB, GT	NA	0.09–0.27 nM Ba/F3 cells	20 mg/kg, IP, HepG2 xenografts	[425, 426]
Cetuximab	Ab	MAb to EGFR	pY, DM, NT, DB, GT	NA	NA	0.2–0.5 mg/mice, IP, A431 xenografts	[427]
KDI1/KDI3/ KDI4	AP	EGFR intracellular domain amino acids 688–821, interacting aptamers	pY, DM, DB, NT, GT	NA	NA	NA	[38]
Xanthohumol	SM	EGFR inhibitor	Py, DM, NT, DB, GT	~5–10^E µM, pSTAT3, PANC-1	~10^E µM, pancreatic cancer cells	25 mg/kg, IP, 27d, PANC-1 xenografts	[428, 429]

Note: Information for Pre-clinical animal models consist of Dose, route of administration, duration (if available) and animal model used. Abbreviations: *E* estimated from descriptive data on inhibition, from corresponding reference, *NA* not available, *Ab* antibody, *SM* small molecule, *pY* STAT3 phosphorylation at Tyr-705, *DM* dimerization, *NT* nuclear translocation, *DB* DNA-binding, *GT* gene transcription, *IG* intra-gastrical, *TK* tyrosine kinase, *IC* intra-cranial, *PO* per Os (by mouth), *IP* intra-Peritoneal, *MAb* monoclonal Ab, *AP* aptamer

Table 5.3 Direct STAT3 inhibitors in development

Inhibitors	Type	Description	Blocks	IC50 STAT3 inhibition (assay)	Kd (STAT3 binding)	IC50 Cell growth inhibition, cells	Pre-clinical animal models	Ref
Inhibitors targeting STAT3 SH2 domain								
PY*LKTK(-mts)	P	Phosphopeptide derived from STAT3 (vicinity of Y-705)	DM, DB, GT	235 µM, STAT3-hSIE binding EMSA	NA	>500 µM, NIH 3T3/vSrc colony	NA	[45]
PY*L	P	Minimal STAT3 p-peptide required for STAT3 inhibition	DM, DB, GT	182 µM, STAT3-hSIE binding EMSA	NA	NA	NA	[45]
ISS 610	PM	Peptidomimetics developed replacing P by 4-cyanobenzoate	DM, DB, GT	42 µM, STAT3-hSIE binding EMSA	NA	>1000 µM, NIH 3T3/vSrc colony	NA	[45, 49, 430, 431]
PDP/ Phosphododeca peptide(-mts)	P	p-peptides Y1068 + p/LPVPE(pY) INQSVP & Y992 + p/TDSNF(pY) RALMDE from STAT3 binding sequence of EGFR	pY, DM, DB, GT	350–750 µM, IL6/ EGFR stimulated STAT3 binding EMSA, HepG2/ UM-SCC-23	NA	~750 µM, A431	NA	[25
Ac-Y*LPQTV	P	p-peptide from STAT3 binding sequence of gp130	DM, DB, GT	0.15 µM, STAT3-hSIE binding EMSA	NA	NA	NA	[44, 52]
Hydrocinnamoyl-Tyr(PO3H2)-L-cis-3,4-methanoPQ-NHBn	P	p-peptide from STAT binding sequence of gp130	DM, DB, GT	0.125 µM, STAT3-hSIE binding EMSA	NA	NA	NA	[44, 52]
CJ-1383	PM	PM developed from Ac-Y*LPQTV	pY, DM, DB, GT	~10 µM^E, pSTAT3, MDA-MB-468	0.95 µM, STAT3 binding, FP	3.6–11.2 µM, MDA-MB-468, MDA-MB-231	NA	[433]
PM-73G	PM	Mimetic developed from Ac-Y*LPQTV	pY, DM, DB, GT	0.1–0.5 µM, pSTAT3-inhibition, cancer cells	NA	≥30 µM, MDA-MB-468, A549	5 mM, IT, MDA-MB-468 xenografts	[53, 54]

APT$_{STAT3}$-9R	AP	Tryptophan zipper scaffold attached to a STAT3-binding peptide and cell-penetrating motif	pY, DM, DB, GT	NA	231 nM STAT3 binding, SPR	10–20 µM, A549	8 mg/kg, IT, A549 xenografts	[55]
Recombinant STAT3 inhibitory peptide aptamer (rS3-PA)	AP	Recognizes dimerization domain and inhibits STAT3 function	Py, DM, NT, DB, GT	NA	1–4^E µM, ligand-stimulated pSTAT3, HepG2	1–4^E µM, various cancer cell lines	7.5 mg/kg, IV 15d, Tu9648 xenografts	[56–59]
DD1/DD2/DD3	AP	STAT3-DD (amino acid positions 655–755) binding aptamers DD-1: PPLVCIRSWCPLMVPHSA DLGPASQWLCHRVASIALLPRYSS DD-2: VGWTWMSVLVCCDGSGLV PEGPVVVQAGGAVPISGSVALMTD DD-3: SPISIPIGFVVRHCALHMAV GPLSWPARVSGYSFALEVLTNF	Py, DM, NT, DB, GT	NA	NA	NA	NA	[163]
Dipicclylamine copper complexes 1,2,3	PM	Phosphate binders e.g. Lewis acidic metal–picolyamine complexes acting as SH2-proteomimetics, disrupt phosphopeptide–STAT3 complexes	DM, DB, GT	15–128 µM, F*pYLPQTV gp130p-STAT3 binding, FP	8–100 µM, pY-LKTK STAT3p binding, IGT	77/11/100 µM, DU145 73/11/100 µM, OCI-AML2 115/5/56 µM, MDA-MB-468	NA	[60]
S31-M2001	SM	Developed from ISS-610 peptidomimetic	pY, DM, DB, GT	79 µM, STAT3-hSIE binding EMSA	NA	~100 µM	5–20 mg/kg, IV, MDA-MB-231 xenografts	[50]
STA-21	SM	Structure-based virtual screening and screening for STAT3-luciferase yielded STA-21	DM, NT, DB, GT	20–30^E µM, STAT3-hSIE binding EMSA	NA	12.2/18.7 µM, DU145, PC3,	NA	[61–63]

(continued)

Table 5.3 (continued)

Inhibitors	Type	Description	Blocks	IC50 STAT3 inhibition (assay)	Kd (STAT3 binding)	IC50 Cell growth inhibition, cells	Pre-clinical animal models	Ref
LLL-3	SM	Structural analogue of STA-21	DM, NT, DB, GT	~40^E μM, STAT3-hSIE binding EMSA, SJSA cell	NA	6.3 μM/K562, 10–20 μM, U87, U251, U373; 11.3 μM, DU145	50 mg/kg, IT, intra-cranial U87 xenografts	[64, 434, 435]
LLL-12	SM	Derived by replacing acetyl group of LLL-3 with sulfonamide to	pY, DM, NT, DB, GT	0.16–3.09 μM, pSTAT3, various cancer cells	NA	0.3–0.8 μM, U2Os, SAOS2, SJSA 0.97–3.1 μM, MDA-M231, SKBR3,		[65–73]
Stattic	SM	Hit from HT fluorescence polarization screen for binding to STAT3 SH2 domain	pY, DM, DB, GT	5.1 $\pm$ 0.8 μM, gp130-derived p-peptide binding to Stat3 SH2 domain	NA	0.43–2.6 μM, C, MM, G cells 4.3–5.6 μM, Nasopharyngeal cancer cells	50 mg/kg, PO (UM-SCC-17B orthotopic xenografts	[74–76]
S31-201/NSC 74859	SM	Structure based virtual screening of NCI chemical libraries with computer model of SH2-pYpeptide interaction	pY, DM, NT, DB, GT	86 μM, STAT3-hSIE binding EMSA	NA	300 μM, LNCaP	5 mg/kg, once/2day, 16d, IV, MDA-MB-231 xenografts	[81, 82]
S31-201.1066/SF-1066	SM	Resulted from molecular modeling of the pTyr–SH2 interaction combined with in silico structural analysis of S31-201	pY, DM, NT, DB, GT	35 μM, STAT3-hSIE binding EMSA 23μM, pY-peptide STAT3 binding, SPR	2.7 μM, pY-peptide STAT3 binding, SPR	35/48/37 μM, NIH3T3/v-Src, Panc-1, MDA-MB-231	5 mg/kg, once/2day, 17d, IV, MDA-MB-231 xenografts	[83, 84]

BP-1-102/17o	SM	Screening of salicyclic acid-containing STAT3 SH2-inhibitors	pY, DM, NT, DB, GT	6.8 µM, STAT3-hSIE binding EMSA	Ki 13 µM, pY-peptide STAT3 binding, SPR	10.9–22.7 µM, MDA-MB-468, DU145, JJN3	1/3 mg/kg, once/2day, 15d, IV or PO, MDA-MB-231,A549 xenografts	[87, 88]
SH4-54	SM	Screening BP-1-102 analogues for anti-STAT3 and anti-tumor functions	pY, DM, NT, DB, GT	4.7 µM, STAT3-hSIE binding EMSA	Kd 0.3–2.4 µM, direct binding to STAT3, SPR	0.07–0.2 µM, 25EF, 67EF, 73E, 84EF, and 127EF	10 mg/kg, 15d, IP/PO, BT73 xenografts	[91, 92]
						1.9–9.6 µM, vSrc, 231, DU145, Panc-1, U251MG, U87MG, U373MG, SF295		
SH5-07	SM	Screening BP-1-102 analogues for anti-STAT3 and anti-tumor functions	pY, DM, NT, DB, GT	3.9 µM, STAT3-hSIE binding EMSA	Kd 2.4 µM, direct binding to STAT3, SPR	1.1–10.3 µM, growth, vSrc, 231, DU145, Panc-1, U251MG, U87MG, U373MG, SF295	5 mg/kg, 15d, IP or 3 mg/kg, OD, PO, U251/ MDA-MB-231 xenografts	[92]
S3I-V3-31/32/33/34	SM	GOLD and 3D-pharmacophore analysis with known STAT3 inhibitors and subsequent wet lab screening	pY, DM, NT, DB, GT	27–84 µM STAT3-hSIE binding EMSA	0.8–12 µM pY-peptide STAT3 binding, SPR	41–80 µM, various cancers	NA	[89]
C188	SM	Virtual ligand screening, by docking 920,000 small molecules into the pY-binding pocket of the STAT3 SH2 domain and further high-throughput screens	pY, DM, NT, DB, GT	7.5–20 µM, pY-peptide STAT3 binding, SPR	Ki 37.3 nM, pY-peptide STAT3 binding, SPR	0.7–3.9 µM, ED50, apoptosis MDA-MB-468/ MDA-MB-231	12.5 mg/kg, 14d, IP, chemoresistant PDX models	[93, 94, 96]
				16.2 µM, G-CSF-stimulated pSTAT3, Kasumi-1, Luminex			50 mg/kg, 14d, IP, UM-SCC-17B xenografts	

(continued)

Table 5.3 (continued)

Inhibitors	Type	Description	Blocks	IC50 STAT3 inhibition (assay)	Kd (STAT3 binding)	IC50 Cell growth inhibition, cells	Pre-clinical animal models	Ref
C188-9	SM	2D similarity screening using scaffold of C188, and 3D pharmacophore analysis in a hit-to-lead program identified C188-9	pY, DM, NT, DB, GT	2.5 µM, pY-peptide STAT3 binding, SPR	Ki 12.4 nM, pY-peptide STAT3 binding, SPR;	0.7–14.8 µM, growth, HNSCC cells, MTT	100 mg/kg, 14d, IP, UM-SCC-17B xenografts	[95–98, 231]
				3.7 µM, G-CSF-stimulated pSTAT3, Kasumi-1, Luminex	Kd 4.7 nM, STAT3-binding, MST	0.8–25 µM, ED50, apoptosis in primary AML		
Cryptotanshinone	SM	Screen of natural compound library with HT STAT-luciferase screen	pY, DM, NT, DB, GT	4.6 µM, STAT3-luciferase	NA	7 µM, DU145; 5.8–15.1 µM, growth AML, colon cancer, breast cancer cells	NA	[100–105]
STX-0119	SM	In-silico docking and screening through biochemical methods	DM, NT, DB, GT	4.6 µM, STAT3-luciferase	NA	1.4–18.3 µM, growth, hematological cancer cells,	40 mg/kg, 5d, IP, SCC-3, GBM-SC xenografts	[110–113]
C48	SM	Hit from VLS screen using entire STAT3 SH2 domain	pY, DM, DB, GT	3–10 µM, OSM-induced STAT3-dependent luciferase activity	NA	10–20 µM, apoptosis induction MDA-MB-468	200 mg/kg, IP, MDA-MB-468 xenografts in nude mice	[79]
							100–200 mg/kg, syngeneic C3L5 mouse model	

Name	Type	Description	Methods	Cell activity	Binding	Growth/IC50	In vivo	Ref
Piperlongumine	SM	High throughput screen of a repositioning library for inhibitor of STAT3 nuclear translocation	pY, DM, NT, DB, GT	0.9–2.7 µM, IL6/sIL6R-induced pSTAT3, luminex	Ki 68 nM, STAT3-pY-peptide binding, SPR	0.2–4.6 µM, growth, breast cancer cell, MTT	15 mg/kg, 21d, MDA-MB-468 xenografts	[115]
OPB-31121	SM	Very potent SH2 domain inhibitor with activity in low nM range	pY, DM, NT, DB, GT	3–10 µM, OSM-induced STAT3-dependent luciferase activity	Kd 10 nM STAT3 binding	Low nM range IC50, STAT-addictive oncokinases (SAO)+ve cells from various cancers	100–300 mg/kg, IP, xenografts in nude mice. Reduction of tumor by 79–95%	[273–278]
Withacnistin	SM	Stops STAT3/5 recruitment to EGFR and gp130. Doesn't affect upstream kinases, most probably targeting SH2	pY, DM, NT, DB, GT	1.4 µM, constitutive pSTAT3 MD-MB-468	NA	1–3^E µM, colony MD-MB-468	20 mg/Kg, IP, FVB/N--Tg(MMTV neu)202Mul/J) mice; 0.5 mg/kg A549.v -Src/3 T3 xenografts	[395, 436]
XZH-5	SM	Peptide mimicking small molecule design from known STAT3 inhibitor knowledge	pY, DM, NT, DB, GT	~20^E µM, constitutive pSTAT3, HCC cells	NA	15–50 µM, growth, breast, pancreatic, HCC, rhabdomyosarcoma, MTT	NA	[119–121]
T2, T3, Celecoxib	SM	FBDD using MLSD and drug repositioning screen	pY, DM, NT, DB, GT	~20–50^E µM, constitutive pSTAT3, HCT-116 cells	NA	9.7/10.1/43.3 µM, HCT-116, growth, MTT	NA	[123]

(continued)

Table 5.3 (continued)

Inhibitors	Type	Description	Blocks	IC50 STAT3 inhibition (assay)	Kd (STAT3 binding)	IC50 Cell growth inhibition, cells	Pre-clinical animal models	Ref
HJC0123	SM	FBDD based on structure of niclosamide and other STAT3 inhibitors	pY, DM, NT, DB, GT	~1^E µM, constitutive pSTAT3, MDA-MB-231 cells	NA	0.1–1.2 µM, breast and pancreatic cancer cells, growth, MTT	50 mg/kg, PO, MDA-MB-231 xenografts	[119, 125, 126]
Ly5	SM	FBDD. By inking naphthalene-5.8-dione-1-sulphoneamide fragment of LLL12 as binding moiety to pTyr705 of STAT3-SH2 domain	pY, DM, NT, DB, GT	~0.5–1.4 µM, stimulated STAT3, MDA-MB-231 cells	NA	0.5–1.39 µM U2OS/RD2, growth, MTT; 0.32–0.48 µM, UW288-1, UW426, and DAOY	NA	[127, 437–439]
T40214/T40231	GQ-ODN	G-quartet oligonucleotide binds to STAT3 SH2 domain	pY, DB, GT	5 µM: STAT3 DNA-binding, prostate, breast, HNSCC cells	NA	NA	10 mg/kg, IP, NSCLC, HNSCC, prostate, breast xenografts	[144, 145, 147, 440–443]
Inhibitors targeting STAT3 DBD								
Decoy ODN	ODN	Sense: 5' C*A*T*TTCCCGTTA*A*T*C 3' AS: 5' G*A*T*TTACGGGAA*A*T*G 3', "*" denotes phosphorothioated sites)	NT, DB, GT	NA	NA	~12.5^E µM, 1483 cell growth MTT; 8 nM, HUVEC and 137 nM, HDMEC	25 µg, IT, 1483 xenografts	[133, 140, 292, 444, 445]
13410/13410A/ SeqD	ODN	Oligonucleotide decoy, modification of consensus STAT3-binding sequence	NT, DB, GT	NA	NA	40–200 nM, apoptosis DU-145	NA	[137, 446]
CPA-7	SM	Platinum (IV) complexes	DB, DM, DB, GT	1.5 µM, DNA binding EMSA	NA	2.9–23.7 µM, GL26, SMA560, CNS1, IN859, U251, HF2303	5.5 mg/kg, tail-vein, GL26 xenografts	[149, 151]

IS3 295	SM	Platinum (IV) compound screened from NCI 2000 diversity set, non-competitive	DB, DM, DB, GT	NA	1.4 µM, DNA binding EMSA	NA	<10 µM^E (colony formation Src/NIH3T3)	NA	[149]
inS3-54	SM	Virtual screening for binding to DBD of STAT3	DB, DM, DB, GT	NA	20 µM, DNA binding EMSA	NA	3.2–5.4 µM (MDA-MB-468, MDA-MB-231, A549, H1299	NA	[154]
inS3-54A18	SM	Activity-guided hit optimization and mechanistic characterization from inS3-54	DB, DM, DB, GT	NA	11 µM, STAT3 dependent luciferase	NA	3.2–4.7 µM, MDA-MB-468, MDA-MB-231, A549, H1299	8 mg/kg, OG, A549 xenografts in nude mice	[150]
HO-3857	SM	Conjugation of a diarylidenyl-piperidone (DAP) backbone to N-hydroxypyrroline (-NOH) group	pY, DM, NT, DB, GT	NA	<10 µM, constitutive pSTAT3, HO-3867	NA	3–5 µM, BRCA-1 mutated ovarian cancer cells	50/100 ppm, in feed, A2780 xenografts	[156–158, 447, 448]
Galiellalactone	SM	Fungal metabolite, co-valent modifier	DM, DB, GT	NA	~4 µM^E, DNA binding DU145, EMSA	NA	3.4 µM, DU-145 cell growth, MTT	5 mg/kg, IP DU-145-Luc xenografts	[160–162]
DBD-1/DBD-1-9R	AP	STAT3-DBD (aa 322–483) binding aptamer, p-seq: PLTAVFWLIYVLAKALVTVC	DM, DB, GT	NA	NA	NA	180–369 nM^E, U266	NA	[38, 163]
Inhibitors targeting STAT3 ND									
Hel2K-Pen/ST3-HA2A	SM	Cell permeable analogs of the STAT3 second helix	DM, NT, DB, GT	NA	NA	NA	0.7–3.5^E, Du145, LNCap, PC3	NA	[151, 288, 407]

Note: Information for Pre-clinical animal models consist of Dose, route of administration, duration (if available) and animal model used

Abbreviations: *E* estimated from descriptive data on inhibition, from corresponding reference, *NA* not available, *Ab* antibody, *SM* small molecule, *pY* STAT3 phosphorylation at Tyr-705, *DM* dimerization, *NT* nuclear translocation, *DB* DNA-binding, *GT* gene transcription, *IG* intra-gastrical, *TK* tyrosine kinase, *IC* intra-cranial, *PO* per Os (by mouth), *OG* oral gavage, *FP* fluorescence polarization. *IP* Intra-Peritoneal, *MAb* Mcnoclonal Ab, *P* peptide, *PM* peptidomimetic, *AP* aptamer, *GQ-ODN* G-quartet oligonucle-otide, *ppm* parts per million

5.3.4.1 Peptides and Peptidomimetics

Elucidation of the crystal structure of STAT3β-STAT3β-DNA complex [43] and subsequent studies [25, 44–46] indicated that the SH2 domain facilitates binding to specific pY-peptide motifs within receptor complexes and mediates dimerization of two STAT3 monomers via reciprocal interaction between the SH2 of one monomer and pY-peptide motif, ^{702}AAPY*LKTKFI^{711}, on the other. Strategies to target STAT3 by identifying pY-peptide inhibitors of STAT3 SH2 binding to pY-peptide ligands have been pursued by several groups (Table 5.3) [47]. Turkson et al. showed that pY-peptides based on the sequence PY*LKTK surrounding Y705 within STAT3, inhibited STAT3 DNA binding ($IC_{50}=235$ μM) and pulled down STAT3 from lysates of unstimulated cells [45]. Alongside the usual limitations of the peptide approaches, e.g. low cell permeability, instability, and the consequential low biological activities, the requirement for the phosphorylation on Tyr for the inhibitory activity presented another challenge to making this approach biologically useful. Covalently attaching a membrane-translocating sequence (mts) of hydrophobic amino acids (AAVLLPVLLAAP) to the C-terminus of the peptide improved membrane permeability and PY*LKTKmts inhibited STAT3-mediated gene transcription and malignant transformation, and induced apoptosis in v-Src-transformed NIH3T3 fibroblasts albeit at 1 mM concentration [45, 48], underscoring the potential difficulty of converting this approach into an effective therapeutic modality. The exploration of peptidomimetic and phosphotyrosine (pY) mimic approaches led to the identification of ISS 610, a peptidomimetic analog of the tripeptide, PY*L [49], the minimal peptide from PY*LKTK that was required for STAT3 inhibition ($IC_{50}=182$ μM). PY*L mimic, ISS 610, better disrupted STAT3 DNA-binding activity ($IC_{50}=42$ μM) [45, 49], and had increased STAT3 selectivity, (STAT1 $IC_{50}=310$ μM; STAT5 $IC_{50}=285$ μM) but still had weak intracellular inhibitory properties ($IC_{50}=1$ mM), due to poor membrane permeability. The abysmal intracellular performance of the peptide forced the group to employ computational modeling to probe the binding of ISS 610 to the STAT3 SH2 domain, which led to generation of the oxazole-based small molecule S3I-M2001 having increased membrane permeability but similar STAT3 DNA binding inhibition ($IC_{50}=79$ μM), loss of specificity (STAT1 $IC_{50}=159$ μM), but improved intracellular activity [50]. S3I-M2001 reduced pY-STAT3 levels, DNA-binding, nuclear translocation, and transcriptional activity in NIH3T3/v-Src fibroblasts and human breast carcinoma cells at 50–100 μM. Cell growth inhibition ability was still weak ($IC_{50}=100$ μM), including inhibition of cell growth, survival, and metastasis of NIH3T3/v-Src fibroblasts and human breast and pancreatic carcinoma cells with increased pY-STAT3. But importantly, it showed a significant regression of MDA-MB-231 xenografts at 5–20 mg/kg [50].

Another peptide-based approach used pY-peptides derived from STAT3 SH2 domain interacting growth factor or cytokine receptors, e.g. EGFR and gp130, to block SH2-pY-peptide ligand interaction. Shao et al. showed that a phosphododecapeptide (PDP) based on the sequence surrounding Y1068 within the EGFR could directly bind non-phosphorylated STAT3 and inhibit pY-STAT3 DNA binding, ligand-stimulated STAT3 activation, and TGFα/EGFR-mediated autocrine growth in cancer cells [25]. Examining the structural basis for the specificity of STAT3-SH2 for pYXXQ peptides revealed that only pY-peptides containing +3 Q (not L, M. E or R) bound to wild-type STAT3-SH2 which required its K591 or R609 residues, whose side-chains interact with the peptide pY, and E638, whose amide hydrogen bonds with oxygen within the +3 Q side-chain when the peptide ligand assumes a β turn [25, 51].

Another approach found gp130-derived STAT3-inhibitory pY-peptide Y*LPQTV and several modified versions, including hydrocinnamoyl-Tyr (PO3 H2)-Leu-*cis*-3,4-methanoPro-Gln-NHBn [44, 52], that showed potent inhibition of STAT3 DNA-binding activity (IC_{50}=0.15–0.29 µM). The peptidomimetic CJ-1383 developed from these, inhibited constitutive pY-STAT3 and inhibited growth of breast cancer cell lines (IC_{50}=3.6–11.2 µM). PM-73G, another peptidomimetic developed from Y*LPQTV, also showed a low micromolar IC_{50} of pY-STAT3 reduction in cancer cells, inhibited their growth, and blocked xenografts formation [53, 54].

The peptide aptamer APT_{STAT3}-9R, which has a tryptophan zipper scaffold attached to a STAT3-binding peptide and a cell-penetrating motif, was screened from a randomized peptide library [55]; it specifically interacted in SPR assays with the STAT3 dimerization domain (K_d=231 nM), reduced levels of pY-STAT3, DNA binding, and transcriptional activity [55] and blocked the growth of A549 cells *in vitro* (IC_{50}=10–20 µM) and *in vivo*. Another aptamer, the recombinant STAT3 inhibitory peptide aptamer (rS3-PA) also decreased pY-STAT3 levels, inhibited growth of cancer cells *in vitro*, and reduced Tu9648 xenograft growth [56–59]. Although partly a peptide, these aptamers differ in their mode of action from peptide inhibitors [47].

A phosphate binder, e.g. Lewis acidic metal–picolylamine complex, was shown to act as a SH2-proteomimetic and disrupt pY-peptide–STAT3 complexes and also was potent in its anti-STAT3 activity (IC_{50}=15–128 µM) as well it ability to inhibit growth of various cancer cells (IC_{50}=11–100 µM) [60].

5.3.4.2 Small-Molecules

Despite having potent STAT3-inhibitory activity, peptides and peptidomimetics continue to suffer the limitations of *in vivo* instability and poor membrane permeability. Most of the peptides have not been tested in xenograft models and those that were tried, with the exception of rS3-PA, had to be administered intratumorally (IT), limiting their effective use *in vivo* [47]. Nevertheless, these studies provided the proof of concept that the STAT3-SH2/pY-peptide interaction was amenable to targeting and provided the impetus for many programs engaged in designing small molecules for this purpose.

SH2 inhibitors resulting from rational design or high-throughput screens. A structure-based virtual screening of ~425,000 compounds from four different chemical libraries followed by examination of 100 of the first 200 compounds in an *in vitro* STAT3-luciferase assay identified STA-21, a deoxytetrangomycin, with potent cell growth inhibitory activities (IC_{50}=12.2/18.7 µM in DU145/PC3, respectively).

Modeling studies suggested that STA-21 binds to the SH2 domain of STAT3 and forms a number of hydrogen bonds with residues that form the pocket that binds the pY residue, including Arg-595, Arg-609, and Ile-634, and thus inhibits STAT3 dimerization, nuclear translocation, DNA-binding, gene transcription, and inhibits growth of breast and soft tissue sarcoma cell lines [61–63] with constitutively activated STAT3. Unexpectedly, STA-21 only minimally reduces levels of constitutively phosphorylated STAT3. The group also identified Compound1, a derivative of STA-21 [61], with similar STAT3 and cell growth inhibitory properties. Another slightly more potent structural analogue LLL-3 had better cellular permeability than STA-21 and inhibited growth of glioblastoma ($IC_{50} = 10$–20 µM), prostate cancer ($IC_{50} = 11.3$ µM), and CML cells (IC50 = 6.3 µM). Intratumoral injection of LLL-3 also inhibited intracranial glioblastoma xenografts in nude mice and increased their survival [64]. The acetyl group of LLL-3 was then replaced with sulfonamide to develop another STAT3 inhibitor, LLL-12 [65–73]. LLL-12 reduces pY-STAT3 levels ($IC_{50} = 0.16$–3.09 µM) and the growth of various cancer cell lines *in vitro* including osteosarcoma cell lines U2Os, SAOS2, and SJSA ($IC_{50} = 0.3$–0.8 µM,), breast cancer cell lines MDA-MB-231 and SKBR3 ($IC_{50} = 0.97$–3.1 µM,), pancreatic cancer cell lines HPAC and Panc-1 ($IC_{50} = 0.16$–0.29 µM), glioblastoma cell lines U87MG and U373MG ($IC_{50} = 0.21$–0.86 µM) and myeloma cell lines U266 and ARH-77 ($IC_{50} = 0.49$–1.9 µM), as well as their xenografts [66, 69, 70, 72].

Stattic (*Stat t*hree *i*nhibitory *c*ompound) was another early small molecule STAT3 inhibitor discovered by high-throughput screening of chemical libraries [74]. Stattic selectively inhibited STAT3 binding to pY-peptide (GY*LPQTV; $IC_{50} = 5.1$ µM) and blocked IL-6-induced STAT3 activation, nuclear accumulation, and DNA-binding activity (IC50 = 20 µM). It efficiently blocked the growth [74–76] of several cancer cell lines with increased levels of pY-STAT3 ($IC_{50} = 0.43$–5.6 µM), as well as UM-SCC-17B orthotopic xenografts [76]. Stattic was used as an adjuvant to sensitize radioresistant esophageal squamous cell carcinoma (ESCC) cells and xenografts to radiation [77], and to sensitize ovarian cancer cells to cisplatin [78]. A structure-activity relationship (SAR) analysis revealed that saturation of the vinyl sulfone leads to loss in activity. In addition, the presence of 2 mM dithiothreitol (DTT), a nucleophile donor, abrogated STAT3 inhibitory activity of Stattic, suggesting the nucleophilic attack of the sulphonic double bond by a cysteine in the STAT3 SH2 domain [74]. Recently, MS-based studies using high quantities of Stattic (800 µM; 10 µM of pY-STAT3) suggested that eight molecules of Stattic bind to one pY-STAT3 scaffold and identified Cys468 as one possible alkylation site [79]. However, a more recent paper [75] reported covalent binding of nine Stattic molecules to one unphosphorylated core STAT3 protein molecule at a lower concentration (50 µM/10 µM STAT3). Four or five of the nine covalently-modified residues are cysteines, but Cys468 and Cys542 were not among these [75]. A recent report by Sanseverino et al. indicated that Stattic targets other STAT proteins, including STAT1 and STAT5 [80].

Another STAT3 inhibitor resulting from structure-based high-throughput virtual screening of the National Cancer Institute (NCI) chemical libraries was S3I-201/NSC74859. In modeling studies, S3I-201 docked to the pTyr binding site of STAT3-SH2 domain through its salicylic acid moiety, inhibited STAT3

DNA-binding (IC_{50} = 86 μM), and inhibited proliferation of several cancer cell lines, including hepatocellular carcinoma, breast cancer, and prostate cancer albeit with high IC_{50}s (100–300 μM) [81, 82]. However, it successfully inhibited growth of MDA-MB-231 xenografts at a dose of 5 mg/kg [82]. Genetic Optimization for Ligand Docking (GOLD) studies suggested suboptimal interaction between S31-201 and STAT3. To improve this interaction, several molecules were subsequently developed [83, 84], many of which showed higher potency in STAT3 DNA binding inhibition assays (IC_{50} = 18.7–51.9 μM) and disruption of STAT3–pY-peptide interactions (Ki = 15.5–41 μM). S3I-201.1066 (or SF-1066) was the most potent in this series; it was demonstrated to directly bind STAT3 (K_d = 2.7 μM) and to inhibit growth of multiple cancer cell lines with greater potency than S3I-201 (IC_{50} = 35–48 μM) [85, 86]. Sixteen novel sulfonamide analogues of SF-1066 were subsequently characterized; of these, BP-1-102 [87, 88] effectively inhibited STAT3 DNA binding (IC_{50} = 6.8 μM), which was a 5-fold improvement over SF-1066 [83, 84], resulting in better cell growth inhibition (IC_{50} = 10.9–22.7 μM). BP-1-102 was orally bioavailable and effectively limited growth of STAT3-dependent tumor xenografts [88]. Known STAT3 dimerization-disrupting small-molecules, including S3I-201, were then subjected to GOLD analysis and a 3D quantitative structure-activity relationship (QSAR) pharmacophore model adopted to predict optimized STAT3 inhibitors. This analysis identified 2,6,9-trisubstituted purine scaffolds [89] as a promising choice of structural scaffold for projecting functionality into the three corners of the most important SH2-domain subpocket A, which contains the key pTyr705-binding residues and is composed of the polar residues Lys591, Ser611, Ser613 and Arg609 [90]. Select purine scaffolds, e.g. S3I-V3-31, S3I-V3-32, S3I-V3-33, S3I-V3-34, and S3I-V4-01, showed good affinities (K_D, 0.8 – 12 μM) for purified, non-phosphorylated STAT3, inhibited STAT3 DNA-binding (IC_{50} = 27 – 84 μM) and intracellular phosphorylation (IC_{50} = 20 – 60 μM) and suppressed growth of transformed cells (IC_{50} = 41 – 80 μM) with increased constitutive STAT3 activity [89]. Recently, another S3I-201 analog, S3I-1757, was described that was capable of inhibiting STAT3-pYpeptide binding (IC_{50} = 13 μM); however, it had only modest potency for decreasing levels of nuclear pY-STAT3 and STAT3-DNA binding ($IC_{50} \geq$ 50 μM) [86].

A library of BP-1-102 analogues containing prodrugs, potential bioisosterses, and salicylic acid mimics was screened for anti-STAT3 and blood-brain barrier permeability properties, which identified 4 inhibitors—SH4-54, SH5-07, SH5-19, and SH5-23. Each had nanomolar IC_{50}s for inhibiting STAT3 binding to pY-peptide [91]. Of these, SH4-54, in which the hydroxyl substituent of the salicyclic acid moiety of BP-1-102 was removed and replaced with hydrogen [91], bound most strongly to STAT3 (K_D = 300 nM). SH4-54 also reduced levels of pY-STAT3 and its downstream transcriptional targets at low nM concentrations and potently targeted glioblastoma brain cancer stem cells (IC_{50} = 0.07–0.2 μM). SH-4-54 crossed the blood–brain barrier, reduced pY-STAT3 levels, and controlled glioma tumor growth *in vivo*. In a more recent study, SH4-54 and SH5-07 were tested in gliomas and breast cancer cells [92]. They were found to have increased ability to inhibit STAT3

DNA binding activity compared to BP-1-102 (IC_{50}=3.9 and 4.7 μM, respectively) and inhibited DNA-binding in cells at 1–3 μM; however, their ability to reduce levels of pY-STAT3 in cells was much less pronounced (significant reduction not observed below 10 μM) and did not correlate with the ability to block DNA-binding and/or STAT3-regulated gene expression. This lack of correlation within the context of constitutively-active STAT3 was explained by suggesting that disruption of pre-existing STAT3:STAT3 dimers, which directly leads to lower DNA-binding activity, has a non-linear relationship with the turnover of disrupted pY-STAT3 molecules and by suggesting that SH4-54 and SH5-07 could act by binding directly to the STAT3 DBD [92]. In fact NMR data showed that these compounds bind to both SH2 domain and DBD of STAT3, in the later case, most probably to a hydrophobic pocket formed by residues Leu411, Ile386, and Ile439 [92].

Using computer-based ligand screening, our group docked 920,000 compounds from 8 chemical libraries into the p-Y-peptide pocket within the STAT3 SH2 domain and identified three hits, C3, C30, and C188 [93]. C188 demonstrated the greatest activity of the three [93–95] and inhibited STAT3-pY-peptide binding in an SPR-based assay (IC_{50}=7.5–20 μM; calculated K_i=37.3 nM), inhibited G-CSF-stimulated increased pY-STAT3 levels in Kasumi-1 cells (IC_{50}=16.2 μM) and induced apoptosis in pY-STAT3-high breast cancer cells (ED_{50}=0.7–3.9 μM) [93, 94, 96]. Hit-to-lead strategies focused on C188 [93–96] led to C188-9, which demonstrated improved potency and was non-toxic and orally bioavailable [95–98]. C188-9 binds to STAT3 with high affinity (K_D=4.7±0.4 nM) in microscale thermophoresis assays and potently inhibited STAT3 binding to its pY-peptide ligand (IC_{50}=2.5 μM, SPR; K_i=12.4 nM), inhibited G-CSF-stimulated increased pY-STAT3 levels (IC_{50}=3.7 μM), and reduced constitutive pY-STAT3 levels ($IC_{50}\sim$4 nM) in A549 cells [99].

Shin et al. searched a library of natural compounds using a STAT3-luciferase assay and identified Cryptotanshinone as a STAT3 inhibitor. Cryptotanshinone is derived from the roots of *Salvia miltiorrhiza*, known as Bunge or Danshen. Cryptotanshinone reduced levels of pY-STAT3 in HCT 116 colon cancer cells (IC_{50}=4.6 μM) and in breast, prostate, and cervical cancer cell lines [100]. Cryptotanshinone inhibited growth of multiple cancer cell lines, including myeloma, glioma, NSCLC, colorectal, and pancreas (IC_{50}=5.8–15.1 μM) and induced cancer cell apoptosis [100–105]. It was also found to synergize with various drugs, including imatinib and cisplatin in several cancers [103, 106–109]. Binding studies suggested that cryptotanshinone directly interacted with the STAT3 SH2 domain of STAT3 to inhibit STAT3 phosphotyrosylation and prevent STAT3 dimerization and nuclear translocation [100].

Matsuno et al. [110] identified a *N*-[2-(1,3,4-oxadiazolyl)]-4 quinolinecarboxamide derivative, STX-0119, as a novel STAT3 dimerization inhibitor by virtual screening using a customized version of the DOCK4 program and the STAT3 crystal structure. The top 136 hits identified were examined in a STAT3-dependent luciferase reporter gene assay and a fluorescence resonance energy transfer-based STAT3 dimerization assay. STX-0119 inhibited STAT3-reporter activity (IC_{50}=74 μM), downregulated STAT3-regulated genes, and inhibited growth of multiple hematological cancers (IC_{50}=1.4–18.3 μM), as well as glioblastoma cell lines (IC$_{50}$ = 6.6–44.5 μM) but did not affect STAT3 phosphorylation [110–113]. A docking model of STX-0119 [110] bound to the STAT3-SH2 domain revealed that the 2-Ph ring of STX-0119 inserted into a hydrophobic cleft in proximity to the pY-peptide binding pocket. Oral administration of STX-0119 effectively abrogated the growth of human lymphoma and glioblastoma xenografts [112, 113].

In another program, 437 of 7000 compounds that docked to a region of a STAT3 distinct from STAT1 in a previous molecular dynamics simulation [114] were further screened on the basis of favorable binding parameters involving ligand buried surface area (>75 %), and van der Waals and hydrogen bond energies. This resulted in identification of 52 compounds that were tested for the ability to block STAT3 DNA binding by EMSA [79]. Of these 52 compounds, C36 was identified as the most potent hit (IC$_{50}$ = 30–50 μM). Subsequent library-screening using C36 as a template yielded another 48 structurally similar compounds. After further screening for STAT3 DNA binding inhibition and elimination of some leads because of low solubility, C48 emerged as the lead (IC$_{50}$ = 10–50 μM); it reduced constitutive pY-STAT3 levels, DNA binding, and transcription of STAT3 gene targets in breast cancer cells leading to growth inhibition and apoptosis of C3L5 murine breast cancer tumors in a syngeneic mouse model [79]. Site-directed mutagenesis and multiple biochemical experiments showed that C48 is a covalent modifier of STAT3 and alkylates Cys468, a residue at the DNA-binding interface.

Our group used a high-throughput fluorescence microscopy search to identify compounds in a drug-repositioning library (Prestwick library) that block ligand-induced nuclear translocation of STAT3 and identified piperlongumine (PL), a natural product isolated from the fruit of the pepper *Piper longum* [115]. PL inhibited STAT3 nuclear translocation (IC$_{50}$ = 0.9–1.7 μM), inhibited ligand-induced (IC$_{50}$ = 0.9–2.7 μM) and constitutive (IC$_{50}$ = 0.4–2.8 μM) STAT3 phosphotyrosylation, and modulated STAT3-regulated genes. SPR revealed that PL directly inhibited binding of STAT3 to its pY-peptide ligand (Ki 68nM). PL inhibited anchorage-independent growth of multiple breast cancer cell lines with increased levels of pY-STAT3 or total STAT3 (IC$_{50}$ = 0.9–1.7 μM), and induced apoptosis. PL also inhibited mammosphere formation by cancer cells in patient-derived xenografts (PDX) and its anti-cancer activity was linked to its STAT3-inhibiting activity. PL was non-toxic in mice up to a dose of 30 mg/kg/day for 14 days and blocked growth of breast cancer cell line xenografts in nude mice.

SH2 inhibitors identified using fragment-based drug design (FBDD). Most of the above molecules resulted from high-throughput screens (HTS) based on rational design followed by lead optimization. Using biophysical methods like NMR and X-ray crystallography, fragment-based drug design (FBDD) has recently emerged as a successful alternative to HTS-based drug discovery [116–118]. Several groups have combined structural motifs of reported STAT3 inhibitors as part of a fragment-based drug design (FBDD) program to develop more potent STAT3 inhibitors. These and other FBDD STAT3 inhibitor programs are described below.

The intention of one such program was to design peptidomimetics that would bind to the pTyr705-binding site and a side pocket within the STAT3 SH2 domain. A urea linker was used to form H-bonds with residues between the two sites, which are rich in

H-bond acceptors and donors. Ten compounds were designed and XZH-5 emerged as the most promising. The features of XZH-5 were: (i) a carboxylate group that mimics the pTyr705 phosphate group; (ii) a fluorobenzene group able to form hydrophobic interactions with the side pocket; and (iii) a combination of urea and peptidyl linkers that spanned the right distance and were capable of forming H-bonds. XZH-5 was shown in a docking model to bind to the SH2 domain of STAT3 and prevent STAT3 phosphorylation at Tyr705, leading to inhibition of downstream STAT3 activities and apoptosis in multiple cancer cell lines including breast, pancreatic, hepatocellular and rhabdomyosarcoma ($IC_{50} \approx 15$–$50\ \mu M$) [119–121].

Li et al. used a novel approach combining Multiple Ligand Simultaneous Docking (MLSD), drug scaffolds, and drug repositioning to find potent STAT3 inhibitors. Briefly, their approach consisted of: (i) building a small library of drug scaffolds for the binding hot spots within the STAT3 SH2 domain; (ii) MLSD screening of privileged drug scaffolds to identify optimal fragment combinations; (iii) linking of the fragment hits to generate possible hit compounds as templates; and (iv) similarity searches of template compounds in drug databases [122] to identify existing drugs as possible inhibitors of STAT3. The above process successfully identified two synthetic compounds T2 and T3 and the repositioning search yielded celecoxib. Each reduced the growth of HCT-116 ($IC_{50} = 9.0$, 10.1 or 43.3 μM, respectively). Further lead optimization produced 5 analogues [123] that were more potent in inhibiting cancer cell line growth ($IC_{50} = 6.5\ \mu M$ for a breast cancer cell line; 7.6 μM for pancreatic cancer cell lines).

Niclosamide, an FDA-approved anticestodal drug with a very low bioavailability in humans, was identified to inhibit STAT3 activation, nuclear translocation and transactivation [124]. FBDD based on the structure of niclosamide and other STAT3 inhibitors yielded a series of orally bioavailable STAT3 inhibitors including HJC0152 and HJC0123 [125, 126]. HJC0123 inhibited STAT3 activation and promoter activity, growth of breast and pancreatic cancer cell lines *in vitro* ($IC_{50} = 0.1$–1.2 μM) and MDA-MB-231 xenografts [125] and also potentiated doxorubicin- and gemcitabine-mediated killing [119].

More recently Yu et al. developed another STAT3 dimerization inhibitor by utilizing FBDD. They linked the naphthalene-5,8-dione-1-sulphoneamide fragment of LLL-12 (thought to bind to the pTyr705-binding pocket within the STAT3 SH2 domain) to a dimethyl amine that contained various R groups and generated 5 different compounds. LY5, the most potent compound, inhibited growth of U2OS and RD2 cancer cells ($IC_{50} = 0.5$–1.39 μM) better than parent compound LLL-12; it also was easy to synthesize and possessed more drug-like properties than LLL-12 [127].

5.3.5   Inhibitors Targeting the STAT3 DNA-Binding Domain (DBD)

Recognition of specific DNA elements is one of the cardinal features of transcription factors (TFs). The DBD of STAT3 is known to bind two types of DNA elements within promoter sites to mediate its transcriptional activities — serum-inducible elements (SIE) and gamma-activated sequences (GAS) [22, 128]. Concerted efforts at blocking this interaction have been underway for some time. The following sections describe these efforts (Table 5.3).

5.3.5.1 Decoy Oligonucleotides

Decoy oligonucleotides are double-stranded or duplex DNAs that mimic TF promoter elements. Their use was first described by Bielinska et al. in 1990 as a way of modulating gene transcriptional activity in the cell [129]. Duplex ODNs act by competitively inhibiting TF binding to their endogenous promoter elements. This strategy has been used to target aberrant TF signaling in various diseases and currently represents an active area of research [130, 131]. Following successful demonstration of STAT6 inhibition using this method [132], Leong et al. reported the use of a 15-mer duplex ODN modeled on the c-fos promoter sequence (SIE) to target STAT3 [133]. They demonstrated reduction in STAT3 mediated gene expression that led to growth inhibition of head and neck cancer cells. Other researchers also have shown similar results with other STAT3-associated cancers including, ovarian cancer, glioma, prostate cancer and hepatocellular carcinoma. [134–138]. Although duplex ODNs appeared to have minimal toxicity in primate models [139], instability in plasma was a limitation to their *in vivo* efficacy. To overcome these limitations, the Grandis lab developed a cyclic STAT3 decoy ODN linked to hexa–ethylene glycol. This ODN showed improved stability and retained antitumor efficacy with minimal toxicity when administered intravenously in a preclinical head and neck cancer models [140]. Creating a peptide nucleic acid (PNA) by adding a novel cell-penetrating peptide (CPP) consisting of a glutamate peptide linked to the N-terminus of the nuclear localization signal (NLS) from Oct6 transcription factor, to the minimal 15-mer linear ODN 13410A (Glu-Oct6-13410A) required for inducing cell apoptosis [137, 141] showed better cell-uptake and better apoptosis inducing capacity [141].

5.3.5.2 G-Quartet Oligonucleotides

G-quartet oligonucleotides (GQ-ODN) constitute another approach that is mechanistically analogous to ODNs in inhibiting the transcriptional activity of STAT3. G-quartets oligonucleotides are random coils outside the cell that complex with K^+ ions within the cell form stable box-like structures composed of stacks of 4 G-bases that are hydrogen bonded via hoogensteen pairings [142]. These structures are normally found in telomeres and promoter regions of many genes. G-Quartets are known to associate with DNA binding proteins [143], thus, making them ideal candidates to be used for targeting DNA binding activity of TFs. In 2003, Jing et al. developed a GQ-ODN, that inhibited IL-6 induced DNA binding activity of STAT3 and suppressed expression of STAT3 mediated genes [144]. Subsequent work showed that GQ-ODNs inhibited proliferation in a wide variety of tumor cell lines, including prostrate, breast, head and neck, non-small cell lung cancer, and T-cell leukemia with IC_{50}s ranging from 5 to 7 μM [145, 146]. Although initial studies predicted that GQ-ODN destabilized dimer formation, the mechanism by which GQ-ODN disrupt and abrogate STAT3 activity remains unclear since subsequent work appeared to show that the GQ-ODN inhibited STAT3 transcriptional activity by preferentially binding to its DNA binding domain rather than the SH2 domain [147]. Nevertheless, it is clear that they show promise as targeted anti-cancer agents. GQ-ODN have not garnered as much interest as small molecules, perhaps due not having properties suitable for systemic delivery. However, this may change as novel nucleic acid delivery systems currently being developed based upon siRNA therapeutics are employed [148].

5.3.5.3 Platinum-Based Inhibitors

The antitumor effects of most platinum compounds are thought to result from their ability to combine with DNA and form complexes that are toxic to cells. In contrast, platinum IV compounds—CPA-1, CPA-7, and platinum (IV) tetra-chloride, were shown to inhibit STAT3 DNA binding activity in an EMSA assay [149]. Importantly, IS3 295, a member of the same group identified from a screen of the NCI 2000 diversity set of compounds, was reported to bind STAT3 and prevent its interaction with specific DNA response elements in a dose dependent manner with an IC_{50} of 1.4 μM [150]. All platinum IV compounds mentioned here preferentially inhibit STAT3 and to some extend STAT1 DNA binding, but showed no activity against STAT5 DNA binding, reducing the possibility that this is a nonspecific DNA targeting effect. The compound suppressed STAT3 dependent gene activation and showed antiproliferative effects against v-Src transformed fibroblast and a variety of breast cancer cells. Of note, CPA-7 also was recently shown to be effective against both gliomas and melanomas in mouse tumor models [151]. Biochemical data also suggests that inhibition of DNA binding by IS3 295 is irreversible, which is not surprising because platinum compounds are known to react with thiol groups [152]. The fact that IS3 295 is selective for STAT3 over STAT5 suggests that covalent modification involves a unique site within STAT3 to which the compounds first binds non-covalently prior to crosslinking. It is important to note that this kind of selectivity implies a "hotspot" within the DNA binding domain [153]. It would therefore be interesting to pinpoint the reactive thiol groups at the DNA interface. This could yield important information that would help drive the development of other compounds directed at STAT3 DNA binding. It remains to be seen what proteins other than STAT3 this class of compounds also targets in order to better assess the possibility of unacceptable levels of off-target effects.

5.3.5.4 Small Molecule Targeting

In contrast to the SH2 binding domain, which presents a well-defined pY binding site that is amenable to targeted small-molecule inhibition, the DNA binding domain has historically been considered challenging, partly due to the belief that disrupting DNA binding would not achieve the desired level of selectivity necessary to discriminate among TFs. In addition, protein DNA interactions of TFs were conventionally deemed undruggable due to the lack of obvious targetable pockets within their binding interfaces. Using high quality structural data of the DBD of STAT3 [43], Huang et al. applied an improved virtual ligand screen to identify a small molecule called InS3-54 (4-[(3E)-3-[(4-nitrophenyl)-methylidene]-2-oxo-5-phenylpyrrol-1-yl] benzoic acid) that non-covalently binds to the DBD of STAT3, thereby competitively inhibiting its DNA-binding activity [154]. To ensure selectivity towards STAT3, top scoring molecules from the initial screen were docked on to the DBD of STAT1. InS3-54 was selected as the most selective compounds that had the ability to inhibit STAT3 dependent gene expression in a luciferase reporter assay. In addition, InS3-54 was demonstrated to inhibit DNA binding of pY-STAT3 dimer ($IC_{50} = 20$ μM) by non-covalently binding to the DBD of STAT3. Although efficacious in inhibiting proliferation of various cancer cell lines, the IC_{50} (<6 μM) was markedly lower than that for its inhibition of DNA binding, which suggested the possibility of off-target effects. To address this issue, Zhan's group made further activity guided hit-to-lead optimizations that resulted in InS3-54A18, a compound that showed improved IC_{50} for growth inhibition, better specificity, and more favorable pharmacological properties [155]. When orally administered, inS3-54A18 effectively inhibited STAT3 activity in mice leading to a reduction in lung xenograft tumor growth.

Another example of a small molecule presumed to work by the directly targeting the STAT3 DBD is a synthetic analog of curcumin, HO-3867, that has been shown to inhibit DNA binding activity in an ELISA assay [156]. HO-3867 inhibited STAT3 transcriptional activity, was preferentially active in a dose dependent manner in inhibiting growth of cancer vs. normal cell lines, and inhibited xenograft tumor growth. However, this compound appears to have minimal selectivity and was shown to inhibit upstream kinases [157, 158]. To advance further, the specificity of HO-3867 likely will need to be improved.

Galiellalactone, a fungal metabolite from the ascomycete, *Galiella rufa*, inhibited the IL-6/STAT3 signaling pathway [159, 160]. Galiellalactone inhibited STAT3-mediated luciferase induction ($IC_{50} \sim 5$ μM), reduced STAT3-regulated gene induction, and blocked the growth of various cancer cell lines e.g. DU145, *in vitro* ($IC_{50} = 3.4$ μM) and *in vivo* [160–162]. Galiellalactone did not prevent dimerization of the STAT3 monomers and showed no significant inhibition of phosphorylation; it appears to mediate its STAT3 inhibitory effect by covalently modifying residues Cys-367, Cys-468, and Cys-542 in the DBD and directly blocking the binding of STAT3 to DNA [162].

5.3.5.5 Peptides and Aptamers

Like STAT3 SH2-directed aptamers, DBD-directed peptide aptamer DBD-1 and its protein transduction domain (PTD)-fused analog, DBD-1-9R could also target STAT3 and reduce growth of STAT3-dependent cells [163].

5.3.6 Inhibitors Targeting the STAT3 N-Terminal Domain

Although tyrosine phosphorylation precedes STAT3 activation, it has been shown that even nonphosphorylated STAT3 contributes to carcinogenesis through regulation of gene expression [164–166]. In addition, protein–protein interactions between STAT3 and other transcription factors also can affect the repertoire of transcribed genes and contribute to tumorigenesis [167]. The N-terminal domain mediates protein–protein interactions during binding of STAT3 dimers to DNA and in the assembly of the transcriptional machinery, including the interactions between two STAT3 dimers to form a tetramer, as well as with other transcriptional factors and regulators [43, 168, 169]. The N-terminal domain interaction with other transcription factors/cofactors leads to formation of enchanceosomes [170] and its interaction with histone-modifier proteins induces changes in chromatin structure [171]. These complex interactions together maximize STAT3-dependent transcriptional control in normal and cancer cells [167]. Moreover, the NTD also has been implicated in the interaction of STAT3 with peptide hormone receptors and the nuclear translocation of STAT3 [172–174]. Short peptides (Table 5.3) derived from helices within the N-terminal domain, especially helix-2 (ST3-H2A2), recognized and bound to STAT3, but not to other STAT members, and inhibited STAT3 transcriptional activity without affecting levels of pY-STAT3 [169, 175, 176]. The cell-permeable form of this peptide (Hel2K-Pen), generated by its fusion with Penetratin (a protein transduction motif with sequence RQIKIWFPNRR-Nle-KWKK-NH2), selectively induced cell growth inhibition and apoptosis of human MDA-MB-231, MDA-MB-435, and MCF-7 breast cancer cells (IC$_{50}$~10 μM) through robust induction of pro-apoptotic genes, as a result of altered STAT3 chromatin binding [175–177]. Issues of peptide stability and bioavailability still remain major challenges to be overcome for this unique approach to STAT3 inhibition to advance.

5.3.7 Inhibitors that Target Endogenous STAT3 Negative Regulators

In normal cells, the level and duration of STAT3 activation is controlled by a variety of mechanisms including dephosphorylation of receptor complexes and nuclear STAT3 dimers by protein phosphatases (PTPases), interaction of activated STAT3 with members of the protein inhibitors of activated STAT (PIAS) family, and the actions of suppressor of cytokine signaling (SOCS) protein members that inhibit and/or degrade JAKs [178, 179]. Many different STAT3 inhibitors seem to work through modulating the activity of these endogenous regulators (Table 5.4).

Several protein tyrosine phosphatases, including members of the Src homology 2 (SH2)-domain containing tyrosine phosphatase family (SHP-1 and SHP-2) and protein tyrosine phosphatase 1B (PTP-1B) [180–182] can deactivate STAT3 signaling through direct dephosphorylation of pY-STAT3, thus, are useful targets [183]. In many cancer cells, loss of regulation by these, lead to constitutive STAT3 activation,

Table 5.4 Other STAT3 inhibitors with varying modes of action

Inhibitors	Type	Description	Blocks	IC50 STAT3 inhibition (assay)	IC50 cell growth inhibition, cell	Pre-clinical animal models	Ref
Endogenous STAT3 inhibitor modulators							
AdCN305-cppSOCS3	RV	Recombinant adenovirus encoding SOCS3	pY, DM, DB, GT	NA	NA	5×10^8 PFU/dose, alternate day$\times$4, SW620, BEL7404 xenografts	[206, 207]
Calyculin A	SM	PP2A inhibitor, increases pS-STAT3, decreases pY-STAT3	pY, GT	80 nM^E, constitutive pSTAT3, T lymphoma	NA	NA	[208–210]
SC-1/SC-43/SC-49	SM	Increases SHP1 activity to reduce pSTAT3	pY, DM, DB, GT	1–5^E µM, constitutive pSTAT3, HCC and breast cancer cells	2–5^E µM, HCC and breast cancer cells	10 mg/kg, 28d, PO, MDA-MB-468 xenografts	[186, 188, 189]
TPA	SM	Phorbol ester, activates PKC-regulated phosphatase and inhibits pSTAT3	pY, DM, DB, GT	NA	NA	NA	[211]
PF4 (Platelet Factor 4)	CK	Angiostatic cytokine upregulates SOCS3 and inhibits pSTAT3	pY, DB, GT	NA	NA	200 ng, 3/wk, 6 wks, IV, OPM2 xenografts in nude mice	[449, 450]
Nucleotide based inhibitors							
Anti-Sense (AZD9150) (70, NCT01839604)	ASO	16 oligonucleotide antisense molecule (ASO) targeting the 3′ untranslated part of STAT3	pY, DM, DB, GT	0.011 µM, STAT3 mRNA A431	0.05 µM, A431	25 mg/kg, A431 xenografts	[293]
CTLA4apt-STAT3 siRNA	AP-ASO	CTLA4apt fused to a STAT3-targeting siRNA, internalized into tumor-associated CD8+ T cells and silencing of STAT3	NA	0.5 nM, STAT3 mRNA in CD8 T cells	NA	782.5 pmol/dose/mouse, IV, melanoma, RCC, lymphoma colon carcinoma xenografts	[225]

(continued)

Table 5.4 (continued)

Inhibitors	Type	Description	Blocks	IC50 STAT3 inhibition (assay)	IC50 cell growth inhibition, cell	Pre-clinical animal models	Ref
Other inhibitors with novel mechanism							
Capsaicin, N-vanillyl-8-methyl-1--nonenamide	SM	Hot-pepper ingredient blcoks IL6-stimulated pSTAT3 by translational inhibition of gp130	pY, DM, DB, GT	−5–7^E μM, const pSTAT3, U266	0.05 μM, A431	1 mg/kg, 3/wk, IP, U266 xenografts	[232, 235, 451]
PF4 (Platelet Factor 4)	CK	Angiostatic cytokine upregulates SOCS3 and inhibits pSTAT3	pY, DB, GT	~4^E μM, const pSTAT3, OPM2, U266	2–4 μM, OPM2, NCI-H929 and U266, growth, MTT	200 ng, 3/wk, 6 wks, IV, OPM2 xenografts in nude mice	[449, 450]
ML116	SM	Novel inhibitor (PubChem CID-2100018) belongs to the thienopyrimidine scaffold	DM, DB, GT	4.2 μM, IL6-stimulated STAT3 luciferase assay	0.8–33.1 μM, glioma cells	15 mg/kg, IP, intracranial GL26 xenografts	[452]

Note: Information for Pre-clinical animal models consist of Dose, route of administration, duration (if available) and animal model used. Information for Pre-clinical animal models consist of Dose, route of administration, duration (if available) and animal model used

Abbreviations: *E* estimated from descriptive data on inhibition, from corresponding reference, *NA* not available, *Ab* antibody, *SM* small molecule, *pY* STAT3 phosphorylation at Tyr-705, *DM* dimerization, *NT* nuclear translocation, *DB* DNA-binding, *GT* gene transcription, *IG* intra-gastrical, *TK* tyrosine kinase, *IC* intra-cranial, *PO* per Os (by mouth), *CK* cytokine, *IP* intra-peritoneal, *AP* aptamer, *ASO* anti-sense oligonucleotide, *RV* recombinant virus

e.g. loss of SHP-1 enhances JAK3/STAT3 signaling in ALK-positive anaplastic large-cell lymphoma and in cutaneous T cell lymphoma [184, 185]. Many chemical agents also appear to up regulate SHP-1 activity/expression. As shown in Table 5.4, sorafenib derivatives lacking Raf-1 kinase activity, e.g. SC-1, SC-43, and SC-49 [186–189], appear to reduce levels of constitutive pY-STAT3 ($IC_{50}=1$–5 μM) by upregulation of SHP1 leading to inhibition of cancer cell growth *in vitro* ($IC_{50}=2$–5 μM) and inhibition of xenografts growth in mice. Many other known JAK/STAT3 inhibitors e.g. betulinic acid [190], guggulsterone [191], 5-azacytidine [192], SC-2001 [193], sorafenib [194], beta-caryophyllene [195], boswellic acid [196], capillarisin [197]. Honokiol [198], dovitinib [199], 1′-acetoxychavicol [200], gambogic acid [201], dihydroxypentamethoxyflavone [202], butein [203], icariside II (a flavonoid icariin derivative) [204] and 5-hydroxy-2-methyl-1,4-naphthoquinone (a vitamin K3 analogue) [205] can enhance the SHP-1 pathway (either by induction of SHP-1 expression or by increase of SHP-1 activity) and show anti-cancer potential.

Adenovirus mediated transduction of the SOCS3 gene also can reduce levels of pY-STAT3 and thereby reduce SW620 and BEL704 xenograft growth [206, 207]. Other known negative STAT3-regulators also could be modulated in a similar way to reduce STAT3 activity.

Woetmann et al. [208] showed that calyculin A, an inhibitor of serine phosphatases and the protein phosphatases (PPs) PP1yPP2A, induces (i) phosphorylation of STAT3 on serine and threonine residues, (ii) inhibition of STAT3 tyrosine phosphorylation and DNA binding activity, and (iii) relocation of STAT3 from the nucleus to the cytoplasm. Similar results were obtained with other PP2A inhibitors (okadaic acid and endothall thioanhydride) but not with inhibitors of PP1 (tautomycin) or PP2B (cyclosporine). There are other reports of a similar inhibition of STAT3 activity by calyculin A [209, 210] but observations with some of the other PP2A inhibitors [209] could not be repeated.

STAT3 activity is, in part, positively regulated by c-Src and negatively regulated by a PKC-activated PTPase(s) in melanoma cells. The tumor-promoting phorbol ester 12-O-tetradecanoylphorbol-13-acetate (TPA) was shown to inhibit melanoma cell growth by suppression of STAT3 activity through upregulation of PTPase(s) and upregulation of PKC [211], which led to a decrease in STAT3 DNA-binding, STAT3 target gene transcription, and inhibition of growth of melanoma cells [211].

5.3.8 Inhibitors with Other Mechanisms of Action

There are numerous examples of agents (Table 5.4) that inhibit STAT3 activity/oncogenic function, that do not necessarily belong to any of the above groups of indirect or direct STAT3-interacting compounds. These will be discussed in this section.

5.3.8.1 siRNA-Based Inhibitors

Apart from the ODNs, which block the ability of STAT3 DBD to bind the STAT3-responsive sequence containing DNA, there also have been concerted efforts at targeting STAT3 mRNA using siRNA and shRNA based methods as outlined below.

Anti-sense therapy. Many antisense oligonucleotide (ASO)-based drugs, which bind to messenger RNA (mRNAs) and inhibit the production of disease-causing proteins, are at various phases of clinical trials. An ASO complementary to apolipoprotein B-100 mRNA, mipomersen sodium (Kynamro), received FDA approval in January 2013 as an adjunct to statin-based lipid lowering therapy [212, 213]. AZD9150 (ISIS-STAT3Rx or ISIS 481464) is a synthetic ASO against STAT3. Information about its pre-clinical development is scant but its testing in clinical trials is summarized below. RNA interference (RNAi) is a natural post-transcriptional gene-silencing (PTGS) mechanism for silencing unwanted genes. The process is initiated by the presence of double-stranded RNA, not a constituent of the normal cell cytoplasm. The dsRNAs are cleaved by dicer, an endonuclease, into 20–25 nucleotide dsRNAs, referred to as short or small interfering RNAs (siRNAs). The RNA-induced silencing complex (RISC) separates the two strands, and one of these strands then serves as a guide for sequence-specific degradation of complementary mRNA. The utility of this approach is limited due to the short half-life of transfected RNAs. This problem can be circumvented using a DNA-directed RNA interference technique in which a short hairpin RNA (shRNA, a double stranded RNA) is expressed in the cell after insertion of a DNA construct into the nucleus. These shRNAs then enter the RNAi pathway and gene silencing can last for as long as the cell continues to produce the shRNA [214, 215]. This strategy is under evaluation in several clinical trials for the treatment of several diseases including cancers (#NCT01591356, #NCT00363714, #NCT00689065, #NCT00938574). However, data regarding siRNA targeted silencing of STAT genes for cancer therapy are limited to *in vitro* studies and *in vivo* studies of animal models only [216–224].

Intracellular therapeutic targets that define tumor immunosuppression in both tumor cells and T cells remain intractable [225]. Administration of a covalently linked siRNA to an aptamer (apt) that selectively binds cytotoxic T lymphocyte-associated antigen 4 [CTLA4(apt)] allowed gene silencing in exhausted CD8+ T cells and Tregs in tumors as well as CTLA4-expressing malignant T cells [225]. CTLA4(apt) fused to a STAT3-targeting siRNA [CTLA4(apt)-STAT3 siRNA] resulted in internalization into tumor-associated CD8+ T cells overexpressing CTLA-4 [226] and silencing of STAT3, which activated tumor antigen-specific T cells in murine models [225]. Both local and systemic administration of CTLA4(apt)-STAT3 siRNA dramatically reduced tumor-associated Tregs and potently inhibited tumor growth and metastasis in various mouse tumor models [225].

5.3.8.2 Inhibitors Targeting Nuclear Translocation

The role of activated STAT3 as a DNA-binding transcription factor relies on the ability of homodimers to traffic from the cytoplasm to the nucleus [178, 227–231]. Preventing this shuttle of STAT3 dimers could be a way to block STAT3 activity [229]. Importins $\alpha 3$, $\alpha 5$, $\alpha 7$, and β, are involved in passage of STAT3 through the nuclear pore [26, 229]. Once within the nucleus, TC45 dephosphorylates pY-STAT3, which then becomes a substrate for exportin-1–mediated export [229]. Inhibition of exportin 1 by leptomycin B or ratjadone A, has been shown to interfere with nuclear export of STAT3; it reduces pY-STAT3 and STAT3-mediated transcription and causes cells to undergo apoptosis [229]. Although interesting, any small-molecule that inhibits general trafficking across the nuclear membrane is likely to be toxic [229]. Whether an inhibitor of nuclear pore transit can be developed with sufficient STAT3 selectivity remains to be determined.

5.3.8.3 Inhibitor with Novel Modes of Action

There are a few inhibitors, which have very novel mechanisms of action, mostly by way of modulating proteins or pathways indirectly regulating the STAT3 signaling pathway (Table 5.4). E.g. capsaicin has been shown to have anti-carcinogenic effects on various tumor cells through multiple mechanisms including STAT3 inhibition [232–234]. Lee et al. showed that capsaicin treatment of glial tumors induced downregulation of the IL-6 receptor gp130 by translation inhibition, and was associated with activation of endoplasmic reticulum (ER) stress [235]. The depletion of the intracellular pool of gp130 by capsaicin combined with the ER stress inducer led to an immediate loss of the IL-6 response due to short half-life of membrane-localized gp130 [235].

Platelet factor 4 (PF4) is an angiostatic chemokine that suppresses tumor growth and metastasis and is frequently lost in multiple myeloma. Exogenous PF4 treatment not only suppressed myeloma-associated angiogenesis, but also inhibited growth and induced apoptosis in myeloma cells. It has been shown that PF4 negatively regulated STAT3 by inhibiting its phosphorylation and transcriptional activity. Overexpression of constitutively activated STAT3 could rescue PF4-induced apoptotic effects. Furthermore, PF4 induced the expression of SOCS3, an endogenous STAT3 inhibitor, and gene silencing of SOCS3 abolished its ability to inhibit STAT3 activation, suggesting a critical role of SOCS3 in PF4-induced STAT3 inhibition.

5.3.8.4 Other Inhibitors that May Act by Targeting STAT3

There are numerous reports of various compounds, most naturally occurring, that are known to exert powerful anti-tumor effects, through their action on STAT3. However, the mechanistic basis for their anti-STAT3 action is unknown. Some examples are protoepigenone/RY10-4 [236], shikonin [237], paclitaxel [238–240], vinrelbin [238–240], nifuroxazide [241], icaritin [242–245], and epigallocatechin-3 [246]. These are potent inhibitors that can reduce STAT3 activation and induce growth inhibition and/or apoptosis and in many cases have been proven, in pre-clinical animal models to reduce tumor growth. Further studies are necessary to elucidate their exact mechanism of action.

In considering this group of compounds, as well as others listed above, it is important to recall that proteases play an important role in STAT3 biochemistry, including its posttranslational modulation [247, 248] and degradation. STAT3 pro-teases include caspases, calpain, and the proteasome complex. Many compounds induce cell cycle arrest and apoptosis accompanied by reduced pY-STAT3 levels. It is frequently concluded that these compounds target STAT3 but the precise mecha-nism of STAT3 targeting is not determined. A number of compounds proposed as STAT3 inhibitors exert their antitumor effects by promoting STAT3 protein degra-dation in cancer cells [249–251]. In addition, pY-STAT3 has been shown to undergo caspase-dependent proteolytic cleavage [252]. Because cysteine proteases, such as caspases and calpain, are well known intracellular effectors of apoptosis, the ability of some purported STAT3 inhibitors to reduce pY-STAT may not be due to direct targeting of STAT3, but rather a reflection of compound-induced apoptosis in which pY-STAT3 levels are reduced by effector proteases within the apoptosis pathway.

5.3.9 Allosteric Effects of STAT3 Inhibitors

Namanja et al. [253] found that pY-peptide interactions with the SH2 domain of STAT3 cause structural and dynamics changes in its LD and DBD. This inter-domain allosteric effect likely is mediated by the flexibility within the hydrophobic core of STAT3. In addition, a mutation (I568F) in the LD, identified in a patient with autosomal-dominant hyper IgE syndrome (AD-HIES) induced NMR chemical shift perturbations in the SH2 domain, the DBD and the CCD domain of STAT3, sug-gesting conformational changes in these domains mediated by a point mutation in a separate domain. Furthermore, they showed that the conformational changes in the SH2 domain seen in the mSTAT3 I568F mutant was accompanied by the reduced affinity of this mSTAT3 for pY-peptide. This effect may help explain the ability of some compounds that bind domains other than the SH2 domain to affect STAT3-pY-peptide binding. The recent paper by Mathew et al. [254] using a rhodium-(II)-catalyzed, proximity-driven modification approach identified the STAT3 coiled-coil domain (CCD) as a novel binding site for a newly described naphthalene sulfon-amide inhibitor, MM-206. Despite binding to the CCD, this compound reduces STAT3 binding to pY-peptide and has structural features of C188, previously shown to reduce STAT3 binding to pY-peptide [93, 94, 96], and BP-1-102, thought to bind to the STAT3 SH2 domain. Findings with MM-206 [254] and STAT3 proteins con-taining substitutions within the CCD, such as Asp170 [174], suggest that the CCD, like the LD, also may engage in interdomain allosteric effects. Based on these find-ings, one might need to reconsider notions about how STAT3 inhibitors demonstrated to bind to STAT3 and to reduce STAT3 activity actually mediate their effects and may change our approach to designing drugs to target this oncogene. The fact that selectivity and mechanisms of action of established STAT3 inhibitors continue to be revisited and clarified [255, 256] reinforces this concept.

5.4   Entry of STAT3 Inhibitors into the Clinic

Attempts to develop peptide inhibitors [25, 44, 45, 51, 257] that target the pY-peptide binding pocket within the STAT SH2 domain [45] quickly followed the elucidation of the crystal structure of STAT3β homodimer [43] and confirmation that STAT3 was an oncoprotein [8]. However, due to their lack of membrane permeability and stability, non-peptidic small molecule inhibitors of STAT3 moved to the forefront of this drug discovery area [61]. Although showing promising pre-clinical activity *in vivo*, many compounds in this category show activity in the medium-to-high micromolar range, indicating the need for additional optimization before transitioning to clinical trials involving systemic administration. STA-21 has completed phase I/II trials in patients with psoriasis [258] with effective concentrations being achieved at affected skin sites through topical application. Several agents that systemically target the IL-6R/JAK/STAT3 signaling pathway are at various stages of clinical trials (Table 5.5) for a cancer indication. STAT3 upstream antagonists include the IL-6-neutralizing MAb siltuximab [259], the IL6R-anatgonist MAb tocilizumab [260, 261], the JAK inhibitor ruxolitinib [262–268], AZD1480 [41, 269–272], OPB-31121 [273–278], fedratinib/SAR302503 [279–282], BSE-SFN [283], pacritinib/SB1518 [284, 285], and the dual JAK2/gp130 inhibitors WP1066 [286–290] and OPB-51602 [291]. Direct STAT3 inhibitors include the STAT3-decoys [292] and the STAT3-antisense oligonucleotide based inhibitor ISIS-STAT3Rx (AZD9150) [293]. The third group of compounds includes two re-purposed drugs that also inhibit STAT3—the antiparasitic drug pyrimethamine [283] and the HMG-CoA inhibitor Simvastatin [294–296].

The importance of the IL-6/JAK/STAT signaling pathway in many human malignancies has, in part, spurred development of several IL-6 and IL-6 receptor inhibitors for cancer treatment [297–299]. Siltuximab (CNTO 328), the chimeric anti-IL-6 MAb has been approved by the FDA in 2014 for the treatment of patients with HIV-negative and HHV-8-negative multicentric Castleman's disease (MCD), a lymphoproliferative disorder with germinal center hyperplasia and high morbidity, at a dose of 11 mg/kg every 3 weeks [259, 300]. In a Phase I study, 18 of 23 patients (78%) had complete response, and 12 patients (52%) demonstrated objective tumor response [301]. In a Phase II study, with HIV-negative and HHV-8-seronegative patients with symptomatic MCD (n = 140), durable tumor and symptomatic responses occurred in 18 of 53 patients (34%) in the siltuximab group and none of 26 in the placebo group [302]. A Japanese Phase 1 trial [303] in multiple myeloma patients showed some responses, but in other studies the 11 mg/kg dose did not improve progression-free survival or achieve other measures of response [259]. Out of the 16

Table 5.5 STAT3 inhibitors at various stages of clinical trials

Inhibitor	Target	Indications	Phase	Goals/results	Ref
Siltuximab (CNTO-328)	IL6	Ovarian, pancreatic, colorectal, head and neck, and lung cancer, Castleman's disease, MM[c]	Phase I, Phase II	FDA-approved for Multicentric Castleman's disease (MCD), a lymphoproliferative disorder with germinal center hyperplasia	[259]
Tocilizumab	IL6R	KSHV-associated multi-centric Castleman's disease, MM (combined with allo-SCT), recurrent ovarian cancer (with chemo)	Phase 0, Phase I, Phase II	As both an anti-myeloma therapy and as a method to reduce GvHD, as chemo-sensitizer in recurrent ovarian cancer	[260, 261]
Ruxolitinib (INCB018424)	JAK1/2, STAT3	Chronic myeloproliferative disorders, leukemia, myelodysplastic syndrome, myeloproliferative neoplasms, unspecified childhood solid tumor, metastatic HER2+ BC, TNIBC (with pre-op chemo), HER2-BC (+ capecitabine)	Phase I, Phase II, Phase III	Encouraging results in myelofibrosis, decreasing not only disease symptoms but also JAK2 c.1849G>T (p.V617F) mutation burden. Toxicity remains an issue	[305]
AZD1480	JAK, STAT3	Metastatic cancer, pancreatic cancer, myeloproliferative diseases	Phase I	Pharmacodynamic analysis of circulating granulocytes demonstrated maximum phosphorylated STAT3 (pSTAT3) inhibition. Trial had to be eliminated because of toxicity	[41]
OPB-31121	JAK, STAT3	Advanced solid tumor, Hodgkin's lymphoma, non-Hodgkin's lymphoma, HCC	Phase I	Insufficient antitumor activity for HCC	[273]
Fedratinib (SAR302503)	JAK, STAT3	Advanced cancer, myelofibrosis	Phase I	Fedratinib treatment led to reduced STAT3 phosphorylation but no meaningful change in JAK2V617F allele burden in MF	[280, 282]
BSE-SFN	JAK2, STAT3	Atypical nevi	Phase 0	Evaluation of sulforaphane from Broccoli Sprout Extract (BSE-SFN) as a candidate natural chemopreventive agent able to modulate key steps in melanoma progression and STAT3 mediated gene transcription	[307, 308]
Pacritinib (SB1518)	JAK2, FLT3, STAT3/5	Myelofibrosis, AML (combined with decitabine/cytarabine)	Phase II	Active drug in myelofibrosis. Going in the AML patients for safety and efficacy as a STAT3 inhibitor in combination with decitabine/cytarabine	[284, 285]

WP1066	JAK2, gp130, STAT3	Advanced solid tumor, melanoma and recurrent glioblastoma	Phase I	Find the highest tolerable dose of WP1066 that can be given to patients with recurrent cancerous brain tumors or melanoma that has spread to the brain	[453, 454]
OPB-51602	JAK2, gp130, STAT3	Advanced solid tumor, glioblastoma multiforme, melanoma, relapsed/refractory hematological malignancies	Phase I	Recommended dose 4 mg, rapidly absorbed, accumulated with 4 weeks of treatments. No clear therapeutic response was observed in patients with relapsed/refractory hematological malignancies. Those with relapsed/refractory solid tumors, showed low pSTAT3 in PBMC	[291, 455]
STAT3 decoy	STAT3 DBD	HNSCC	Phase 0	Expression levels of STAT3 target genes were decreased in head and neck cancer patients following intra-tumoral injection	[292]
ISIS-STAT3Rx (AZD9150)	STAT3	Advanced metastatic HCC, Advanced cancer, malignant lymphoma, people with malignant ascites, adult subjects with diffuse large B-cell lymphoma, relapsed metastatic HNSCC (with MEDI4736)	Phase I/Phase Ib	AZD9150 (ISIS-STAT3Rx) showed single-agent antitumor activity in patients with highly treatment-refractory lymphoma and NSCLC	[293]
Pyrimethamine	STAT3	Relapsed chronic lymphocytic leukemia, small lymphocytic lymphoma	Phase I, Phase II	Phase I: to determine the maximum tolerated dose and recommended Phase II dose of pyrimethamine in relapsed CLL/SLL	[283]
Simvastatin	HMG-CoA, JAK2, STAT3, AKT, ERK	Refractory and/or relapsed solid or CNS tumors of childhood	Phase I	Define toxicity and evaluate cholesterol levels and IL-6/STAT3 pathway changes as biomarkers of patient response	[294–296]

E estimated from descriptive data on inhibition from corresponding reference, *NA* not available, *Ab* antibody, *SM* small molecule, *pY* STAT3 phosphorylation at Tyr-705, *DM* dimerization, *NT* nuclear translocation, *DB* DNA-binding, *GT* gene transcription

C indicates completed, *MM* Multiple Myeloma, *HNSCC* head and neck cell squamous cell carcinoma, *BC* breast cancer, *GvHD* Graft vs Host disease, *BSE-SFN* Brocholi Sprout Extract-sulforaphane

studies undertaken in various cancers with this agent, six have been completed, five are still ongoing, and five have been either terminated or withdrawn because of lack of efficacy. IL-6 signaling inhibition using the IL-6R monoclonal antibody, tocilizumab, has shown promising results in rheumatoid arthritis and related diseases in approximately 230 trials [304] and is being evaluated in patients with cancers, including multiple myeloma, both as an anti-myeloma therapy and as a method to reduce GvHD after allogeneic stem cell transplant (SCT), as well as in recurrent ovarian cancer as adjuvant with carboplatin/doxorubicin [260, 261]. Preliminary analysis of the ongoing trial shows that immune reconstitution was preserved in recipients of tocilizumab and there was a reduced incidence of grade 2–4 acute GvHD [261]. A completed phase I trial combining carboplatin/doxorubicin with tocilizumab and IFNα2b in patients with recurrent epithelial ovarian cancer (EOC) revealed that functional IL-6R blockade is feasible and safe in EOC patients treated with carboplatin/doxorubicin, using 8 mg/kg tocilizumab [260], and the combination was recommended for phase II evaluation based on immune parameters.

Approximately 50 trials with the JAK inhibitor, ruxolitinib, in many different cancer indications are underway and a few completed ones show some encouraging results in myelofibrosis [305], but toxicity remains an issue. In phase III clinical studies, ruxolitinib provided rapid and durable improvement of myelofibrosis-related splenomegaly and symptoms irrespective of mutation status, and was associated with a survival advantage compared with placebo or best available therapy. But because of dose-dependent cytopenias, blood count monitoring and dose titrations were recommended [266]. The JAK2 mutation (c.1849G>T; p.V617F) causes constitutive activation of Janus kinase (JAK)2 and dysregulated JAK signaling in myelofibrosis (MF), polycythemia vera (PV), and essential thrombocythemia (ET). Interestingly, in the phase III Controlled Myelofibrosis Study, patients with MF not only achieved significant reductions in splenomegaly and improvements in symptoms with ruxolitinib vs. placebo but 26/236 patients carrying the allele, also had their mutation burden lowered [306]; 20 achieved partial and 6 achieved complete molecular responses, with median times to response of 22.2 and 27.5 months [306]. The phase I study [41] with AZD1480, a JAK inhibitor, in 38 patients with advanced solid tumors, revealed rapid absorption and elimination with minimal accumulation after repeated daily or twice daily dosing. Pharmacodynamic analysis of circulating granulocytes demonstrated maximal reduction of pY-STAT3 within 1–2 h after dose, coincident with C_{max}, and greater reduction at higher doses. The average reduction in pY-STAT3 levels in granulocytes at the highest dose tested (70 mg daily), was 56% at steady-state drug levels. Dose-limiting toxicities (DLTs) included pleiotropic neurologic adverse events (AEs), like dizziness, anxiety, ataxia, memory loss, hallucinations, and behavior changes. The trial had to be stopped because of toxicity.

Another JAK inhibitor that showed the best potency in pre-clinical studies, OPB-31121 [274–276], demonstrated insufficient antitumor activity in patients with hepatocellular carcinoma (HCC) in a clinical trial [273]. In an open-label, dose-escalation, and pharmacokinetic study of OPB-31121 in subjects with advanced solid tumor observed that twice-daily administration of OPB-31121 was feasible up to doses of 300 mg. The pharmacokinetic profile, however, was unfavorable and no objective responses were observed [273]. A similar study in advanced HCC also came up with the same result [273]. Furthermore, peripheral nervous system-related toxicities were experienced, which may limit long-term administration of OPB-31121 [273].

A very recent interventional study will evaluate the effect of sulforaphane from broccoli sprout extract (BSE-SFN) as a candidate natural chemopreventive agent which is known to modulate key steps in melanoma progression and STAT3 mediated gene transcription [307, 308] in melanocytic and stromal elements of 18 melanoma patients with at least two atypical nevi of ≥ 4 mm diameter and those who have not received any form of systemic antineoplastic treatment for melanoma within the last year before recruitment, The primary outcomes that will be measured are (i) adverse events associated with oral sulforaphane, (ii) visual changes of atypical nevi size, border and color and (iii) the cellular changes.

Another new trial examines the safety and efficacy of the JAK2 inhibitor, pacritinib, for patients with AML in combination with either decitabine or cytarabine. Pacritinib has been shown to work through inhibition of STAT3 and STAT5 [284]. Pacritinib is an active agent in patients with myelofibrosis (MF), offering a potential treatment option for patients with preexisting anemia and thrombocytopenia. It demonstrated a favorable safety profile with promising efficacy in phase I studies in patients with primary and secondary MF. A subsequent multicenter phase II study demonstrated efficacy [285]. Out of 26 evaluable patients who either had clinical splenomegaly poorly controlled with standard therapies or were newly diagnosed with intermediate- or high-risk Lille score, 8 patients (31%) achieved a $\geq 35\%$ decrease in spleen volume (MRI) and 42% on the whole attained a $\geq 50\%$ reduction in spleen size by physical examination. Grade 1 or 2 diarrhea (69%) and nausea (49%) were the most common treatment-emergent adverse events. The study drug was discontinued in 9 patients (26%) due to adverse events (4 severe).

STAT3-decoy oligonucleotides (ODN) targeting the STAT3 DBD [292] and STAT3 siRNA based formulations [293] are the only direct STAT3 inhibitors that are in clinical trial for a cancer indication. Expression levels of STAT3 target genes were decreased in head and neck cancer patients following intratumoral injection with the STAT3 decoy compared with tumors receiving saline control in a phase 0 trial [292]. While intratumoral administration clearly shows target inhibition, it should be noted that there is no clear evidence that the same level of efficacy would be attained if the ODN were systemically administered. Therefore, it would be interesting to assess the effectiveness of this and the subsequent cyclic ODNs, on tumor STAT3 activity when delivered systemically in patients. Considering that effective and safe systemic intracellular delivery remains a challenge in this field it appears that there still remain some obstacles that have to be overcome before ODNs realize their full clinical potential as STAT3-targeting therapeutic agents.

STAT3 antisense based AZD9150 (ISIS-STAT3Rx) showed single-agent antitumor activity in patients with highly treatment-refractory lymphoma and NSCLC in a phase 1 dose escalation study. Of the 25 patients enrolled (12 advanced lymphoma; 7 with DLBCL, 2 Hodgkin's lymphoma, 2 follicular non-Hodgkin's lymphoma, 1 mantle cell lymphoma), 44% (11/25) achieved stable disease (SD) or a partial response (PR); three of six patients (50 %) with treatment-refractory DLBCL had evidence of tumor shrinkage and two patients (33 %) achieved a confirmed durable PR [293]. The only NSCLC patient evaluated showed evidence of near-complete resolution of highly treatment refractory NSCLC liver metastasis upon first restaging, with additional stabilization of mediastinal lymph nodes in response to AZD9150 treatment (3 mg/kg) [293]. The maximum tolerated dose (MTD) of AZD9150 was determined to be 3 mg/kg. A rapidly evolving thrombocytopenia (in the first month of dosing) was observed in two of nine patients at 4 mg/kg and was considered the dose-limiting toxicity (DLT). A more chronic slowly progressing thrombocytopenia also occurred after 4–6 months of dosing at 2 and 3 mg/kg (and for most patients at 4 mg/kg) and was effectively managed with pauses and dose frequency adjustments. The slowly progressing thrombocytopenia seen in patients at or below the MTD is consistent with the reported role of STAT3 in megakaryo-poiesis [309, 310], whereas the rapidly progressing thrombocytopenia seen above the MTD was of uncertain etiology. Other drug-related adverse events included aspartate aminotransferase (AST) elevation (44 %), alanine aminotransferase (ALT) elevation (44 %). Responses have also been seen in the DLBCL study. Dose escalation continues in the HCC study and knockdown of STAT3 in peripheral blood mononuclear cells (PBMCs) has been shown. IONIS-STAT3Rx, a variant of AZD9150 is also being examined for safety in patients with advanced cancers.

Tumor-induced STAT3 generates an immunosuppressive microenvironment and, therefore, has become a promising target for cancer therapy. Based on this premise, an ongoing clinical trial is investigating the effects of the antiparasitic drug, pyrimethamine, an inhibitor of STAT3 [283], in chronic lymphocytic leuke-mia (CLL) patients. Interestingly, pyrimethamine does not affect STAT3 phosphor-ylation [283] but does affect transcription of STAT3 gene targets.

Another re-purposed STAT3-inhibitor, simvastatin, an inhibitor of 3-hydroxy-3-methylglutaryl-coenzyme A (HMG-CoA) [294–296] is being tested in a phase I trial in combination with topotecan and cyclophosphamide for refractory and/or relapsed solid or CNS tumors of childhood. HMG-CoA reductase inhibitors, or "statins", lower LDL (low density lipoprotein) cholesterol by inhibiting cholesterol biosynthesis. Statins also have been found to decrease the incidence of cancer [311, 312]. Statins have been shown to inhibit IL-6 mediated STAT3 activation and pre-vent recruitment of pro-inflammatory cells to injured heart tissue [313].

In conclusion, most of the inhibitors in trial, which target STAT3 in various can-cer indications, belong to the upstream and repurposed inhibitors groups. None of the direct small-molecule STAT3 inhibitors under development has entered clinical trials. Since the pharmacokinetic properties of many of these are not well elabo-rated, it is difficult to comment on their preparedness to go to the clinics. The most promising in this regard is C188-9. Pharmacokinetic (PK) and toxicity studies in mice, rats, and dogs demonstrated that C188-9 provides excellent plasma exposures following oral administration and revealed no toxicity detectable by gross, microscopic or clinical laboratory evaluations when administered up to a dose of 100 mg/kg/day for 28 days in dogs, and up to a dose of 200 mg/kg/day for 28 days in rats [96]. Tumor PK studies of C188-9 in mice at 10 mg/kg demonstrated tumor levels twice those of plasma levels and nearly 3 times the IC_{50} for pSTAT3 inhibition [96]. C188-9 inhibits growth and survival of many types of cancer cells *in vitro*, including AML [95, 97], NSCLC [99], breast cancer (Dobrolecki et al. 2016, manuscript in preparation), and HNSCC [96] and inhibits the growth of NSCLC and HNSCC xenografts *in vivo* [96, 99].

5.5   Conclusion

Due to the essential contributions of STAT3 to virtually all the hallmarks of cancer, numerous approaches have been applied to identify molecules that effectively block STAT3 signaling to treat and/or prevent cancer, including peptidomimicry, *de novo* rational design, screening chemical libraries *in silico* and *in vitro*, and FBDD. Despite these efforts, few specific and selective STAT3 inhibitors with optimal anti-STAT3 activity have garnered the requisite pharmacokinetic and pharmacodynamic credentials to proceed to clinical trials. Some authors have stated that, unlike small enzymatic clefts, the STAT3:STAT3 dimer represents a protein-protein interaction that involves too large a surface area [86] to be effectively targeted by small, drug-like molecules [314]. These interaction surfaces and others involved in STAT3 protein-protein and protein-DNA interaction also are shallow and relatively featureless, as opposed to the well-defined binding pockets seen in enzyme active sites, thereby making the designing difficult [315]. In addition, the binding regions of STAT3 protein–protein or DNA–protein interactions are often non-contiguous, making mimicry of these domains difficult to accomplish for simple peptides or peptidomimetics [314]. Yet, several small-molecule STAT3 inhibitors are under development, which have good binding affinity for STAT3, potent STAT3 inhibitory activities, and a good safety profile. If these compounds fail to progress into drugs, efforts need to continue in this area of drug development as the impact of having an effective STAT3 inhibitor available in the clinic to treat and/or prevent many cancers will be substantial. Future strategies directed toward the identification of new small-molecule STAT3 probes should combine conventional screening-based strategies with FBDD and structural analytical tools, such as NMR analysis.

References

1. Darnell JEJ (2002) Transcription factors as targets for cancer therapy. Nat Rev Cancer 2(10):740–749
2. Banerjee K, Resat H (2015) Constitutive activation of STAT3 in breast cancer cells: a review. Int J Cancer 138(11):2570–2578
3. Vogt M, Domoszlai T, Kleshchanok D et al (2011) The role of the N-terminal domain in dimerization and nucleocytoplasmic shuttling of latent STAT3. J Cell Sci 124(Pt 6):900–909
4. Sriuranpong V, Park JT, Amornphimoltham P et al (2003) Epidermal growth factor receptor-independent constitutive activation of STAT3 in head and neck squamous cell carcinoma is

mediated by the autocrine/paracrine stimulation of the interleukin 6/gp130 cytokine system. Cancer Res 63(11):2948–2956

5. Ulaganathan VK, Sperl B, Rapp UR et al (2015) Germline variant FGFR4 p.G388R exposes a membrane-proximal STAT3 binding site. Nature 528(7583):570–574
6. Banerjee K, Resat H (2015) Constitutive activation of STAT3 in breast cancer cells: a review. Int J Cancer 138(11):2570–2578
7. Yuan J, Zhang F, Niu R (2015) Multiple regulation pathways and pivotal biological functions of STAT3 in cancer. Sci Rep 5:17663
8. Bromberg JF, Wrzeszczynska MH, Devgan G et al (1999) Stat3 as an oncogene. Cell 98(3):295–303
9. Gritsko T, Williams A, Turkson J et al (2006) Persistent activation of stat3 signaling induces survivin gene expression and confers resistance to apoptosis in human breast cancer cells. Clin Cancer Res 12(1):11–19
10. Doucette TA, Kong L-Y, Yang Y et al (2012) Signal transducer and activator of transcription 3 promotes angiogenesis and drives malignant progression in glioma. Neuro Oncol 14(9):1136–1145
11. Xiong H, Hong J, Du W et al (2012) Roles of STAT3 and ZEB1 proteins in E-cadherin down-regulation and human colorectal cancer epithelial–mesenchymal transition. J Biol Chem 287(8):5819–5832
12. Sherry MM, Reeves A, Wu JK et al (2009) STAT3 is required for proliferation and maintenance of multipotency in glioblastoma stem cells. Stem Cells 27(10):2383–2392
13. Yu H, Kortylewski M, Pardoll D (2007) Crosstalk between cancer and immune cells: role of STAT3 in the tumour microenvironment. Nat Rev Immunol 7(1):41–51
14. Kortylewski M, Kujawski M, Wang T et al (2005) Inhibiting Stat3 signaling in the hematopoietic system elicits multicomponent antitumor immunity. Nat Med 11(12):1314–1321
15. Nabarro S, Himoudi N, Papanastasiou A et al (2005) Coordinated oncogenic transformation and inhibition of host immune responses by the PAX3-FKHR fusion oncoprotein. J Exp Med 202(10):1399–1410
16. Marzec M, Zhang Q, Goradia A et al (2008) Oncogenic kinase NPM/ALK induces through STAT3 expression of immunosuppressive protein CD274 (PD-L1, B7-H1). Proc Natl Acad Sci U S A 105(52):20852–20857
17. Lee H-J, Zhuang G, Cao Y et al (2014) Drug resistance via feedback activation of Stat3 in oncogene-addicted cancer cells. Cancer Cell 26(2):207–221
18. Szakacs G, Paterson JK, Ludwig JA et al (2006) Targeting multidrug resistance in cancer. Nat Rev Drug Discov 5(3):219–234
19. Real PJ, Sierra A, De Juan A et al (2002) Resistance to chemotherapy via Stat3-dependent overexpression of Bcl-2 in metastatic breast cancer cells. Oncogene 21(50):7611–7618
20. Huang S, Chen M, Shen Y et al (2012) Inhibition of activated Stat3 reverses drug resistance to chemotherapeutic agents in gastric cancer cells. Cancer Lett 315(2):198–205
21. Zhao C, Li H, Lin H-J et al (2016) Feedback activation of STAT3 as a cancer drug-resistance mechanism. Trends Pharmacol Sci 37(1):47–61
22. Darnell JEJ, Kerr IM, Stark GR (1994) Jak-STAT pathways and transcriptional activation in response to IFNs and other extracellular signaling proteins. Science 264(5164): 1415–1421
23. Zhong Z, Wen Z, Darnell JEJ (1994) Stat3: a STAT family member activated by tyrosine phosphorylation in response to epidermal growth factor and interleukin-6. Science 264(5155):95–98
24. Ram PT, Iyengar R (2001) G protein coupled receptor signaling through the Src and Stat3 pathway: role in proliferation and transformation. Oncogene 20(13):1601–1606
25. Shao H, Xu X, Mastrangelo MA, Jing N, Cook RG, Legge GB, Tweardy DJ (2004) Structural requirements for signal transducer and activator of transcription 3 binding to phosphotyrosine ligands containing the YXXQ motif. J Biol Chem 30;279(18):18967–73
26. Liu L, McBride KM, Reich NC (2005) STAT3 nuclear import is independent of tyrosine phosphorylation and mediated by importin-alpha3. Proc Natl Acad Sci U S A 102(23): 8150–8155

27. Cimica V, Chen H-C, Iyer JK et al (2011) Dynamics of the STAT3 transcription factor: nuclear import dependent on Ran and importin-beta1. PLoS One 6(5):e20188
28. Reich NC (2013) STATs get their move on. JAKSTAT 2(4):e27080
29. Ma J, Zhang T, Novotny-Diermayr V et al (2003) A novel sequence in the coiled-coil domain of Stat3 essential for its nuclear translocation. J Biol Chem 278(31):29252–29260
30. Pranada AL, Metz S, Herrmann A et al (2004) Real time analysis of STAT3 nucleocytoplasmic shuttling. J Biol Chem 279(15):15114–15123
31. Paulson M, Pisharody S, Pan L et al (1999) Stat protein transactivation domains recruit p300/CBP through widely divergent sequences. J Biol Chem 274(36):25343–25349
32. Giraud S, Bienvenu F, Avril S et al (2002) Functional interaction of STAT3 transcription factor with the coactivator NcoA/SRC1a. J Biol Chem 277(10):8004–8011
33. Quesnelle KM, Boehm AL, Grandis JR (2007) STAT-mediated EGFR signaling in cancer. J Cell Biochem 102(2):311–319
34. Silva CM (2004) Role of STATs as downstream signal transducers in Src family kinase-mediated tumorigenesis. Oncogene 23(48):8017–8023
35. Garcia R, Bowman TL, Niu G et al (2001) Constitutive activation of Stat3 by the Src and JAK tyrosine kinases participates in growth regulation of human breast carcinoma cells. Oncogene 20(20):2499–2513
36. Buchert M, Burns CJ, Ernst M (2015) Targeting JAK kinase in solid tumors: emerging opportunities and challenges. Oncogene 35(8):939–951
37. Guo Y, Xu F, Lu T et al (2012) Interleukin-6 signaling pathway in targeted therapy for cancer. Cancer Treat Rev 38(7):904–910
38. Buerger C, Nagel-Wolfrum K, Kunz C et al (2003) Sequence-specific peptide aptamers, interacting with the intracellular domain of the epidermal growth factor receptor, interfere with Stat3 activation and inhibit the growth of tumor cells. J Biol Chem 278(39):37610–37621
39. Balabanov S, Braig M, Brummendorf TH (2014) Current aspects in resistance against tyrosine kinase inhibitors in chronic myelogenous leukemia. Drug Discov Today Technol 11:89–99
40. Norman P (2014) Selective JAK inhibitors in development for rheumatoid arthritis. Expert Opin Investig Drugs 23(8):1067–1077
41. Plimack ER, Lorusso PM, McCoon P et al (2013) AZD1480: a phase I study of a novel JAK2 inhibitor in solid tumors. Oncologist 18(7):819–820
42. Vultur A, Villanueva J, Krepler C et al (2014) MEK inhibition affects STAT3 signaling and invasion in human melanoma cell lines. Oncogene 33(14):1850–1861
43. Becker S, Groner B, Muller CW (1998) Three-dimensional structure of the Stat3beta homodimer bound to DNA. Nature 394(6689):145–151
44. Ren Z, Cabell LA, Schaefer TS et al (2003) Identification of a high-affinity phosphopeptide inhibitor of Stat3. Bioorg Med Chem Lett 13(4):633–636
45. Turkson J, Ryan D, Kim JS et al (2001) Phosphotyrosyl peptides block Stat3-mediated DNA binding activity, gene regulation, and cell transformation. J Biol Chem 276(48):45443–45455
46. Wiederkehr-Adam M, Ernst P, Muller K et al (2003) Characterization of phosphopeptide motifs specific for the Src homology 2 domains of signal transducer and activator of transcription 1 (STAT1) and STAT3. J Biol Chem 278(18):16117–16128
47. Yue P, Turkson J (2009) Targeting STAT3 in cancer: how successful are we? Expert Opin Investig Drugs 18(1):45–56
48. Vultur A, Cao J, Arulanandam R et al (2004) Cell-to-cell adhesion modulates Stat3 activity in normal and breast carcinoma cells. Oncogene 23(15):2600–2616
49. Turkson J, Kim JS, Zhang S et al (2004) Novel peptidomimetic inhibitors of signal transducer and activator of transcription 3 dimerization and biological activity. Mol Cancer Ther 3(3):261–269
50. Siddiquee KA, Gunning PT, Glenn M et al (2007) An oxazole-based small-molecule Stat3 inhibitor modulates Stat3 stability and processing and induces antitumor cell effects. ACS Chem Biol 2(12):787–798

51. Shao H, Xu X, Jing N et al (2006) Unique structural determinants for Stat3 recruitment and activation by the granulocyte colony-stimulating factor receptor at phosphotyrosine ligands 704 and 744. J Immunol 176(5):2933–2941

52. Coleman DR, Ren Z, Mandal PK et al (2005) Investigation of the binding determinants of phosphopeptides targeted to the SRC homology 2 domain of the signal transducer and activator of transcription 3. Development of a high-affinity peptide inhibitor. J Med Chem 48(21):6661–6670

53. Auzenne EJ, Klostergaard J, Mandal PK et al (2012) A phosphopeptide mimetic prodrug targeting the SH2 domain of Stat3 inhibits tumor growth and angiogenesis. J Exp Ther Oncol 10(2):155–162

54. Mandal PK, Gao F, Lu Z et al (2011) Potent and selective phosphopeptide mimetic prodrugs targeted to the Src homology 2 (SH2) domain of signal transducer and activator of transcription 3. J Med Chem 54(10):3549–3563

55. Kim D, Lee IH, Kim S et al (2014) A specific STAT3-binding peptide exerts antiproliferative effects and antitumor activity by inhibiting STAT3 phosphorylation and signaling. Cancer Res 74(8):2144–2151

56. Borghouts C, Delis N, Brill B et al (2012) A membrane penetrating peptide aptamer inhibits STAT3 function and suppresses the growth of STAT3 addicted tumor cells. JAKSTAT 1(1):44–54

57. Mack L, Brill B, Delis N et al (2012) Stat3 is activated in skin lesions by the local application of imiquimod, a ligand of TLR7, and inhibited by the recombinant peptide aptamer rS3-PA. Horm Mol Biol Clin Investig 10(2):265–272

58. Schoneberger H, Weiss A, Brill B et al (2011) The integration of a Stat3 specific peptide aptamer into the thioredoxin scaffold protein strongly enhances its inhibitory potency. Horm Mol Biol Clin Investig 5(1):1–9

59. Weber A, Borghouts C, Delis N et al (2012) Inhibition of Stat3 by peptide aptamer rS3-PA enhances growth suppressive effects of irinotecan on colorectal cancer cells. Horm Mol Biol Clin Investig 10(2):273–279

60. Drewry JA, Fletcher S, Yue P et al (2010) Coordination complex SH2 domain proteomimetics: an alternative approach to disrupting oncogenic protein-protein interactions. Chem Commun (Camb) 46(6):892–894

61. Bhasin D, Cisek K, Pandharkar T et al (2008) Design, synthesis, and studies of small molecule STAT3 inhibitors. Bioorg Med Chem Lett 18(1):391–395

62. Chen CL, Loy A, Cen L et al (2007) Signal transducer and activator of transcription 3 is involved in cell growth and survival of human rhabdomyosarcoma and osteosarcoma cells. BMC Cancer 7:111

63. Song H, Wang R, Wang S et al (2005) A low-molecular-weight compound discovered through virtual database screening inhibits Stat3 function in breast cancer cells. Proc Natl Acad Sci U S A 102(13):4700–4705

64. Fuh B, Sobo M, Cen L et al (2009) LLL-3 inhibits STAT3 activity, suppresses glioblastoma cell growth and prolongs survival in a mouse glioblastoma model. Br J Cancer 100(1):106–112

65. Ball S, Li C, Li PK et al (2011) The small molecule, LLL12, inhibits STAT3 phosphorylation and induces apoptosis in medulloblastoma and glioblastoma cells. PLoS One 6(4):e18820

66. Bid HK, Oswald D, Li C et al (2012) Anti-angiogenic activity of a small molecule STAT3 inhibitor LLL12. PLoS One 7(4):e35513

67. Couto JI, Bear MD, Lin J et al (2012) Biologic activity of the novel small molecule STAT3 inhibitor LLL12 against canine osteosarcoma cell lines. BMC Vet Res 8:244

68. Jain R, Kulkarni P, Dhali S et al (2014) Quantitative proteomic analysis of global effect of LLL12 on U87 cell's proteome: an insight into the molecular mechanism of LLL12. J Proteomics 113:127–142

69. Lin L, Benson DM Jr, DeAngelis S et al (2012) A small molecule, LLL12 inhibits constitutive STAT3 and IL-6-induced STAT3 signaling and exhibits potent growth suppressive activity in human multiple myeloma cells. Int J Cancer 130(6):1459–1469
70. Lin L, Hutzen B, Li PK et al (2010) A novel small molecule, LLL12, inhibits STAT3 phosphorylation and activities and exhibits potent growth-suppressive activity in human cancer cells. Neoplasia 12(1):39–50
71. Liu A, Liu Y, Li PK et al (2011) LLL12 inhibits endogenous and exogenous interleukin-6-induced STAT3 phosphorylation in human pancreatic cancer cells. Anticancer Res 31(6):2029–2035
72. Onimoe GI, Liu A, Lin L et al (2012) Small molecules, LLL12 and FLLL32, inhibit STAT3 and exhibit potent growth suppressive activity in osteosarcoma cells and tumor growth in mice. Invest New Drugs 30(3):916–926
73. Wei CC, Ball S, Lin L et al (2011) Two small molecule compounds, LLL12 and FLLL32, exhibit potent inhibitory activity on STAT3 in human rhabdomyosarcoma cells. Int J Oncol 38(1):279–285
74. Schust J, Sperl B, Hollis A et al (2006) Stattic: a small-molecule inhibitor of STAT3 activation and dimerization. Chem Biol 13(11):1235–1242
75. Heidelberger S, Zinzalla G, Antonow D et al (2013) Investigation of the protein alkylation sites of the STAT3:STAT3 inhibitor Stattic by mass spectrometry. Bioorg Med Chem Lett 23(16):4719–4722
76. Pan Y, Zhou F, Zhang R et al (2013) Stat3 inhibitor Stattic exhibits potent antitumor activity and induces chemo- and radio-sensitivity in nasopharyngeal carcinoma. PLoS One 8(1):e54565
77. Zhang Q, Zhang C, He J et al (2015) STAT3 inhibitor stattic enhances radiosensitivity in esophageal squamous cell carcinoma. Tumour Biol 36(3):2135–2142
78. Ji T, Gong D, Han Z et al (2013) Abrogation of constitutive Stat3 activity circumvents cisplatin resistant ovarian cancer. Cancer Lett 341(2):231–239
79. Buettner R, Corzano R, Rashid R et al (2011) Alkylation of cysteine 468 in Stat3 defines a novel site for therapeutic development. ACS Chem Biol 6(5):432–443
80. Sanseverino I, Purificato C, Gauzzi MC et al (2012) Revisiting the specificity of small molecule inhibitors: the example of stattic in dendritic cells. Chem Biol 19(10): 1213–1214
81. Gurbuz V, Konac E, Varol N et al (2014) Effects of AG490 and S3I-201 on regulation of the JAK/STAT3 signaling pathway in relation to angiogenesis in TRAIL-resistant prostate cancer cells. Oncol Lett 7(3):755–763
82. Siddiquee K, Zhang S, Guida WC et al (2007) Selective chemical probe inhibitor of Stat3, identified through structure-based virtual screening, induces antitumor activity. Proc Natl Acad Sci U S A 104(18):7391–7396
83. Fletcher S, Page BD, Zhang X et al (2011) Antagonism of the Stat3-Stat3 protein dimer with salicylic acid based small molecules. Chem Med Chem 6(8):1459–1470
84. Zhang X, Yue P, Fletcher S et al (2010) A novel small-molecule disrupts Stat3 SH2 domain-phosphotyrosine interactions and Stat3-dependent tumor processes. Biochem Pharmacol 79(10):1398–1409
85. Fletcher S, Singh J, Zhang X et al (2009) Disruption of transcriptionally active Stat3 dimers with non-phosphorylated, salicylic acid-based small molecules: potent in vitro and tumor cell activities. Chembiochem 10(12):1959–1964
86. Furtek SL, Backos DS, Matheson CJ, Reigan P (2016) Strategies and approaches of targeting STAT3 for cancer treatment. ACS Chem Biol. 9;11(2):308–318
87. Page BD, Fletcher S, Yue P et al (2011) Identification of a non-phosphorylated, cell permeable, small molecule ligand for the Stat3 SH2 domain. Bioorg Med Chem Lett 21(18):5605–5609
88. Zhang X, Yue P, Page BD et al (2012) Orally bioavailable small-molecule inhibitor of transcription factor Stat3 regresses human breast and lung cancer xenografts. Proc Natl Acad Sci U S A 109(24):9623–9628

89. Shahani VM, Yue P, Haftchenary S et al (2011) Identification of purine-scaffold small-molecule inhibitors of Stat3 activation by QSAR studies. ACS Med Chem Lett 2(1):79–84
90. Fletcher S, Turkson J, Gunning PT (2008) Molecular approaches towards the inhibition of the signal transducer and activator of transcription 3 (Stat3) protein. ChemMedChem 3(8):1159–1168
91. Haftchenary S, Luchman HA, Jouk AO et al (2013) Potent targeting of the STAT3 protein in brain cancer stem cells: a promising route for treating glioblastoma. ACS Med Chem Lett 4(11):1102–1107
92. Yue P, Lopez-Tapia F, Paladino D et al (2016) Hydroxamic acid and benzoic acid-based STAT3 inhibitors suppress human glioma and breast cancer phenotypes in vitro and in vivo. Cancer Res 76(3):652–663
93. Xu X, Kasembeli MM, Jiang X et al (2009) Chemical probes that competitively and selectively inhibit Stat3 activation. PLoS One 4(3):e4783
94. Dave B, Landis MD, Tweardy DJ et al (2012) Selective small molecule Stat3 inhibitor reduces breast cancer tumor-initiating cells and improves recurrence free survival in a human-xenograft model. PLoS One 7(8):e30207
95. Redell MS, Ruiz MJ, Alonzo TA et al (2011) Stat3 signaling in acute myeloid leukemia: ligand-dependent and -independent activation and induction of apoptosis by a novel small-molecule Stat3 inhibitor. Blood 117(21):5701–5709
96. Bharadwaj U, Eckols TK, Xu X, Kasembeli MM, Chen Y, Adachi M, Song Y, Mo Q, Lai SY, Tweardy DJ (2016) Small-molecule inhibition of STAT3 in radioresistant head and neck squamous cell carcinoma. Oncotarget 7(18):26307–26330
97. Redell MS, Ruiz MJ, Gerbing RB et al (2013) FACS analysis of Stat3/5 signaling reveals sensitivity to G-CSF and IL-6 as a significant prognostic factor in pediatric AML: a Children's Oncology Group report. Blood 121(7):1083–1093
98. Zhang L, Pan J, Dong Y et al (2013) Stat3 activation links a C/EBPdelta to myostatin pathway to stimulate loss of muscle mass. Cell Metab 18(3):368–379
99. Lewis KM, Bharadwaj U, Eckols TK et al (2015) Small-molecule targeting of signal transducer and activator of transcription (STAT) 3 to treat non-small cell lung cancer. Lung Cancer 90(2):182–190
100. Shin DS, Kim HN, Shin KD et al (2009) Cryptotanshinone inhibits constitutive signal transducer and activator of transcription 3 function through blocking the dimerization in DU145 prostate cancer cells. Cancer Res 69(1):193–202
101. Ge Y, Yang B, Chen Z et al (2015) Cryptotanshinone suppresses the proliferation and induces the apoptosis of pancreatic cancer cells via the STAT3 signaling pathway. Mol Med Rep 12(5):7782–7788
102. Li W, Saud SM, Young MR et al (2015) Cryptotanshinone, a Stat3 inhibitor, suppresses colorectal cancer proliferation and growth in vitro. Mol Cell Biochem 406(1-2):63–73
103. Liu P, Xu S, Zhang M et al (2013) Anticancer activity in human multiple myeloma U266 cells: synergy between cryptotanshinone and arsenic trioxide. Metallomics 5(7):871–878
104. Lu L, Li C, Li D et al (2013) Cryptotanshinone inhibits human glioma cell proliferation by suppressing STAT3 signaling. Mol Cell Biochem 381(1–2):273–282
105. Yu HJ, Park C, Kim SJ et al (2014) Signal transducer and activators of transcription 3 regulates cryptotanshinone-induced apoptosis in human mucoepidermoid carcinoma cells. Pharmacogn Mag 10(Suppl 3):S622–S629
106. Ge Y, Yang B, Xu X et al (2015) Cryptotanshinone acts synergistically with imatinib to induce apoptosis of human chronic myeloid leukemia cells. Leuk Lymphoma 56(3):730–738
107. Jung JH, Kwon TR, Jeong SJ et al (2013) Apoptosis induced by tanshinone IIA and cryptotanshinone is mediated by distinct JAK/STAT3/5 and SHP1/2 signaling in chronic myeloid leukemia K562 cells. Evid Based Complement Alternat Med 2013:805639
108. Xia C, Bai X, Hou X et al (2015) Cryptotanshinone reverses cisplatin resistance of human lung carcinoma A549 cells through down-regulating Nrf2 pathway. Cell Physiol Biochem 37(2):816–824
109. Zhu Z, Zhao Y, Li J, Tao L, Shi P, Wei Z, Sheng X, Shen D, Liu Z, Zhou L, Tian C, Fan F, Shen C, Zhu P, Wang A, Chen W, Zhao Q, Lu Y (2015) Cryptotanshinone, a novel tumor

angiogenesis inhibitor, destabilizes tumor necrosis factor-α mRNA via decreasing nuclear-cytoplasmic translocation of RNA-binding protein HuR. Mol Carcinog 55(10):1399–1401

110. Matsuno K, Masuda Y, Uehara Y et al (2010) Identification of a new series of STAT3 inhibitors by virtual screening. ACS Med Chem Lett 1(8):371–375

111. Ashizawa T, Akiyama Y, Miyata H et al (2014) Effect of the STAT3 inhibitor STX-0119 on the proliferation of a temozolomide-resistant glioblastoma cell line. Int J Oncol 45(1):411–418

112. Ashizawa T, Miyata H, Iizuka A et al (2013) Effect of the STAT3 inhibitor STX-0119 on the proliferation of cancer stem-like cells derived from recurrent glioblastoma. Int J Oncol 43(1):219–227

113. Ashizawa T, Miyata H, Ishii H et al (2011) Antitumor activity of a novel small molecule STAT3 inhibitor against a human lymphoma cell line with high STAT3 activation. Int J Oncol 38(5):1245–1252

114. Lin J, Buettner R, Yuan YC et al (2009) Molecular dynamics simulations of the conformational changes in signal transducers and activators of transcription, Stat1 and Stat3. J Mol Graph Model 28(4):347–356

115. Bharadwaj U, Eckols TK, Kolosov M et al (2014) Drug-repositioning screening identified piperlongumine as a direct STAT3 inhibitor with potent activity against breast cancer. Oncogene 34(11):1341–1353

116. Fukunishi Y (2010) Post processing of protein-compound docking for fragment-based drug discovery (FBDD): in-silico structure-based drug screening and ligand-binding pose prediction. Curr Top Med Chem 10(6):680–694

117. Murray CW, Rees DC (2016) Opportunity knocks: organic chemistry for fragment-based drug discovery (FBDD). Angew Chem Int Ed Engl 55(2):488–492

118. Whittaker M (2009) Picking up the pieces with FBDD or FADD: invest early for future success. Drug Discov Today 14(13–14):623–624

119. Liu A, Liu Y, Jin Z et al (2012) XZH-5 inhibits STAT3 phosphorylation and enhances the cytotoxicity of chemotherapeutic drugs in human breast and pancreatic cancer cells. PLoS One 7(10):e46624

120. Liu A, Liu Y, Xu Z et al (2011) Novel small molecule, XZH-5, inhibits constitutive and interleukin-6-induced STAT3 phosphorylation in human rhabdomyosarcoma cells. Cancer Sci 102(7):1381–1387

121. Liu Y, Liu A, Xu Z et al (2011) XZH-5 inhibits STAT3 phosphorylation and causes apoptosis in human hepatocellular carcinoma cells. Apoptosis 16(5):502–510

122. Law V, Knox C, Djoumbou Y et al (2014) DrugBank 4.0: shedding new light on drug metabolism. Nucleic Acids Res 42(Database issue):D1091–D1097

123. Daka P, Liu A, Karunaratne C et al (2015) Design, synthesis and evaluation of XZH-5 analogues as STAT3 inhibitors. Bioorg Med Chem 23(6):1348–1355

124. Ren X, Duan L, He Q et al (2010) Identification of niclosamide as a new small-molecule inhibitor of the STAT3 signaling pathway. ACS Med Chem Lett 1(9):454–459

125. Chen H, Yang Z, Ding C et al (2013) Fragment-based drug design and identification of HJC0123, a novel orally bioavailable STAT3 inhibitor for cancer therapy. Eur J Med Chem 62:498–507

126. Chen H, Yang Z, Ding C et al (2013) Discovery of -alkylamino tethered niclosamide derivatives as potent and orally bioavailable anticancer agents. ACS Med Chem Lett 4(2):180–185

127. Yu W, Xiao H, Lin J et al (2013) Discovery of novel STAT3 small molecule inhibitors via in silico site-directed fragment-based drug design. J Med Chem 56(11):4402–4412

128. Seidel HM, Milocco LH, Lamb P et al (1995) Spacing of palindromic half sites as a determinant of selective STAT (signal transducers and activators of transcription) DNA binding and transcriptional activity. Proc Natl Acad Sci U S A 92(7):3041–3045

129. Bielinska A, Shivdasani RA, Zhang LQ et al (1990) Regulation of gene expression with double-stranded phosphorothioate oligonucleotides. Science 250(4983):997–1000

130. Mann MJ, Dzau VJ (2000) Therapeutic applications of transcription factor decoy oligonucleotides. J Clin Invest 106(9):1071–1075

131. Ahmad MZ, Akhter S, Mallik N et al (2013) Application of decoy oligonucleotides as novel therapeutic strategy: a contemporary overview. Current Drug Discov Tech 10(1):71–84

132. Yokozeki H, Wu MH, Sumi K et al (2004) In vivo transfection of a cis element 'decoy' against signal transducers and activators of transcription 6 (STAT6)-binding site ameliorates IgE-mediated late-phase reaction in an atopic dermatitis mouse model. Gene Ther 11(24):1753–1762

133. Leong PL, Andrews GA, Johnson DE et al (2003) Targeted inhibition of Stat3 with a decoy oligonucleotide abrogates head and neck cancer cell growth. Proc Natl Acad Sci U S A 100(7):4138–4143

134. Shen J, Li R, Li G (2009) Inhibitory effects of decoy-ODN targeting activated STAT3 on human glioma growth in vivo. In Vivo 23(2):237–243

135. Zhang X, Liu P, Zhang B et al (2013) Inhibitory effects of STAT3 decoy oligodeoxynucleotides on human epithelial ovarian cancer cell growth in vivo. Int J Mol Med 32(3):623–628

136. Liu M, Wang F, Wen Z et al (2014) Blockage of STAT3 signaling pathway with a decoy oligodeoxynucleotide inhibits growth of human ovarian cancer cells. Cancer Invest 32(1):8–12

137. Lewis HD, Winter A, Murphy TF et al (2008) STAT3 inhibition in prostate and pancreatic cancer lines by STAT3 binding sequence oligonucleotides: differential activity between 5′ and 3′ ends. Mol Cancer Ther 7(6):1543–1550

138. Sun X, Zhang J, Wang L et al (2008) Growth inhibition of human hepatocellular carcinoma cells by blocking STAT3 activation with decoy-ODN. Cancer Lett 262(2):201–213

139. Sen M, Tosca PJ, Zwayer C et al (2009) Lack of toxicity of a STAT3 decoy oligonucleotide. Cancer Chemother Pharmacol 63(6):983–995

140. Sen M, Paul K, Freilino ML et al (2014) Systemic administration of a cyclic signal transducer and activator of transcription 3 (STAT3) decoy oligonucleotide inhibits tumor growth without inducing toxicological effects. Mol Med 20:46–56

141. Lewis HD, Husain A, Donnelly RJ et al (2010) Creation of a novel peptide with enhanced nuclear localization in prostate and pancreatic cancer cell lines. BMC Biotechnol 10:79

142. Williamson JR (1994) G-quartet structures in telomeric DNA. Annu Rev Biophys Biomol Struct 23:703–730

143. Sundquist WI, Klug A (1989) Telomeric DNA dimerizes by formation of guanine tetrads between hairpin loops. Nature 342(6251):825–829

144. Jing N, Li Y, Xu X et al (2003) Targeting Stat3 with G-quartet oligodeoxynucleotides in human cancer cells. DNA Cell Biol 22(11):685–696

145. Jing N, Li Y, Xiong W et al (2004) G-quartet oligonucleotides: a new class of signal transducer and activator of transcription 3 inhibitors that suppresses growth of prostate and breast tumors through induction of apoptosis. Cancer Res 64(18):6603–6609

146. Tweardy DJ, Jing N (2006) Enhancing or eliminating signals for cell survival to treat disease. Trans Am Clin Climatol Assoc 117:33–51

147. Weerasinghe P, Garcia GE, Zhu Q et al (2007) Inhibition of Stat3 activation and tumor growth suppression of non-small cell lung cancer by G-quartet oligonucleotides. Int J Oncol 31(1):129–136

148. Zuckerman JE, Davis ME (2015) Clinical experiences with systemically administered siRNA-based therapeutics in cancer. Nat Rev Drug Discov 14(12):843–856

149. Turkson J, Zhang S, Palmer J et al (2004) Inhibition of constitutive signal transducer and activator of transcription 3 activation by novel platinum complexes with potent antitumor activity. Mol Cancer Ther 3(12):1533–1542

150. Turkson J, Zhang S, Mora LB et al (2005) A novel platinum compound inhibits constitutive Stat3 signaling and induces cell cycle arrest and apoptosis of malignant cells. J Biol Chem 280(38):32979–32988

151. Assi HH, Paran C, VanderVeen N et al (2014) Preclinical characterization of signal transducer and activator of transcription 3 small molecule inhibitors for primary and metastatic brain cancer therapy. J Pharmacol Exp Ther 349(3):458–469

152. Heudi O, Brisset H, Cailleux A et al (2001) Chemical instability and methods for measurement of cisplatin adducts formed by interactions with cysteine and glutathione. Int J Clin Pharmacol Ther 39(8):344–349

153. Singh J, Petter RC, Baillie TA et al (2011) The resurgence of covalent drugs. Nat Rev Drug Discov 10(4):307–317

154. Huang W, Dong Z, Wang F et al (2014) A small molecule compound targeting STAT3 DNA-binding domain inhibits cancer cell proliferation, migration, and invasion. ACS Chem Biol 9(5):1188–1196

155. Huang W, Dong Z, Chen Y et al (2015) Small-molecule inhibitors targeting the DNA-binding domain of STAT3 suppress tumor growth, metastasis and STAT3 target gene expression in vivo. Oncogene 35(6):783–792

156. Rath KS, Naidu SK, Lata P et al (2014) HO-3867, a safe STAT3 inhibitor, is selectively cytotoxic to ovarian cancer. Cancer Res 74(8):2316–2327

157. Tierney BJ, McCann GA, Naidu S et al (2014) Aberrantly activated pSTAT3-Ser727 in human endometrial cancer is suppressed by HO-3867, a novel STAT3 inhibitor. Gynecol Oncol 135(1):133–141

158. Selvendiran K, Tong L, Bratasz A et al (2010) Anticancer efficacy of a difluorodiarylidenyl piperidone (HO-3867) in human ovarian cancer cells and tumor xenografts. Mol Cancer Ther 9(5):1169–1179

159. Weidler M, Rether J, Anke T et al (2000) Inhibition of interleukin-6 signaling by galiellalactone. FEBS Lett 484(1):1–6

160. Hellsten R, Johansson M, Dahlman A et al (2008) Galiellalactone is a novel therapeutic candidate against hormone-refractory prostate cancer expressing activated Stat3. Prostate 68(3):269–280

161. Canesin G, Evans-Axelsson S, Hellsten R et al (2015) The STAT3 inhibitor galiellalactone effectively reduces tumor growth and metastatic spread in an orthotopic xenograft mouse model of prostate cancer. Eur Urol 69(3):400–404

162. Don-Doncow N, Escobar Z, Johansson M et al (2014) Galiellalactone is a direct inhibitor of the transcription factor STAT3 in prostate cancer cells. J Biol Chem 289(23):15969–15978

163. Nagel-Wolfrum K, Buerger C, Wittig I et al (2004) The interaction of specific peptide aptamers with the DNA binding domain and the dimerization domain of the transcription factor Stat3 inhibits transactivation and induces apoptosis in tumor cells. Mol Cancer Res 2(3):170–182

164. Yang J, Chatterjee-Kishore M, Staugaitis SM et al (2005) Novel roles of unphosphorylated STAT3 in oncogenesis and transcriptional regulation. Cancer Res 65(3):939–947

165. Yang J, Liao X, Agarwal MK et al (2007) Unphosphorylated STAT3 accumulates in response to IL-6 and activates transcription by binding to NFkappaB. Genes Dev 21(11):1396–1408

166. Yang J, Stark GR (2008) Roles of unphosphorylated STATs in signaling. Cell Res 18(4):443–451

167. Shuai K (2000) Modulation of STAT signaling by STAT-interacting proteins. Oncogene 19(21):2638–2644

168. Furqan M, Akinleye A, Mukhi N et al (2013) STAT inhibitors for cancer therapy. J Hematol Oncol 6:90

169. Timofeeva OA, Gaponenko V, Lockett SJ et al (2007) Rationally designed inhibitors identify STAT3 N-domain as a promising anticancer drug target. ACS Chem Biol 2(12):799–809

170. Zhang X, Darnell JE Jr (2001) Functional importance of Stat3 tetramerization in activation of the alpha 2-macroglobulin gene. J Biol Chem 276(36):33576–33581

171. Zhang Y, Sif S, DeWille J (2007) The mouse C/EBPdelta gene promoter is regulated by STAT3 and Sp1 transcriptional activators, chromatin remodeling and c-Myc repression. J Cell Biochem 102(5):1256–1270

172. Ota N, Brett TJ, Murphy TL et al (2004) N-domain-dependent nonphosphorylated STAT4 dimers required for cytokine-driven activation. Nat Immunol 5(2):208–215

173. Tyler DR, Persky ME, Matthews LA et al (2007) Pre-assembly of STAT4 with the human IFN-alpha/beta receptor-2 subunit is mediated by the STAT4 N-domain. Mol Immunol 44(8):1864–1872

174. Zhang T, Kee WH, Seow KT et al (2000) The coiled-coil domain of Stat3 is essential for its SH2 domain-mediated receptor binding and subsequent activation induced by epidermal growth factor and interleukin-6. Mol Cell Biol 20(19):7132–7139

175. Timofeeva OA, Tarasova NI, Zhang X et al (2013) STAT3 suppresses transcription of pro-apoptotic genes in cancer cells with the involvement of its N-terminal domain. Proc Natl Acad Sci U S A 110(4):1267–1272

176. Zhao Y, Zeng C, Tarasova NI et al (2013) A new role for STAT3 as a regulator of chromatin topology. Transcription 4(5):227–231

177. Timofeeva OA, Chasovskikh S, Lonskaya I et al (2012) Mechanisms of unphosphorylated STAT3 transcription factor binding to DNA. J Biol Chem 287(17):14192–14200

178. Heinrich PC, Behrmann I, Haan S et al (2003) Principles of interleukin (IL)-6-type cytokine signalling and its regulation. Biochem J 374(Pt 1):1–20

179. Kubo M, Hanada T, Yoshimura A (2003) Suppressors of cytokine signaling and immunity. Nat Immunol 4(12):1169–1176

180. Gu F, Dube N, Kim JW et al (2003) Protein tyrosine phosphatase 1B attenuates growth hormone-mediated JAK2-STAT signaling. Mol Cell Biol 23(11):3753–3762

181. Kim HY, Park EJ, Joe EH et al (2003) Curcumin suppresses Janus kinase-STAT inflammatory signaling through activation of Src homology 2 domain-containing tyrosine phosphatase 2 in brain microglia. J Immunol 171(11):6072–6079

182. Tai WT, Cheng AL, Shiau CW et al (2011) Signal transducer and activator of transcription 3 is a major kinase-independent target of sorafenib in hepatocellular carcinoma. J Hepatol 55(5):1041–1048

183. Fan LC, Teng HW, Shiau CW et al (2015) Pharmacological targeting SHP-1-STAT3 signaling is a promising therapeutic approach for the treatment of colorectal cancer. Neoplasia 17(9):687–696

184. Han Y, Amin HM, Franko B et al (2006) Loss of SHP1 enhances JAK3/STAT3 signaling and decreases proteosome degradation of JAK3 and NPM-ALK in ALK+ anaplastic large-cell lymphoma. Blood 108(8):2796–2803

185. Witkiewicz A, Raghunath P, Wasik A et al (2007) Loss of SHP-1 tyrosine phosphatase expression correlates with the advanced stages of cutaneous T-cell lymphoma. Human Pathol 38(3):462–467

186. Chen KF, Chen HL, Shiau CW et al (2013) Sorafenib and its derivative SC-49 sensitize hepatocellular carcinoma cells to CS-1008, a humanized anti-TNFRSF10B (DR5) antibody. Br J Pharmacol 168(3):658–672

187. Liu CY, Tseng LM, Su JC et al (2013) Novel sorafenib analogues induce apoptosis through SHP-1 dependent STAT3 inactivation in human breast cancer cells. Breast Cancer Res 15(4):R63

188. Su TH, Shiau CW, Jao P et al (2015) Sorafenib and its derivative SC-1 exhibit antifibrotic effects through signal transducer and activator of transcription 3 inhibition. Proc Natl Acad Sci U S A 112(23):7243–7248

189. Wang CT, Lin CS, Shiau CW et al (2013) SC-1, a sorafenib derivative, shows anti-tumor effects in osteogenic sarcoma cells. J Orthop Res 31(2):335–342

190. Pandey MK, Sung B, Aggarwal BB (2010) Betulinic acid suppresses STAT3 activation pathway through induction of protein tyrosine phosphatase SHP-1 in human multiple myeloma cells. Int J Cancer 127(2):282–292

191. Ahn KS, Sethi G, Sung B et al (2008) Guggulsterone, a farnesoid X receptor antagonist, inhibits constitutive and inducible STAT3 activation through induction of a protein tyrosine phosphatase SHP-1. Cancer Res 68(11):4406–4415

192. Al-Jamal HA, Mat Jusoh SA, Hassan R et al (2015) Enhancing SHP-1 expression with 5-azacytidine may inhibit STAT3 activation and confer sensitivity in lestaurtinib (CEP-701)-resistant FLT3-ITD positive acute myeloid leukemia. BMC Cancer 15:869

193. Chen KF, Su JC, Liu CY et al (2012) A novel obatoclax derivative, SC-2001, induces apoptosis in hepatocellular carcinoma cells through SHP-1-dependent STAT3 inactivation. Cancer Lett 321(1):27–35

194. Fan LC, Teng HW, Shiau CW et al (2014) SHP-1 is a target of regorafenib in colorectal cancer. Oncotarget 5(15):6243–6251

195. Kim C, Cho SK, Kapoor S et al (2014) beta-Caryophyllene oxide inhibits constitutive and inducible STAT3 signaling pathway through induction of the SHP-1 protein tyrosine phosphatase. Mol Carcinog 53(10):793–806

196. Kunnumakkara AB, Nair AS, Sung B et al (2009) Boswellic acid blocks signal transducers and activators of transcription 3 signaling, proliferation, and survival of multiple myeloma via the protein tyrosine phosphatase SHP-1. Mol Cancer Res 7(1):118–128

197. Lee JH, Chiang SY, Nam D et al (2014) Capillarisin inhibits constitutive and inducible STAT3 activation through induction of SHP-1 and SHP-2 tyrosine phosphatases. Cancer Lett 345(1):140–148

198. Rajendran P, Li F, Shanmugam MK et al (2012) Honokiol inhibits signal transducer and activator of transcription-3 signaling, proliferation, and survival of hepatocellular carcinoma cells via the protein tyrosine phosphatase SHP-1. J Cell Physiol 227(5):2184–2195

199. Tai WT, Cheng AL, Shiau CW et al (2012) Dovitinib induces apoptosis and overcomes sorafenib resistance in hepatocellular carcinoma through SHP-1-mediated inhibition of STAT3. Mol Cancer Ther 11(2):452–463

200. Wang J, Zhang L, Chen G et al (2014) Small molecule 1′-acetoxychavicol acetate suppresses breast tumor metastasis by regulating the SHP-1/STAT3/MMPs signaling pathway. Breast Cancer Res Treat 148(2):279–289

201. Prasad S, Pandey MK, Yadav VR et al (2011) Gambogic acid inhibits STAT3 phosphorylation through activation of protein tyrosine phosphatase SHP-1: potential role in proliferation and apoptosis. Cancer Prev Res (Phila) 4(7):1084–1094

202. Phromnoi K, Prasad S, Gupta SC et al (2011) Dihydroxypentamethoxyflavone downregulates constitutive and inducible signal transducers and activators of transcription-3 through the induction of tyrosine phosphatase SHP-1. Mol Pharmacol 80(5):889–899

203. Pandey MK, Sung B, Ahn KS et al (2009) Butein suppresses constitutive and inducible signal transducer and activator of transcription (STAT) 3 activation and STAT3-regulated gene products through the induction of a protein tyrosine phosphatase SHP-1. Mol Pharmacol 75(3):525–533

204. Kang SH, Jeong SJ, Kim SH et al (2012) Icariside II induces apoptosis in U937 acute myeloid leukemia cells: role of inactivation of STAT3-related signaling. PLoS One 7(4):e28706

205. Sandur SK, Pandey MK, Sung B et al (2010) 5-hydroxy-2-methyl-1,4-naphthoquinone, a vitamin K3 analogue, suppresses STAT3 activation pathway through induction of protein tyrosine phosphatase, SHP-1: potential role in chemosensitization. Mol Cancer Res 8(1):107–118

206. Cui Q, Jiang W, Wang Y et al (2008) Transfer of suppressor of cytokine signaling 3 by an oncolytic adenovirus induces potential antitumor activities in hepatocellular carcinoma. Hepatology 47(1):105–112

207. Wei X, Wang G, Li W et al (2014) Activation of the JAK-STAT3 pathway is associated with the growth of colorectal carcinoma cells. Oncol Rep 31(1):335–341

208. Woetmann A, Nielsen M, Christensen ST et al (1999) Inhibition of protein phosphatase 2A induces serine/threonine phosphorylation, subcellular redistribution, and functional inhibition of STAT3. Proc Natl Acad Sci U S A 96(19):10620–10625

209. Zgheib C, Zouein FA, Chidiac R et al (2012) Calyculin A reveals serine/threonine phosphatase protein phosphatase 1 as a regulatory nodal point in canonical signal transducer and activator of transcription 3 signaling of human microvascular endothelial cells. J Interferon Cytokine Res 32(2):87–94

210. Zhang Q, Raghunath PN, Xue L et al (2002) Multilevel dysregulation of STAT3 activation in anaplastic lymphoma kinase-positive T/null-cell lymphoma. J Immunol 168(1):466–474

211. Oka M, Sumita N, Sakaguchi M et al (2009) 12-O-tetradecanoylphorbol-13-acetate inhibits melanoma growth by inactivation of STAT3 through protein kinase C-activated tyrosine phosphatase(s). J Biol Chem 284(44):30416–30423

212. McGowan MP, Tardif JC, Ceska R et al (2012) Randomized, placebo-controlled trial of mipomersen in patients with severe hypercholesterolemia receiving maximally tolerated lipid-lowering therapy. PLoS One 7(11):e49006

213. Stein EA, Dufour R, Gagne C et al (2012) Apolipoprotein B synthesis inhibition with mipomersen in heterozygous familial hypercholesterolemia: results of a randomized, double-blind, placebo-controlled trial to assess efficacy and safety as add-on therapy in patients with coronary artery disease. Circulation 126(19):2283–2292

214. Rao DD, Senzer N, Cleary MA et al (2009) Comparative assessment of siRNA and shRNA off target effects: what is slowing clinical development. Cancer Gene Ther 16(11):807–809

215. Rao DD, Vorhies JS, Senzer N et al (2009) siRNA vs. shRNA: similarities and differences. Adv Drug Deliv Rev 61(9):746–759

216. Chen JY, Luo B, Guo XB et al (2011) Double suicide gene therapy with RNAi targeting to STAT3 inhibits the growth of colorectal carcinoma cells in vitro. Zhonghua Zhong Liu Za Zhi [Chinese Journal of Oncology] 33(2):91–96

217. Gao LF, Wen LJ, Yu H et al (2006) Knockdown of Stat3 expression using RNAi inhibits growth of laryngeal tumors in vivo. Acta Pharmacol Sin 27(3):347–352

218. Gao Z, Huang C, Qiu ZJ et al (2008) Effect of RNAi-mediated STAT3 gene inhibition on metastasis of human pancreatic cancer cells. Zhonghua Wai Ke Za Zhi [Chinese Journal of Surgery] 46(13):1010–1013

219. Kaymaz BT, Selvi N, Gunduz C et al (2013) Repression of STAT3, STAT5A, and STAT5B expressions in chronic myelogenous leukemia cell line K-562 with unmodified or chemically modified siRNAs and induction of apoptosis. Ann Hematol 92(2):151–162

220. Konnikova L, Kotecki M, Kruger MM et al (2003) Knockdown of STAT3 expression by RNAi induces apoptosis in astrocytoma cells. BMC Cancer 3:23

221. LaPan P, Zhang J, Pan J et al (2008) Single cell cytometry of protein function in RNAi treated cells and in native populations. BMC Cell Biol 9:43

222. Li GH, Wei H, Lv SQ et al (2010) Knockdown of STAT3 expression by RNAi suppresses growth and induces apoptosis and differentiation in glioblastoma stem cells. Int J Oncol 37(1):103–110

223. Wang HR, Li XM, Lu XY (2009) Silencing of signal transducer and activator of transcription 3 gene expression using RNAi enhances the efficacy of radiotherapy for laryngeal carcinoma in vivo. Zhonghua Er Bi Yan Hou Tou Jing Wai Ke Za Zhi 44(7):591–596

224. Zhao SH, Zhao F, Zheng JY et al (2011) Knockdown of stat3 expression by RNAi inhibits in vitro growth of human ovarian cancer. Radiol Oncol 45(3):196–203

225. Ball DP, Lewis AM, Williams D, Resetca D, Wilson DJ, Gunning PT. Signal transducer and activator of transcription 3 (STAT3) inhibitor, S3I-201, acts as a potent and non-selective alkylating agent. Oncotarget. 2016 Apr 12;7(15):20669–20679

226. Shrikant P, Khoruts A, Mescher MF (1999) CTLA-4 blockade reverses CD8+ T cell tolerance to tumor by a CD4+ T cell- and IL-2-dependent mechanism. Immunity 11(4):483–493

227. Frank DA (2007) STAT3 as a central mediator of neoplastic cellular transformation. Cancer Lett 251(2):199–210

228. Germain D, Frank DA (2007) Targeting the cytoplasmic and nuclear functions of signal transducers and activators of transcription 3 for cancer therapy. Clin Cancer Res 13(19):5665–5669

229. Herrmann A, Vogt M, Monnigmann M et al (2007) Nucleocytoplasmic shuttling of persistently activated STAT3. J Cell Sci 120(Pt 18):3249–3261

230. Jing N, Tweardy DJ (2005) Targeting Stat3 in cancer therapy. Anticancer Drugs 16(6):601–607

231. Redell MS, Tweardy DJ (2005) Targeting transcription factors for cancer therapy. Curr Pharm Des 11(22):2873–2887

232. Bhutani M, Pathak AK, Nair AS et al (2007) Capsaicin is a novel blocker of constitutive and interleukin-6-inducible STAT3 activation. Clin Cancer Res 13(10):3024–3032

233. Oyagbemi AA, Saba AB, Azeez OI (2010) Capsaicin: a novel chemopreventive molecule and its underlying molecular mechanisms of action. Indian J Cancer 47(1):53–58

234. Pramanik KC, Fofaria NM, Gupta P et al (2015) Inhibition of beta-catenin signaling suppresses pancreatic tumor growth by disrupting nuclear beta-catenin/TCF-1 complex: critical role of STAT-3. Oncotarget 6(13):11561–11574

235. Lee HK, Seo IA, Shin YK et al (2009) Capsaicin inhibits the IL-6/STAT3 pathway by depleting intracellular gp130 pools through endoplasmic reticulum stress. Biochem Biophys Res Commun 382(2):445–450
236. Xue P, Zhao Y, Liu Y et al (2014) A novel compound RY10-4 induces apoptosis and inhibits invasion via inhibiting STAT3 through ERK-, p38-dependent pathways in human lung adenocarcinoma A549 cells. Chem Biol Interact 209:25–34
237. Xu Y, Xu X, Gao X et al (2014) Shikonin suppresses IL-17-induced VEGF expression via blockage of JAK2/STAT3 pathway. Int Immunopharmacol 19(2):327–333
238. Walker SR, Chaudhury M, Frank DA (2011) STAT3 inhibition by microtubule-targeted drugs: dual molecular effects of chemotherapeutic agents. Mol Cell Pharmacol 3(1):13–19
239. Walker SR, Chaudhury M, Nelson EA et al (2010) Microtubule-targeted chemotherapeutic agents inhibit signal transducer and activator of transcription 3 (STAT3) signaling. Mol Pharmacol 78(5):903–908
240. Zhang L, Xu X, Yang R et al (2015) Paclitaxel attenuates renal interstitial fibroblast activation and interstitial fibrosis by inhibiting STAT3 signaling. Drug Des Devel Ther 9:2139–2148
241. Nelson EA, Walker SR, Kepich A et al (2008) Nifuroxazide inhibits survival of multiple myeloma cells by directly inhibiting STAT3. Blood 112(13):5095–5102
242. Li S, Priceman SJ, Xin H et al (2013) Icaritin inhibits JAK/STAT3 signaling and growth of renal cell carcinoma. PLoS One 8(12):e81657
243. Wu T, Wang S, Wu J et al (2015) Icaritin induces lytic cytotoxicity in extranodal NK/T-cell lymphoma. J Exp Clin Cancer Res 34:17
244. Zhao H, Guo Y, Li S et al (2015) A novel anti-cancer agent Icaritin suppresses hepatocellular carcinoma initiation and malignant growth through the IL-6/Jak2/Stat3 pathway. Oncotarget 6(31):31927–31943
245. Zhu S, Wang Z, Li Z et al (2015) Icaritin suppresses multiple myeloma, by inhibiting IL-6/JAK2/STAT3. Oncotarget 6(12):10460–10472
246. Jung JH, Yun M, Choo EJ et al (2015) A derivative of epigallocatechin-3-gallate induces apoptosis via SHP-1-mediated suppression of BCR-ABL and STAT3 signalling in chronic myelogenous leukaemia. Br J Pharmacol 172(14):3565–3578
247. Chakraborty A, Tweardy DJ (1998) Granulocyte colony-stimulating factor activates a 72-kDa isoform of STAT3 in human neutrophils. J Leuk Biol 64(5):675–680
248. Oda A, Wakao H, Fujita H (2002) Calpain is a signal transducer and activator of transcription (STAT) 3 and STAT5 protease. Blood 99(5):1850–1852
249. Nie XH, Ou-yang J, Xing Y et al (2015) Paeoniflorin inhibits human glioma cells via STAT3 degradation by the ubiquitin-proteasome pathway. Drug Des Devel Ther 9:5611–5622
250. Fu J, Chen D, Zhao B et al (2012) Luteolin induces carcinoma cell apoptosis through binding Hsp90 to suppress constitutive activation of STAT3. PLoS One 7(11):e49194
251. Darnowski JW, Goulette FA, Guan YJ et al (2006) Stat3 cleavage by caspases: impact on full-length Stat3 expression, fragment formation, and transcriptional activity. J Biol Chem 281(26):17707–17717
252. Matthews JR, Watson SM, Tevendale MC et al (2007) Caspase-dependent proteolytic cleavage of STAT3alpha in ES cells, in mammary glands undergoing forced involution and in breast cancer cell lines. BMC Cancer 7:29
253. Namanja AT, Wang J, Buettner R et al (2016) Allosteric communication across STAT3 domains associated with STAT3 function and disease-causing mutation. J Mol Biol 428(3):579–589
254. Minus MB, Liu W, Vohidov F et al (2015) Rhodium(II) proximity-labeling identifies a novel target site on STAT3 for inhibitors with potent anti-leukemia activity. Angew Chem Int Ed Engl 54(44):13085–13089
255. Ball DP, Lewis AM, Williams D, Resetca D, Wilson DJ, Gunning PT (2016) Signal transducer and activator of transcription 3 (STAT3) inhibitor, S3I-201, acts as a potent and non-selective alkylating agent. Oncotarget 7(15):20669–20679. doi:10.18632/oncotarget.7838
256. Morlacchi P, Robertson FM, Klostergaard J et al (2014) Targeting SH2 domains in breast cancer. Future Med Chem 6(17):1909–1926

257. Shao H, Xu X, Mastrangelo MA et al (2004) Structural requirements for signal transducer and activator of transcription 3 binding to phosphotyrosine ligands containing the YXXQ motif. J Biol Chem 279(18):18967–18973
258. Miyoshi K, Takaishi M, Nakajima K et al (2011) Stat3 as a therapeutic target for the treatment of psoriasis: a clinical feasibility study with STA-21, a Stat3 inhibitor. J Invest Dermatol 131(1):108–117
259. Chen R, Chen B (2015) Siltuximab (CNTO 328): a promising option for human malignancies. Drug Des Dev Ther 9:3455–3458
260. Dijkgraaf EM, Santegoets SJ, Reyners AK et al (2015) A phase I trial combining carboplatin/doxorubicin with tocilizumab, an anti-IL-6R monoclonal antibody, and interferon-alpha2b in patients with recurrent epithelial ovarian cancer. Ann Oncol 26(10):2141–2149
261. Kennedy GA, Varelias A, Vuckovic S et al (2014) Addition of interleukin-6 inhibition with tocilizumab to standard graft-versus-host disease prophylaxis after allogeneic stem-cell transplantation: a phase 1/2 trial. Lancet Oncol 15(13):1451–1459
262. Patel KP, Newberry KJ, Luthra R et al (2015) Correlation of mutation profile and response in patients with myelofibrosis treated with ruxolitinib. Blood 126(6):7907
263. Daver N, Cortes J, Newberry K et al (2015) Ruxolitinib in combination with lenalidomide as therapy for patients with myelofibrosis. Haematologica 100(8):1058–1063
264. Loh ML, Tasian SK, Rabin KR et al (2015) A phase 1 dosing study of ruxolitinib in children with relapsed or refractory solid tumors, leukemias, or myeloproliferative neoplasms: A Children's Oncology Group Phase 1 Consortium Study (ADVL1011). Pediatr Blood Cancer 62(10):1717–1724
265. Mead AJ, Milojkovic D, Knapper S et al (2015) Response to ruxolitinib in patients with intermediate-1-, intermediate-2-, and high-risk myelofibrosis: results of the UK ROBUST Trial. Br J Haematol 170(1):29–39
266. Arana Yi C, Tam CS, Verstovsek S (2015) Efficacy and safety of ruxolitinib in the treatment of patients with myelofibrosis. Future Oncol 11(5):719–733
267. Pemmaraju N, Kantarjian H, Kadia T et al (2015) A phase I/II study of the Janus kinase (JAK)1 and 2 inhibitor ruxolitinib in patients with relapsed or refractory acute myeloid leukemia. Clin Lymphoma Myeloma Leuk 15(3):171–176
268. Santos FP, Verstovsek S (2014) Efficacy of ruxolitinib for myelofibrosis. Expert Opin Pharmacother 15(10):1465–1473
269. Hedvat M, Huszar D, Herrmann A et al (2009) The JAK2 inhibitor AZD1480 potently blocks Stat3 signaling and oncogenesis in solid tumors. Cancer Cell 16(6):487–497
270. Suryani S, Bracken LS, Harvey RC et al (2015) Evaluation of the in vitro and in vivo efficacy of the JAK inhibitor AZD1480 against JAK-mutated acute lymphoblastic leukemia. Mol Cancer Ther 14(2):364–374
271. Wang SW, Hu J, Guo QH et al (2014) AZD1480, a JAK inhibitor, inhibits cell growth and survival of colorectal cancer via modulating the JAK2/STAT3 signaling pathway. Oncol Rep 32(5):1991–1998
272. Yan S, Li Z, Thiele CJ (2013) Inhibition of STAT3 with orally active JAK inhibitor, AZD1480, decreases tumor growth in neuroblastoma and pediatric sarcomas in vitro and in vivo. Oncotarget 4(3):433–445
273. Bendell JC, Hong DS, Burris HA 3rd et al (2014) Phase 1, open-label, dose-escalation, and pharmacokinetic study of STAT3 inhibitor OPB-31121 in subjects with advanced solid tumors. Cancer Chemother Pharmacol 74(1):125–130
274. Brambilla L, Genini D, Laurini E et al (2015) Hitting the right spot: mechanism of action of OPB-31121, a novel and potent inhibitor of the signal transducer and activator of transcription 3 (STAT3). Mol Oncol 9(6):1194–1206
275. Hayakawa F, Sugimoto K, Harada Y et al (2013) A novel STAT inhibitor, OPB-31121, has a significant antitumor effect on leukemia with STAT-addictive oncokinases. Blood Cancer J 3:e166

276. Kim MJ, Nam HJ, Kim HP et al (2013) OPB-31121, a novel small molecular inhibitor, disrupts the JAK2/STAT3 pathway and exhibits an antitumor activity in gastric cancer cells. Cancer Lett 335(1):145–152
277. Oh DY, Lee SH, Han SW et al (2015) Phase I study of OPB-31121, an oral STAT3 inhibitor, in patients with advanced solid tumors. Cancer Res Treat 47(4):607–615
278. Okusaka T, Ueno H, Ikeda M et al (2015) Phase 1 and pharmacological trial of OPB-31121, a signal transducer and activator of transcription-3 inhibitor, in patients with advanced hepatocellular carcinoma. Hepatol Res 45(13):1283–1291
279. Pardanani A, Harrison C, Cortes JE et al (2015) Safety and efficacy of Fedratinib in patients with primary or secondary myelofibrosis: a randomized clinical trial. JAMA Oncol 1(5):643–651
280. Pardanani A, Tefferi A, Jamieson C et al (2015) A phase 2 randomized dose-ranging study of the JAK2-selective inhibitor fedratinib (SAR302503) in patients with myelofibrosis. Blood Cancer J 5:e335
281. Polverelli N, Catani L, Vianelli N et al (2015) Ruxolitinib- but not fedratinib-induced extreme thrombocytosis: the combination therapy with hydroxyurea and ruxolitinib is effective in reducing platelet count and splenomegaly/constitutional symptoms. Ann Hematol 94(9):1585–1587
282. Zhang M, Xu CR, Shamiyeh E et al (2014) A randomized, placebo-controlled study of the pharmacokinetics, pharmacodynamics, and tolerability of the oral JAK2 inhibitor fedratinib (SAR302503) in healthy volunteers. J Clin Pharmacol 54(4):415–421
283. Takakura A, Nelson EA, Haque N et al (2011) Pyrimethamine inhibits adult polycystic kidney disease by modulating STAT signaling pathways. Hum Mol Genet 20(21):4143–4154
284. Derenzini E, Younes A (2013) Targeting the JAK-STAT pathway in lymphoma: a focus on pacritinib. Expert Opin Investig Drugs 22(6):775–785
285. Komrokji RS, Seymour JF, Roberts AW et al (2015) Results of a phase 2 study of pacritinib (SB1518), a JAK2/JAK2(V617F) inhibitor, in patients with myelofibrosis. Blood 125(17):2649–2655
286. Huang Y, Zhou X, Liu A et al (2014) Signal transducer and activator of transcription-3 inhibitor WP1066 affects human tongue squamous cell carcinoma proliferation and apoptosis in vitro and in vivo. Zhonghua Kou Qiang Yi Xue Za Zhi 49(5):308–313
287. Lu K, Fang XS, Feng LL et al (2015) The STAT3 inhibitor WP1066 reverses the resistance of chronic lymphocytic leukemia cells to histone deacetylase inhibitors induced by interleukin-6. Cancer Lett 359(2):250–258
288. Verstovsek S, Manshouri T, Quintas-Cardama A et al (2008) WP1066, a novel JAK2 inhibitor, suppresses proliferation and induces apoptosis in erythroid human cells carrying the JAK2 V617F mutation. Clin Cancer Res 14(3):788–796
289. Zhou X, Ren Y, Liu A et al (2014) STAT3 inhibitor WP1066 attenuates miRNA-21 to suppress human oral squamous cell carcinoma growth in vitro and in vivo. Oncol Rep 31(5):2173–2180
290. Zhou X, Ren Y, Liu A et al (2014) WP1066 sensitizes oral squamous cell carcinoma cells to cisplatin by targeting STAT3/miR-21 axis. Sci Rep 4:7461
291. Ogura M, Uchida T, Terui Y et al (2015) Phase I study of OPB-51602, an oral inhibitor of signal transducer and activator of transcription 3, in patients with relapsed/refractory hematological malignancies. Cancer Sci 106(7):896–901
292. Sen M, Thomas SM, Kim S et al (2012) First-in-human trial of a STAT3 decoy oligonucleotide in head and neck tumors: implications for cancer therapy. Cancer Discov 2(8):694–705
293. Hong D, Kurzrock R, Kim Y et al (2015) AZD9150, a next-generation antisense oligonucleotide inhibitor of STAT3 with early evidence of clinical activity in lymphoma and lung cancer. Sci Transl Med 7(314):314ra185
294. Banes-Berceli AK, Shaw S, Ma G et al (2006) Effect of simvastatin on high glucose- and angiotensin II-induced activation of the JAK/STAT pathway in mesangial cells. Am J Physiol Renal Physiol 291(1):F116–F121

295. Fang Z, Tang Y, Fang J et al (2013) Simvastatin inhibits renal cancer cell growth and metastasis via AKT/mTOR, ERK and JAK2/STAT3 pathway. PLoS One 8(5):e62823
296. Oh B, Kim TY, Min HJ et al (2013) Synergistic killing effect of imatinib and simvastatin on imatinib-resistant chronic myelogenous leukemia cells. Anticancer Drugs 24(1):20–31
297. Chang Q, Daly L, Bromberg J (2014) The IL-6 feed-forward loop: a driver of tumorigenesis. Semin Immunol 26(1):48–53
298. Fisher DT, Appenheimer MM, Evans SS (2014) The two faces of IL-6 in the tumor microenvironment. Semin Immunol 26(1):38–47
299. Heo TH, Wahler J, Suh N (2016) Potential therapeutic implications of IL-6/IL-6R/gp130-targeting agents in breast cancer. Oncotarget 7(13):15460–15473
300. Markham A, Patel T (2014) Siltuximab: first global approval. Drugs 74(10):1147–1152
301. van Rhee F, Fayad L, Voorhees P et al (2010) Siltuximab, a novel anti-interleukin-6 monoclonal antibody, for Castleman's disease. J Clin Oncol 28(23):3701–3708
302. van Rhee F, Wong RS, Munshi N et al (2014) Siltuximab for multicentric Castleman's disease: a randomised, double-blind, placebo-controlled trial. Lancet Oncol 15(9):966–974
303. Suzuki K, Ogura M, Abe Y et al (2015) Phase 1 study in Japan of siltuximab, an anti-IL-6 monoclonal antibody, in relapsed/refractory multiple myeloma. Int J Hematol 101(3):286–294
304. Doggrell SA (2008) Is tocilizumab an option for the treatment of arthritis? Expert Opin Pharmacother 9(11):2009–2013
305. Ganetsky A (2013) Ruxolitinib: a new treatment option for myelofibrosis. Pharmacotherapy 33(1):84–92
306. Deininger M, Radich J, Burn TC et al (2015) The effect of long-term ruxolitinib treatment on JAK2p.V617F allele burden in patients with myelofibrosis. Blood 126(13):1551–1554
307. Hahm ER, Singh SV (2010) Sulforaphane inhibits constitutive and interleukin-6-induced activation of signal transducer and activator of transcription 3 in prostate cancer cells. Cancer Prev Res (Phila) 3(4):484–494
308. Hutzen B, Willis W, Jones S et al (2009) Dietary agent, benzyl isothiocyanate inhibits signal transducer and activator of transcription 3 phosphorylation and collaborates with sulforaphane in the growth suppression of PANC-1 cancer cells. Cancer Cell Int 9:24
309. Kirito K, Osawa M, Morita H et al (2002) A functional role of Stat3 in in vivo megakaryopoiesis. Blood 99(9):3220–3227
310. Mantel C, Messina-Graham S, Moh A et al (2012) Mouse hematopoietic cell-targeted STAT3 deletion: stem/progenitor cell defects, mitochondrial dysfunction, ROS overproduction, and a rapid aging-like phenotype. Blood 120(13):2589–2599
311. Arnaud C, Burger F, Steffens S et al (2005) Statins reduce interleukin-6-induced C-reactive protein in human hepatocytes: new evidence for direct antiinflammatory effects of statins. Arterioscler Thromb Vasc Biol 25(6):1231–1236
312. Ivanov VN, Hei TK (2011) Regulation of apoptosis in human melanoma and neuroblastoma cells by statins, sodium arsenite and TRAIL: a role of combined treatment versus monotherapy. Apoptosis 16(12):1268–1284
313. Omoigui S (2007) The Interleukin-6 inflammation pathway from cholesterol to aging--role of statins, bisphosphonates and plant polyphenols in aging and age-related diseases. Immun Ageing 4:1
314. Lavecchia A, Di Giovanni C, Novellino E (2011) STAT-3 inhibitors: state of the art and new horizons for cancer treatment. Curr Med Chem 18(16):2359–2375
315. Yin H, Hamilton AD (2005) Strategies for targeting protein–protein interactions with synthetic agents. Angew Chem Int Ed Engl 44(27):4130–4163
316. Sayed D, Badrawy H, Gaber N et al (2014) p-Stat3 and bcr/abl gene expression in chronic myeloid leukemia and their relation to imatinib therapy. Leuk Res 38(2):243–250
317. Epling-Burnette PK, Liu JH, Catlett-Falcone R et al (2001) Inhibition of STAT3 signaling leads to apoptosis of leukemic large granular lymphocytes and decreased Mcl-1 expression. J Clin Invest 107(3):351–362

318. Andersson EI, Rajala HL, Eldfors S et al (2013) Novel somatic mutations in large granular lymphocytic leukemia affecting the STAT-pathway and T-cell activation. Blood Cancer J 3:e168
319. Frank DA, Mahajan S, Ritz J (1997) B lymphocytes from patients with chronic lymphocytic leukemia contain signal transducer and activator of transcription (STAT) 1 and STAT3 constitutively phosphorylated on serine residues. J Clin Invest 100(12):3140–3148
320. Hazan-Halevy I, Harris D, Liu Z et al (2010) STAT3 is constitutively phosphorylated on serine 727 residues, binds DNA, and activates transcription in CLL cells. Blood 115(14):2852–2863
321. Skinnider BF, Elia AJ, Gascoyne RD et al (2002) Signal transducer and activator of transcription 6 is frequently activated in Hodgkin and Reed-Sternberg cells of Hodgkin lymphoma. Blood 99(2):618–626
322. Khoury JD, Medeiros LJ, Rassidakis GZ et al (2003) Differential expression and clinical significance of tyrosine-phosphorylated STAT3 in ALK+ and ALK- anaplastic large cell lymphoma. Clin Cancer Res 9(10 Pt 1):3692–3699
323. McKenzie RC, Jones CL, Tosi I et al (2012) Constitutive activation of STAT3 in Sezary syndrome is independent of SHP-1. Leukemia 26(2):323–331
324. Zamo A, Chiarle R, Piva R et al (2002) Anaplastic lymphoma kinase (ALK) activates Stat3 and protects hematopoietic cells from cell death. Oncogene 21(7):1038–1047
325. Schlette EJ, Medeiros LJ, Goy A et al (2004) Survivin expression predicts poorer prognosis in anaplastic large-cell lymphoma. J Clin Oncol 22(9):1682–1688
326. Wu ZL, Song YQ, Shi YF et al (2011) High nuclear expression of STAT3 is associated with unfavorable prognosis in diffuse large B-cell lymphoma. J Hematol Oncol 4(1):31
327. Stewart DA, Bahlis N, Mansoor A (2009) pY-STAT3 and p53 expression predict outcome for poor prognosis diffuse large B-cell lymphoma treated with high dose chemotherapy and autologous stem cell transplantation. Leuk Lymphoma 50(8):1276–1282
328. Ding BB, Yu JJ, Yu RY et al (2008) Constitutively activated STAT3 promotes cell proliferation and survival in the activated B-cell subtype of diffuse large B-cell lymphomas. Blood 111(3):1515–1523
329. Huang X, Meng B, Iqbal J et al (2013) Activation of the STAT3 signaling pathway is associated with poor survival in diffuse large B-cell lymphoma treated with R-CHOP. J Clin Oncol 31(36):4520–4528
330. Berishaj M, Gao SP, Ahmed S et al (2007) Stat3 is tyrosine-phosphorylated through the interleukin-6/glycoprotein 130/Janus kinase pathway in breast cancer. Breast Cancer Res 9(3):R32
331. Diaz N, Minton S, Cox C et al (2006) Activation of stat3 in primary tumors from high-risk breast cancer patients is associated with elevated levels of activated SRC and survivin expression. Clin Cancer Res 12(1):20–28
332. Jiang R, Jin Z, Liu Z et al (2011) Correlation of activated STAT3 expression with clinicopathologic features in lung adenocarcinoma and squamous cell carcinoma. Mol Diagn Ther 15(6):347–352
333. Xu YH, Lu S (2014) A meta-analysis of STAT3 and phospho-STAT3 expression and survival of patients with non-small-cell lung cancer. Eur J Surg Oncol 40(3):311–317
334. Chen CL, Hsieh FC, Lieblein JC et al (2007) Stat3 activation in human endometrial and cervical cancers. Br J Cancer 96(4):591–599
335. Takemoto S, Ushijima K, Kawano K et al (2009) Expression of activated signal transducer and activator of transcription-3 predicts poor prognosis in cervical squamous-cell carcinoma. Br J Cancer 101(6):967–972
336. Qin J, Yang B, Xu BQ et al (2014) Concurrent CD44s and STAT3 expression in human clear cell renal cellular carcinoma and its impact on survival. Int J Clin Exp Pathol 7(6):3235–3244
337. Lin L, Amin R, Gallicano GI et al (2009) The STAT3 inhibitor NSC 74859 is effective in hepatocellular cancers with disrupted TGF-beta signaling. Oncogene 28(7):961–972

338. Yang SF, Wang SN, Wu CF et al (2007) Altered p-STAT3 (tyr705) expression is associated with histological grading and intratumour microvessel density in hepatocellular carcinoma. J Clin Pathol 60(6):642–648

339. Dokduang H, Techasen A, Namwat N et al (2014) STATs profiling reveals predominantly-activated STAT3 in cholangiocarcinoma genesis and progression. J Hepatobiliary Pancreat Sci 21(10):767–776

340. Morikawa T, Baba Y, Yamauchi M et al (2011) STAT3 expression, molecular features, inflammation patterns, and prognosis in a database of 724 colorectal cancers. Clin Cancer Res 17(6):1452–1462

341. Savarese TM, Campbell CL, McQuain C et al (2002) Coexpression of oncostatin M and its receptors and evidence for STAT3 activation in human ovarian carcinomas. Cytokine 17(6):324–334

342. Silver DL, Naora H, Liu J et al (2004) Activated signal transducer and activator of transcription (STAT) 3: localization in focal adhesions and function in ovarian cancer cell motility. Cancer Res 64(10):3550–3558

343. Huang C, Huang R, Chang W et al (2012) The expression and clinical significance of pSTAT3, VEGF and VEGF-C in pancreatic adenocarcinoma. Neoplasma 59(1):52–61

344. Lee TL, Yeh J, Van Waes C et al (2006) Epigenetic modification of SOCS-1 differentially regulates STAT3 activation in response to interleukin-6 receptor and epidermal growth factor receptor signaling through JAK and/or MEK in head and neck squamous cell carcinomas. Mol Cancer Ther 5(1):8–19

345. Seethala RR, Gooding WE, Handler PN et al (2008) Immunohistochemical analysis of phosphotyrosine signal transducer and activator of transcription 3 and epidermal growth factor receptor autocrine signaling pathways in head and neck cancers and metastatic lymph nodes. Clin Cancer Res 14(5):1303–1309

346. Masuda M, Suzui M, Yasumatu R et al (2002) Constitutive activation of signal transducers and activators of transcription 3 correlates with cyclin D1 overexpression and may provide a novel prognostic marker in head and neck squamous cell carcinoma. Cancer Res 62(12):3351–3355

347. Shah NG, Trivedi TI, Tankshali RA et al (2006) Stat3 expression in oral squamous cell carcinoma: association with clinicopathological parameters and survival. Int J Biol Markers 21(3):175–183

348. Mizoguchi M, Betensky RA, Batchelor TT et al (2006) Activation of STAT3, MAPK, and AKT in malignant astrocytic gliomas: correlation with EGFR status, tumor grade, and survival. J Neuropathol Exp Neurol 65(12):1181–1188

349. Abou-Ghazal M, Yang DS, Qiao W et al (2008) The incidence, correlation with tumor-infiltrating inflammation, and prognosis of phosphorylated STAT3 expression in human gliomas. Clin Cancer Res 14(24):8228–8235

350. Lo HW, Cao X, Zhu H et al (2008) Constitutively activated STAT3 frequently coexpresses with epidermal growth factor receptor in high-grade gliomas and targeting STAT3 sensitizes them to Iressa and alkylators. Clin Cancer Res 14(19):6042–6054

351. Liu HJ, Moroi Y, Masuda T et al (2006) Expression of phosphorylated Stat3, cyclin D1 and Bcl-xL in extramammary Paget disease. Br J Dermatol 154(5):926–932

352. Dong W, Cui J, Tian X et al (2014) Aberrant sonic hedgehog signaling pathway and STAT3 activation in papillary thyroid cancer. Int J Clin Exp Med 7(7):1786–1793

353. Bos M, Mendelsohn J, Kim YM et al (1997) PD153035, a tyrosine kinase inhibitor, prevents epidermal growth factor receptor activation and inhibits growth of cancer cells in a receptor number-dependent manner. Clin Cancer Res 3(11):2099–2106

354. Kunkel MW, Hook KE, Howard CT et al (1996) Inhibition of the epidermal growth factor receptor tyrosine kinase by PD153035 in human A431 tumors in athymic nude mice. Invest New Drugs 13(4):295–302

355. Li L, Shaw PE (2002) Autocrine-mediated activation of STAT3 correlates with cell proliferation in breast carcinoma lines. J Biol Chem 277(20):17397–17405

356. Fujiwara Y, Komohara Y, Kudo R et al (2011) Oleanolic acid inhibits macrophage differentiation into the M2 phenotype and glioblastoma cell proliferation by suppressing the activation of STAT3. Oncol Rep 26(6):1533–1537
357. Kim HS, Sung HY, Kim MS et al (2013) Oleanolic acid suppresses resistin induction in adipocytes by modulating Tyk-STAT signaling. Nutr Res 33(2):144–153
358. Chen X, Du Y, Nan J et al (2013) Brevilin A, a novel natural product, inhibits janus kinase activity and blocks STAT3 signaling in cancer cells. PLoS One 8(5):e63697
359. Boyle DL, Soma K, Hodge J et al (2015) The JAK inhibitor tofacitinib suppresses synovial JAK1-STAT signalling in rheumatoid arthritis. Ann Rheum Dis 74(6):1311–1316
360. Gao W, McGarry T, Orr C et al (2016) Tofacitinib regulates synovial inflammation in psoriatic arthritis, inhibiting STAT activation and induction of negative feedback inhibitors. Ann Rheum Dis 75(1):311–315
361. Rosengren S, Corr M, Firestein GS et al (2012) The JAK inhibitor CP-690,550 (tofacitinib) inhibits TNF-induced chemokine expression in fibroblast-like synoviocytes: autocrine role of type I interferon. Ann Rheum Dis 71(3):440–447
362. Yoshida H, Kimura A, Fukaya T et al (2012) Low dose CP-690,550 (tofacitinib), a pan-JAK inhibitor, accelerates the onset of experimental autoimmune encephalomyelitis by potentiating Th17 differentiation. Biochem Biophys Res Commun 418(2):234–240
363. Manshouri T, Quintas-Cardama A, Nussenzveig RH et al (2008) The JAK kinase inhibitor CP-690,550 suppresses the growth of human polycythemia vera cells carrying the JAK2V617F mutation. Cancer Sci 99(6):1265–1273
364. Siegelin MD, Raskett CM, Gilbert CA et al (2010) Sorafenib exerts anti-glioma activity in vitro and in vivo. Neurosci Lett 478(3):165–170
365. Couto JP, Almeida A, Daly L et al (2012) AZD1480 blocks growth and tumorigenesis of RET- activated thyroid cancer cell lines. PLoS One 7(10):e46869
366. Gu L, Talati P, Vogiatzi P et al (2014) Pharmacologic suppression of JAK1/2 by JAK1/2 inhibitor AZD1480 potently inhibits IL-6-induced experimental prostate cancer metastases formation. Mol Cancer Ther 13(5):1246–1258
367. Houghton PJ, Kurmasheva RT, Lyalin D et al (2014) Initial solid tumor testing (stage 1) of AZD1480, an inhibitor of Janus kinases 1 and 2 by the pediatric preclinical testing program. Pediatr Blood Cancer 61(11):1972–1979
368. Maenhout SK, Du Four S, Corthals J et al (2014) AZD1480 delays tumor growth in a melanoma model while enhancing the suppressive activity of myeloid-derived suppressor cells. Oncotarget 5(16):6801–6815
369. Scuto A, Krejci P, Popplewell L et al (2011) The novel JAK inhibitor AZD1480 blocks STAT3 and FGFR3 signaling, resulting in suppression of human myeloma cell growth and survival. Leukemia 25(3):538–550
370. Xin H, Herrmann A, Reckamp K et al (2011) Antiangiogenic and antimetastatic activity of JAK inhibitor AZD1480. Cancer Res 71(21):6601–6610
371. Amit-Vazina M, Shishodia S, Harris D et al (2005) Atiprimod blocks STAT3 phosphorylation and induces apoptosis in multiple myeloma cells. Br J Cancer 93(1):70–80
372. Choudhari SR, Khan MA, Harris G et al (2007) Deactivation of Akt and STAT3 signaling promotes apoptosis, inhibits proliferation, and enhances the sensitivity of hepatocellular carcinoma cells to an anticancer agent, Atiprimod. Mol Cancer Ther 6(1):112–121
373. Faderl S, Ferrajoli A, Harris D et al (2007) Atiprimod blocks phosphorylation of JAK-STAT and inhibits proliferation of acute myeloid leukemia (AML) cells. Leuk Res 31(1):91–95
374. Quintas-Cardama A, Manshouri T, Estrov Z et al (2011) Preclinical characterization of atiprimod, a novel JAK2 AND JAK3 inhibitor. Invest New Drugs 29(5):818–826
375. Hamasaki M, Hideshima T, Tassone P et al (2005) Azaspirane (N-N-diethyl-8,8-dipropyl-2-azaspiro [4.5] decane-2-propanamine) inhibits human multiple myeloma cell growth in the bone marrow milieu in vitro and in vivo. Blood 105(11):4470–4476
376. Kim NH, Lee MY, Park SJ et al (2007) Auranofin blocks interleukin-6 signalling by inhibiting phosphorylation of JAK1 and STAT3. Immunology 122(4):607–614

377. Kim NH, Park HJ, Oh MK et al (2013) Antiproliferative effect of gold(I) compound aurano-fin through inhibition of STAT3 and telomerase activity in MDA-MB 231 human breast cancer cells. BMB Rep 46(1):59–64
378. Madeira JM, Gibson DL, Kean WF et al (2012) The biological activity of auranofin: implications for novel treatment of diseases. Inflammopharmacology 20(6):297–306
379. Nakaya A, Sagawa M, Muto A et al (2011) The gold compound auranofin induces apoptosis of human multiple myeloma cells through both down-regulation of STAT3 and inhibition of NF-kappaB activity. Leuk Res 35(2):243–249
380. Kalogris C, Garulli C, Pietrella L et al (2014) Sanguinarine suppresses basal-like breast cancer growth through dihydrofolate reductase inhibition. Biochem Pharmacol 90(3):226–234
381. Sun M, Liu C, Nadiminty N et al (2012) Inhibition of Stat3 activation by sanguinarine suppresses prostate cancer cell growth and invasion. Prostate 72(1):82–89
382. Gu S, Yang XC, Xiang XY et al (2015) Sanguinarine-induced apoptosis in lung adenocarcinoma cells is dependent on reactive oxygen species production and endoplasmic reticulum stress. Oncol Rep 34(2):913–919
383. Blaskovich MA, Sun J, Cantor A et al (2003) Discovery of JSI-124 (cucurbitacin I), a selective Janus kinase/signal transducer and activator of transcription 3 signaling pathway inhibitor with potent antitumor activity against human and murine cancer cells in mice. Cancer Res 63(6):1270–1279
384. Ishdorj G, Johnston JB, Gibson SB (2010) Inhibition of constitutive activation of STAT3 by curcurbitacin-I (JSI-124) sensitized human B-leukemia cells to apoptosis. Mol Cancer Ther 9(12):3302–3314
385. Aribi A, Gery S, Lee DH et al (2013) The triterpenoid cucurbitacin B augments the antiproliferative activity of chemotherapy in human breast cancer. Int J Cancer 132(12):2730–2737
386. Chan KT, Li K, Liu SL et al (2010) Cucurbitacin B inhibits STAT3 and the Raf/MEK/ERK pathway in leukemia cell line K562. Cancer Lett 289(1):46–52
387. Chan KT, Meng FY, Li Q et al (2010) Cucurbitacin B induces apoptosis and S phase cell cycle arrest in BEL-7402 human hepatocellular carcinoma cells and is effective via oral administration. Cancer Lett 294(1):118–124
388. Iwanski GB, Lee DH, En-Gal S et al (2010) Cucurbitacin B, a novel in vivo potentiator of gemcitabine with low toxicity in the treatment of pancreatic cancer. Br J Pharmacol 160(4):998–1007
389. Liu T, Peng H, Zhang M et al (2010) Cucurbitacin B, a small molecule inhibitor of the Stat3 signaling pathway, enhances the chemosensitivity of laryngeal squamous cell carcinoma cells to cisplatin. Eur J Pharmacol 641(1):15–22
390. Thoennissen NH, Iwanski GB, Doan NB et al (2009) Cucurbitacin B induces apoptosis by inhibition of the JAK/STAT pathway and potentiates antiproliferative effects of gemcitabine on pancreatic cancer cells. Cancer Res 69(14):5876–5884
391. Wakimoto N, Yin D, O'Kelly J et al (2008) Cucurbitacin B has a potent antiproliferative effect on breast cancer cells in vitro and in vivo. Cancer Sci 99(9):1793–1797
392. Zheng Q, Liu Y, Liu W et al (2014) Cucurbitacin B inhibits growth and induces apoptosis through the JAK2/STAT3 and MAPK pathways in SHSY5Y human neuroblastoma cells. Mol Med Rep 10(1):89–94
393. Dong Y, Lu B, Zhang X et al (2010) Cucurbitacin E, a tetracyclic triterpenes compound from Chinese medicine, inhibits tumor angiogenesis through VEGFR2-mediated Jak2-STAT3 signaling pathway. Carcinogenesis 31(12):2097–2104
394. Sun C, Zhang M, Shan X et al (2010) Inhibitory effect of cucurbitacin E on pancreatic cancer cells growth via STAT3 signaling. J Cancer Res Clin Oncol 136(4):603–610
395. Sun J, Blaskovich MA, Jove R et al (2005) Cucurbitacin Q: a selective STAT3 activation inhibitor with potent antitumor activity. Oncogene 24(20):3236–3245
396. Fan XX, Li N, Wu JL et al (2014) Celastrol induces apoptosis in gefitinib-resistant non-small cell lung cancer cells via caspases-dependent pathways and Hsp90 client protein degradation. Molecules 19(3):3508–3522

397. Kannaiyan R, Hay HS, Rajendran P et al (2011) Celastrol inhibits proliferation and induces chemosensitization through down-regulation of NF-kappaB and STAT3 regulated gene products in multiple myeloma cells. Br J Pharmacol 164(5):1506–1521

398. Rajendran P, Li F, Shanmugam MK et al (2012) Celastrol suppresses growth and induces apoptosis of human hepatocellular carcinoma through the modulation of STAT3/JAK2 signaling cascade in vitro and in vivo. Cancer Prev Res (Phila) 5(4):631–643

399. Subramaniam A, Shanmugam MK, Ong TH et al (2013) Emodin inhibits growth and induces apoptosis in an orthotopic hepatocellular carcinoma model by blocking activation of STAT3. Br J Pharmacol 170(4):807–821

400. Buettner R, Mesa T, Vultur A et al (2008) Inhibition of Src family kinases with dasatinib blocks migration and invasion of human melanoma cells. Mol Cancer Res 6(11):1766–1774

401. Michels S, Trautmann M, Sievers E et al (2013) SRC signaling is crucial in the growth of synovial sarcoma cells. Cancer Res 73(8):2518–2528

402. Jung JE, Kim HS, Lee CS et al (2007) Caffeic acid and its synthetic derivative CADPE suppress tumor angiogenesis by blocking STAT3-mediated VEGF expression in human renal carcinoma cells. Carcinogenesis 28(8):1780–1787

403. Choi D, Han J, Lee Y et al (2010) Caffeic acid phenethyl ester is a potent inhibitor of HIF prolyl hydroxylase: structural analysis and pharmacological implication. J Nutr Biochem 21(9):809–817

404. Won C, Lee CS, Lee JK et al (2010) CADPE suppresses cyclin D1 expression in hepatocellular carcinoma by blocking IL-6-induced STAT3 activation. Anticancer Res 30(2):481–488

405. Zheng Q, Han L, Dong Y et al (2014) JAK2/STAT3 targeted therapy suppresses tumor invasion via disruption of the EGFRvIII/JAK2/STAT3 axis and associated focal adhesion in EGFRvIII-expressing glioblastoma. Neuro Oncol 16(9):1229–1243

406. Horiguchi A, Oya M, Marumo K et al (2002) STAT3, but not ERKs, mediates the IL-6-induced proliferation of renal cancer cells, ACHN and 769P. Kidney Int 61(3):926–938

407. Horiguchi A, Asano T, Kuroda K et al (2010) STAT3 inhibitor WP1066 as a novel therapeutic agent for renal cell carcinoma. Br J Cancer 102(11):1592–1599

408. Pardanani A, Hood J, Lasho T et al (2007) TG101209, a small molecule JAK2-selective kinase inhibitor potently inhibits myeloproliferative disorder-associated JAK2V617F and MPLW515L/K mutations. Leukemia 21(8):1658–1668

409. Ramakrishnan V, Kimlinger T, Haug J et al (2010) TG101209, a novel JAK2 inhibitor, has significant in vitro activity in multiple myeloma and displays preferential cytotoxicity for CD45+ myeloma cells. Am J Hematol 85(9):675–686

410. Lin L, Deangelis S, Foust E et al (2010) A novel small molecule inhibits STAT3 phosphorylation and DNA binding activity and exhibits potent growth suppressive activity in human cancer cells. Mol Cancer 9:217

411. Lin L, Hutzen B, Zuo M et al (2010) Novel STAT3 phosphorylation inhibitors exhibit potent growth-suppressive activity in pancreatic and breast cancer cells. Cancer Res 70(6):2445–2454

412. Haridas V, Nishimura G, Xu ZX et al (2009) Avicin D: a protein reactive plant isoprenoid dephosphorylates Stat 3 by regulating both kinase and phosphatase activities. PLoS One 4(5):e5578

413. Zhang C, Li B, Gaikwad AS et al (2008) Avicin D selectively induces apoptosis and down-regulates p-STAT-3, bcl-2, and survivin in cutaneous T-cell lymphoma cells. J Invest Dermatol 128(11):2728–2735

414. Nam S, Wen W, Schroeder A et al (2013) Dual inhibition of Janus and Src family kinases by novel indirubin derivative blocks constitutively-activated Stat3 signaling associated with apoptosis of human pancreatic cancer cells. Mol Oncol 7(3):369–378

415. Liu L, Gaboriaud N, Vougogianopoulou K et al (2014) MLS-2384, a new 6-bromoindirubin derivative with dual JAK/Src kinase inhibitory activity, suppresses growth of diverse cancer cells. Cancer Biol Ther 15(2):178–184

416. Abubaker K, Luwor RB, Escalona R et al (2014) Targeted disruption of the JAK2/STAT3 pathway in combination with systemic administration of Paclitaxel inhibits the priming of ovarian cancer stem cells leading to a reduced tumor burden. Front Oncol 4:75

417. Abubaker K, Luwor RB, Zhu H et al (2014) Inhibition of the JAK2/STAT3 pathway in ovarian cancer results in the loss of cancer stem cell-like characteristics and a reduced tumor burden. BMC Cancer 14:317
418. Rhee YH, Jeong SJ, Lee HJ et al (2012) Inhibition of STAT3 signaling and induction of SHP1 mediate antiangiogenic and antitumor activities of ergosterol peroxide in U266 multiple myeloma cells. BMC Cancer 12:28
419. Aftimos PG, Wiedig M, Langouo Fontsa M et al (2013) Sequential use of protein kinase inhibitors potentiates their toxicity to melanoma cells: a rationale to combine targeted drugs based on protein expression inhibition profiles. Int J Oncol 43(3):919–926
420. Quaglino A, Schere-Levy C, Romorini L et al (2007) Mouse mammary tumors display Stat3 activation dependent on leukemia inhibitory factor signaling. Breast Cancer Res 9(5):R69
421. Li SQ, Cheuk AT, Shern JF et al (2013) Targeting wild-type and mutationally activated FGFR4 in rhabdomyosarcoma with the inhibitor ponatinib (AP24534). PLoS One 8(10):e76551
422. Sahu RP, Srivastava SK (2009) The role of STAT-3 in the induction of apoptosis in pancreatic cancer cells by benzyl isothiocyanate. J Natl Cancer Inst 101(3):176–193
423. Guo Y, Nemeth J, O'Brien C et al (2010) Effects of siltuximab on the IL-6-induced signaling pathway in ovarian cancer. Clin Cancer Res 16(23):5759–5769
424. Song L, Smith MA, Doshi P et al (2014) Antitumor efficacy of the anti-interleukin-6 (IL-6) antibody siltuximab in mouse xenograft models of lung cancer. J Thorac Oncol 9(7):974–982
425. Garbers C, Thaiss W, Jones GW et al (2011) Inhibition of classic signaling is a novel function of soluble glycoprotein 130 (sgp130), which is controlled by the ratio of interleukin 6 and soluble interleukin 6 receptor. J Biol Chem 286(50):42959–42970
426. Wan S, Zhao E, Kryczek I et al (2014) Tumor-associated macrophages produce interleukin 6 and signal via STAT3 to promote expansion of human hepatocellular carcinoma stem cells. Gastroenterology 147(6):1393–1404
427. Ung N, Putoczki TL, Stylli SS et al (2014) Anti-EGFR therapeutic efficacy correlates directly with inhibition of STAT3 activity. Cancer Biol Ther 15(5):623–632
428. Dokduang H, Yongvanit P, Namwat N et al (2016) Xanthohumol inhibits STAT3 activation pathway leading to growth suppression and apoptosis induction in human cholangiocarcinoma cells. Oncol Rep 35(4):2065–2072
429. Jiang W, Zhao S, Xu L et al (2015) The inhibitory effects of xanthohumol, a prenylated chalcone derived from hops, on cell growth and tumorigenesis in human pancreatic cancer. Biomed Pharmacother 73:40–47
430. Agrawal S, Febbraio M, Podrez E et al (2007) Signal transducer and activator of transcription 1 is required for optimal foam cell formation and atherosclerotic lesion development. Circulation 115(23):2939–2947
431. Gunning PT, Katt WP, Glenn M et al (2007) Isoform selective inhibition of STAT1 or STAT3 homo-dimerization via peptidomimetic probes: structural recognition of STAT SH2 domains. Bioorg Med Chem Lett 17(7):1875–1878
432. Shao H, Quintero AJ, Tweardy DJ (2001) Identification and characterization of cis elements in the STAT3 gene regulating STAT3 alpha and STAT3 beta messenger RNA splicing. Blood 98(13):3853–3856
433. Chen J, Bai L, Bernard D et al (2010) Structure-based design of conformationally constrained, cell-permeable STAT3 inhibitors. ACS Med Chem Lett 1(2):85–89
434. Fossey SL, Liao AT, McCleese JK et al (2009) Characterization of STAT3 activation and expression in canine and human osteosarcoma. BMC Cancer 9:81
435. Mencalha AL, Du Rocher B, Salles D et al (2010) LLL-3, a STAT3 inhibitor, represses BCR-ABL-positive cell proliferation, activates apoptosis and improves the effects of Imatinib mesylate. Cancer Chemother Pharmacol 65(6):1039–1046
436. Zhang X, Blaskovich MA, Forinash KD et al (2014) Withacnistin inhibits recruitment of STAT3 and STAT5 to growth factor and cytokine receptors and induces regression of breast tumours. Br J Cancer 111(5):894–902
437. Wu X, Xiao H, Wang R, Liu L, Li C, Lin J (2015) Persistent GP130/STAT3 signaling contributes to the resistance of doxorubicin, cisplatin, and MEK inhibitor in human rhabdomyosarcoma cells. Curr Cancer Drug Targets 16(7):631–638

438. Xiao H, Bid HK, Jou D et al (2015) A novel small molecular STAT3 inhibitor, LY5, inhibits cell viability, cell migration, and angiogenesis in medulloblastoma cells. J Biol Chem 290(6):3418–3429

439. Zhao C, Xiao H, Wu X et al (2015) Rational combination of MEK inhibitor and the STAT3 pathway modulator for the therapy in K-Ras mutated pancreatic and colon cancer cells. Oncotarget 6(16):14472–14487

440. Hillion J, Belton AM, Shah SN et al (2014) Nanoparticle delivery of inhibitory signal transducer and activator of transcription 3 G-quartet oligonucleotides blocks tumor growth in HMGA1 transgenic model of T-cell leukemia. Leuk Lymphoma 55(5):1194–1197

441. Jing N, Sha W, Li Y et al (2005) Rational drug design of G-quartet DNA as anti-cancer agents. Curr Pharm Des 11(22):2841–2854

442. Jing N, Zhu Q, Yuan P et al (2006) Targeting signal transducer and activator of transcription 3 with G-quartet oligonucleotides: a potential novel therapy for head and neck cancer. Mol Cancer Ther 5(2):279–286

443. Zhu Q, Jing N (2007) Computational study on mechanism of G-quartet oligonucleotide T40214 selectively targeting Stat3. J Comput Aided Mol Des 21(10-11):641–648

444. Klein JD, Sano D, Sen M et al (2014) STAT3 oligonucleotide inhibits tumor angiogenesis in preclinical models of squamous cell carcinoma. PLoS One 9(1):e81819

445. Xi S, Gooding WE, Grandis JR (2005) In vivo antitumor efficacy of STAT3 blockade using a transcription factor decoy approach: implications for cancer therapy. Oncogene 24(6): 970–979

446. Barton BE, Murphy TF, Shu P et al (2004) Novel single-stranded oligonucleotides that inhibit signal transducer and activator of transcription 3 induce apoptosis in vitro and in vivo in prostate cancer cell lines. Mol Cancer Ther 3(10):1183–1191

447. Selvendiran K, Ahmed S, Dayton A et al (2011) HO-3867, a curcumin analog, sensitizes cisplatin-resistant ovarian carcinoma, leading to therapeutic synergy through STAT3 inhibition. Cancer Biol Ther 12(9):837–845

448. Tierney BJ, McCann GA, Cohn DE et al (2012) HO-3867, a STAT3 inhibitor induces apoptosis by inactivation of STAT3 activity in BRCA1-mutated ovarian cancer cells. Cancer Biol Ther 13(9):766–775

449. Fang S, Liu B, Sun Q et al (2014) Platelet factor 4 inhibits IL-17/Stat3 pathway via upregulation of SOCS3 expression in melanoma. Inflammation 37(5):1744–1750

450. Liang P, Cheng SH, Cheng CK et al (2013) Platelet factor 4 induces cell apoptosis by inhibition of STAT3 via up-regulation of SOCS3 expression in multiple myeloma. Haematologica 98(2):288–295

451. Granato M, Gilardini Montani MS, Filardi M et al (2015) Capsaicin triggers immunogenic PEL cell death, stimulates DCs and reverts PEL-induced immune suppression. Oncotarget 6(30):29543–29554

452. Madoux F, Koenig M, Sessions H, Nelson E, Mercer BA, Cameron M, Roush W, Frank D, Hodder P (2009) Modulators of STAT Transcription Factors for the Targeted Therapy of Cancer (STAT3 Inhibitors). [updated 2011 Mar 25]. Probe Reports from the NIH Molecular Libraries Program [Internet]. Bethesda (MD) (2010) National Center for Biotechnology Information (US). Available from http://www.ncbi.nlm.nih.gov/books/NBK56232/

453. Ferrajoli A, Faderl S, Van Q et al (2007) WP1066 disrupts Janus kinase-2 and induces caspase-dependent apoptosis in acute myelogenous leukemia cells. Cancer Res 67(23):11291–11299

454. Xue ZJ, Shen L, Wang ZY et al (2014) STAT3 inhibitor WP1066 as a novel therapeutic agent for bCCI neuropathic pain rats. Brain Res 1583:79–88

455. Wong AL, Soo RA, Tan DS et al (2015) Phase I and biomarker study of OPB-51602, a novel signal transducer and activator of transcription (STAT) 3 inhibitor, in patients with refractory solid malignancies. Ann Oncol 26(5):998–1005

Chapter 6
Targeting Upstream Janus Kinases

Parisa Rasighaemi and Alister C. Ward

Abstract Janus kinases (JAKs) are the tyrosine kinases that are the principal activators of STAT proteins – particularly downstream of cytokine receptors – during normal development and homeostasis. The JAKs also make a major contribution to the hyperactivation of STATs observed in various malignancies, including through mutation of the JAKs themselves in several neoplastic conditions. These properties have made JAKs attractive targets for the development of small molecule inhibitors based on similar approaches used for other tyrosine kinases. This chapter details the lead JAK inhibitors, which show variable specificity, including multi-kinase inhibitors that have demonstrated excellent clinical efficacy.

Keywords EGFR • IL-6R • VEGF • SRC • ABL • STAT3 • RTK • Inhibitor • Cancer

6.1 Introduction

As discussed in Chap. 1, JAKs represent one of the major activators of STAT proteins during normal development and homeostasis, especially downstream of cytokine receptors. JAKs are similarly involved in the hyperactivation of STATs that is commonly found in a variety of neoplastic states in which they make a significant contribution to the malignant phenotypes observed. Indeed, in a number of cases of hematological neoplasia, mutation of the JAKs themselves — notably JAK2 V617F — represents the key driver of cytokine-independent STAT activation that underpins the pathophysiology of disease. Tyrosine kinases also represent well-characterized targets for small molecule inhibitors. Collectively, these factors have resulted in the development of an array of JAK inhibitors, several of which have shown clinical efficacy.

P. Rasighaemi (✉) • A.C. Ward
School of Medicine, Deakin University, Geelong, VIC, Australia

Centre for Molecular and Medical Research, Deakin University, Geelong, VIC, Australia
e-mail: parisa.rasighaemi@deakin.edu.au; alister.ward@deakin.edu.au

© Springer International Publishing Switzerland 2016   163
A.C. Ward (ed.), *STAT Inhibitors in Cancer*, Cancer Drug
Discovery and Development, DOI 10.1007/978-3-319-42949-6_6

6.2 JAK Selective Inhibitors

A range of alternative inhibitors have been explored that have variable specificity towards individual JAKs (Fig. 6.1). These are at different stages of the drug development pipeline.

6.2.1 Ruxolitinib

Ruxolitinib (INCB018424) is an oral inhibitor of both JAK1 and JAK2, with no selectivity toward mutant forms of JAK2 [1, 2]. This compound has been shown to act by inhibiting downstream STATs, including STAT5 activation in primary cells carrying JAK2 V617F from MPN patients [3] and STAT3 activation in cisplatin-resistant non-small cell lung cancer (NSCLC) cell lines [4]. Ruxolitinib was the first JAK inhibitor to receive FDA approval for the treatment of myeloproliferative

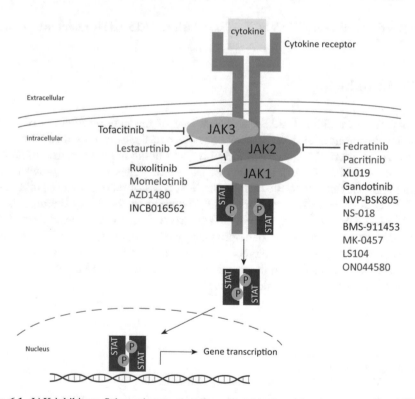

Fig. 6.1 JAK inhibitors. Schematic representation of cytokine/cytokine receptor-mediated STAT activation via JAK kinases, showing the specificity of various JAK inhibitors that act to ablate the STAT activation, with multi-kinase inhibitors displayed in *pink*

neoplasms (MPNs), specifically primary myelofibrosis (MF) and secondary myelofibrosis following polycythemia vera (PV) and essential thrombocythemia (ET), with efficacy demonstrated in several random-controlled trials (RCTs).

The COMFORT I study randomized MF patients to either ruxolitinib or a placebo control. Nearly half of the patients in the ruxolitinib arm demonstrated >50 % decrease in symptoms and >35 % reduction in spleen size at 24 weeks. This correlated with a dramatic decrease in pro-inflammatory, fibrogenic and angiogenic growth factors, as well as abrogation of neoplastic cell proliferation [5, 6]. Importantly, ruxolitinib treated patients showed a significant survival advantage after 28 months compared to those provided with placebo [7]. Interestingly, neither the response rate nor survival advantage were affected by JAK2 V617F mutational status [6, 8].

The COMFORT II trial randomized MF patients to either ruxolitinib or best available therapy (BAT). Over a quarter of patients on ruxolitinib exhibited reduced spleen size at 48 weeks [7–9]. Ruxolitinib treated patients also showed improvement in several clinical symptoms, such as night sweats, itching, weight loss and poor appetite, which correlated with restoration of ferritin and leptin levels as well as a reduction in IL-1Rα. The ruxolitinib and BAT arms showed no statistically significant difference in survival at 48 weeks, but mortality was reduced by 52 % in the ruxolitinib arm at 3 years [10].

Ruxolitinib was also evaluated in PV patients who were either intolerant of, or resistant to, hydroxyl urea (HU). Ruxolitinib elicited rapid and long-lasting clinical improvements, including reduced leucocytosis and thrombocytosis, resolution of splenomegaly and reduced need for phlebotomy, while also being well tolerated [11]. A recent study compared the efficacy and safety of ruxolitinib to BAT in HU-intolerant PV patients and demonstrated that ruxolitinib was more effective that BAT in controling hematocrit, spleen size and disease-related symptoms [12].

A significant proportion of patients administered ruxolitinib experienced grade 3 or 4 anemia and less commonly thrombocytopenia early in the treatment regime, likely due to direct effects on signalling by the cytokines erythropoietin and thrombopoietin. However, these side-effects were typically manageable with transfusions or modification of drug dosage and showed reduced severity over time [7, 8].

Several pre-clinical studies have suggested that ruxolitinib may also be an effective treatment in other cancer settings. For example, this agent was able to induce apoptosis in colorectal cancer cells [13] as well as overcome resistance to cisplatin in NSCLC cell lines [4]. This has provided a rationale for additional RCTs. In patients with refractory metastatic pancreatic cancer, ruxolitinib treatment has yielded clinically significant activity, such as improved survival and reduced tumor burden, particularly in those with systemic inflammation [14]. A phase III of study with 310 subjects are being conducted to confirm the activity of ruxolitinib in these patients (#NCT02117479). Clinical trials investigating the efficacy and safety of this drug in treatment of colorectal cancer (#NCT02119676) and NSCLC (#NCT02119650) are on-going. Ruxolitinib studies in patients with prostate cancer (#NCT00638378) and breast cancer (#NCT01562873) have been terminated due to poor efficacy.

6.2.2   Fedratinib

Fedratinib (SAR302503) is an oral JAK2 inhibitor, which acts on both wild type and mutant forms of JAK2 [15, 16]. This drug was effective in blocking downstream activation of STAT3 and STAT5 in JAK2 mutant cells [15] and peripheral blood leukocytes of patients with MF [17].

In clinical trials with fedratinib, patients with primary MF or MF secondary to PV and ET achieved normalization of leukocyte and thrombocyte counts, reduced spleen size and improved disease related symptoms, including resolution of marrow fibrosis in some cases, with response rates similar to ruxolitinib. Outcomes correlated with significant modulation of key cytokines including decreased loads of TNF-α but increased adiponectin [17–19]. A significant reduction in the JAK2 V617F allele burden was observed particularly in patients with >20 % of this allele, suggesting increased sensitivity of the mutant form of JAK2 [18]. However, this has been contradicted by recent results showing no consistent changes in JAK2 V617F allele burden [17]. Common side effects of fedratinib included myelosuppresion and gastrointestinal toxicity.

Additional studies have examined the efficacy and safety of federatinib in MF patients previously treated with Ruxolitinib with interim results showing clinical beneficial through reduced symptom burden and splenomegaly [17]. A phase I study has also been completed in those with solid tumors (#NCT01836705) although no results have been presented. However, several instances of Wernicke's encephalopathy in federatinib-treated patients has resulted in the halt of all ongoing clinical trials.

6.2.3   Momelotinib

Momelotinib (CYT387) is a selective inhibitor of JAK1 and JAK2 that also exhibits a significantly reduced activity against JAK3. Momelotininb abrogated downstream activation of STAT3 and STAT5 in human erythroleukemia and Ba/F3 cells harbouring the JAK2 V617F mutation [20]. In pre-clinical studies in mice, momelotinib normalized blood counts, spleen size and pro-inflammatory cytokines with no effect on bone marrow hypercellularity or JAK2 V617F mutation burden [21]. Momelotinib also inhibited the erythropoietin-independent proliferation of erythroid colonies from the bone marrow of PV patients [20].

In phase I/II clinical trials with intermediate or high-risk MF patients, momelotinib led to a sustained reduction in spleen size, constitutional symptoms and anemia, with ~70 % of transfusion-dependent patients able to achieve independence. Significantly, patients that had previously failed to respond to ruxolitinib and fedratinib showed clinically significant responses to this compound [22]. The efficacy and safety of this drug is currently being evaluated in MF patients previously treated with ruxolitinib (#NCT02101268). Thrombocytopenia remains the major side-effect observed for momelotinib [18].

6.2.4 Tofacitinib

Tofacitinib (CP-690550) was initially identified as a selective JAK3 inhibitor and has been evaluated primarily in the context of an immunosuppressant in a variety of immune conditions [23–29]. However, this compound also demonstrated activity toward JAK1 and to a lesser extent JAK2, although this was enhanced toward mutant JAK2. Thus, pre-clinical studies identified enhanced anti-proliferative and pro-apoptotic effects in murine factor-dependent cell lines harbouring human JAK2 V617F compared to wild type JAK2. Similarly, erythroid progenitor cells derived from JAK2 V617F-positive PV patients were more sensitive to tofacitinib than those from healthy controls. This was accompanied by decreased STAT5 phosphorylation, reduced JAK2 V617F allele frequency and enhanced erythroid differentiation in treated PV samples [30], supporting further investigation in the context of MPN.

Tofacitinib is currently being evaluated for refractory T-cell large granular lymphocytic leukemia and has demonstrated hematological benefit specifically with regard to neutropenia. However, further studies are required to confirm this study and to examine long term outcomes [31].

6.2.5 AZD1480

AZD1480 is a pyrazole pyrimidine ATP-competitive inhibitor of both JAK1 and JAK2. This agent was shown to inhibit proliferation and survival of JAK2 V617F-positive myeloid and myeloma cell lines, which correlated with suppression of STAT3 and STAT5 phosphorylation [32, 33]. The *in vivo* efficacy of AZD1480 has been demonstrated in various xenograft mouce models, including ETV6-JAK2-positive leukemias and solid tumors such as breast, ovarian and prostate cancer, neuroblastoma, sarcoma and glioblastoma, with inhibition of tumor growth observed that correlated with decreased activation of STAT5 and STAT3 [33–37]. Significantly, AZD1480 was not only able to suppress tumor growth at the primary site but also inhibited both angiogenesis and metastasis [32].

However, despite these very favourable pre-clinical results, a phase I clinical trial investigating the safety and efficacy of AZD1480 in patients with MF and solid tumors resulted in a lack of clinical response due to rapid elimination from plasma, as well as induction of a rare unusual neuropsychiatric dose-limiting toxicity, which resulted in the cessation of the trial [38, 39].

6.2.6 Gandotinib

Gandotinib (LY2784544) is an agent that shows selectivity toward mutant JAK2. This compound was able to inhibit JAK2 V617F and downstream STAT5 signaling at a significantly lower concentration than that required to inhibit wild-type JAK2, and so with the potential to minimize effects on normal hematopoisis [40]. Clinical evaluation of this inhibitor in MPN patients identified reduced spleen size, improved clinical symptoms and decreased bone marrow fibrosis, although no significant changes in mutant allele burden were seen. Gastrointestinal toxicity, increased serum creatinine, hyperuricemia and anemia were the most frequent drug related adverse effect [41]. Several clinical trials using this inhibitor in MPN patients are currently active (#NCT01134120, #NCT01520220, #NCT01594723).

6.2.7   XL019

XL019 is a 4-aryl-2-aminoalkylpyrimidine-based derivative with high selectivity and potency toward JAK2. XL019 administration in a xenograft mice model of erythroleukemia resulted in significant dose-dependent inhibition of STAT1 and STAT3 phosphorylation, reduced tumor growth and vascularization along with increased tumor cell apoptosis [42].

Preliminary results in MF patients identified a reduction in spleen size, blast count and other clinical symptoms in concert with a restoration of hemoglobin in those treated with XL019. However, further clinical studies have been suspended due to high neurologic toxicity [43].

6.2.8   NS-018

NS-018 is a selective JAK2 inhibitor preferential with activity toward constitutively-active JAK2 V617F and its downstream signalling including via STAT3 and STAT5. NS-018 showed anti-proliferative activity in cell lines harboring mutated JAK2 and primary cells from PV patients. *In vivo* administration of NS-018 in mouse models of MF demonstrated improvements in splenomegaly, bone marrow fibrosis, leukocytosis and survival without reducing the platelet or erythrocyte count in peripheral blood. [44, 45]. A clinical trial to test NS-018 in MPN patients is ongoing (#NCT01423851) with preliminary data indicating a safe durable dosing schedule associated with splenic volume reduction and clinical improvement [46].

6.2.9   BMS-911453

BMS-911453 is a selective inhibitor of JAK2 with increased sensitivity toward mutated JAK2. Functionally, it displayed antiproliferative activity in cells harbouring activated JAK2 mutation and in primary progenitor cells from MPN patients that correlated with suppression of constitutive active STAT5 in these cells.

Unexpectedly, this inhibitor also downregulated STAT1 transcripts and phosphory-lation level [47]. However, *in vivo* studies on a murine model of JAK2 V617F-driven MPN revealed limited efficacy of this inhibitor, with suppression of leucocytosis but not erythrocytosis, partial normalization of cytokines such as IL-6, IL-15 and TNF, but without any alteration in MPN histopathology [48]. A phase I/II clinical study to determine the safety and efficacy of this inhibitor in myelofi-brotic patients has completed recently with preliminary results indicating rapid con-trol of constitutional symptoms and splenomegaly in these patients [49].

6.2.10   Other JAK Inhibitors

A variety of other JAK inhibitors are under development, particularly those target-ing JAK2. INCB16562 is a potent inhibitor of both JAK1 and JAK2. This agent was shown to exert a strong anti-proliferative effect in cell lines harbouring JAK1V658F and JAK2 V617F mutations, or with activating mutations in the upstream thrombo-poietin receptor (MPL W515L), as well as in primary hematopoietic cells obtained from PV patients [50, 51]. In a JAK2 V617F murine bone marrow transplantation (BMT) model, treatment with INCB16562 resulted in a reduction in splenomegaly, malignant cell burden and pro-inflammatory cytokines levels, along with increased survival [50]. Furthermore, in a murine MPL W515 BMT model, INCB16562 treat-ment decreased extramedullary hematopoiesis and bone marrow fibrosis and nor-malize white blood cell and platelet counts, but did not alter malignant clone frequency in the BM [51]. INCB16562 has also been demonstrated to inhibit both proliferation and survival of myeloma cell lines and primary BM-derived plasma cells from multiple myeloma patients by inhibiting IL-6-induced STAT3 activation [52]. INCB16562 is yet to be evaluated in clinical trials. NVP-BSK805 is a potent inhibitor of JAK2 that exhibited both anti-proliferative and pro-apoptotic effects in JAK2 V617F-postive cells with concurrent reduction in STAT5 phosphorylation. This compound also showed significant efficacy in a mouse JAK2 V617F transplan-tation model, where it reduced splenomegaly and spread of malignant cells, and was also able to suppress erythropoietin-induced extramedullary erythropoiesis and PV in a rat model [53], but is yet to progress to clinical trials.

6.3   Multi-Kinase Inhibitors

An emerging theme in cancer therapy is the efficacy of broad range inhibitors that can target several tyrosine kinases simultaneously. This has also proven to be the case for several inhibitors for which JAKs are part of their spectrum of activity.

6.3.1 Pacritinib

Pacritinib (SB1518) is an inhibitor of FLT3 and JAK2 that has demonstrated promising efficacy in the context of both myeloid and lymphoid malignancies. Pre-clinical studies of pacritinib have demonstrated dose-dependent inhibition of STAT3 and STAT5 activation with concomitant cell cycle arrest and induction of apoptosis in lymphoid and myeloid cell lines harbouring either wild-type or mutant JAK2. Similarly, in a mouse MPN xenograft model pacritinib suppressed JAK2/STAT5 signaling within tumor tissue concurrently with inhibition of proliferation [54].

In clinical studies, improved splenomegaly and constitutional symptoms was observed in a significant proportion of MF patients treated with pacritinib. Importantly, this agent did not cause significant myelosuppression, indicating it might be particularly amendable to MF patients with baseline cytopenia [55]. Pacritinib was also shown to be well tolerated in patients with relapsed/refractory Hodgkin and non-Hodgkin lymphoma and elicited a decrease in tumor size in >50 % of patients [55, 56]. Two phase III clinical trials are currently underway for this agent comparing pacritinib with BAT in MF patients, either with no platelet count cut off (#NCT01773187) or in patients with thrombocytopenia (#NCT02055781). Gastrointestinal toxicity represents the main side effect of pacritinib [55].

6.3.2 Lestaurtinib

Lestaurtinib (CEP701) is a multi-kinase inhibitor that has significant activity toward TRK family members, FLT3, as well as both JAK2 and JAK3. Lestaurtinib was shown to inhibit the proliferation of primary erythroid cells from MPN patients with concomitant inhibition of JAK2 V617F phosphorylation and activation of downstream effectors, including both STAT3 and STAT5 [57].

In clinical trials, lestaurtinib demonstrated modest efficacy in JAK2 V617F-positive MF patients with a response rate of 27 %, but with no significant changes in bone marrow fibrosis and JAK2 V617F allele burden detected [58]. Lestaurtinib was also trialled in high risk JAK2 V617F-positive PV and ET patients, where administration of this agent resulted in a reduction in spleen volume, amelioration of pruritus, minor reduction in mutant allele burden and a decreased need for phlebotomy [59]. Thrombocytopenia leading to thrombotic events remains the main concern for this agent [58, 59], although both anemia and gastrointestinal symptoms have also been commonly observed [58].

6.3.3 MK-0457

MK-0457 (VX-680) is an inhibitor of Aurora kinase, BCR-ABL and JAK2. This agent displayed significant *in vitro* activity against cells harboring normal and mutated BCR-ABL and also *in vivo* in xenograft models of leukemia, where it led to a block in mitosis and induction of apoptosis in cycling cells [60, 61].

MK-0457 was the first kinase inhibitor to enter the clinic for treatment of chronic myeloid leukemia (CML) patients expressing the BCR-ABL T315I mutation that is responsible for clinical resistance to imantinib [62, 63]. Significant hematological responses were identified in nearly half of the patients, with complete remission observed in around one-third of patients in the blastic phase of the disease. However, MK-0457 failed to elicit a significant response in a variety of other refractory hematological malignancies, including Philadelphia-positive ALL, AML and MF. Febrile neutropenia, transient mucositis and alopecia were the most common toxicities of this drug. However, another clinical limitation of MK-0457 is the requirement to deliver therapy as a continuous infusion compared to other inhibitors that can be taken orally [62].

6.3.4 LS104

LS104 (CR4) is a novel non-ATP inhibitor of several therapeutically important kinases, including BCR-ABL and JAK2. Importantly, it has been shown to inhibit JAK2 autophosphorylation and activation of downstream targets including STAT3 and STAT5 [64]. It is being developed for the treatment of non-CML MPNs and other hematological malignancies, with a significant advantage in treating refractory leukemias harbouring mutations in the ATP binding pocket, since it interacts away from this site. LS104 preferably inhibited the growth and survival of a variety of leukemic cell lines of myeloid and lymphoid origin, while being relatively non-toxic to the growth and differentiation of normal cells [64–66]. The in vivo efficacy of LS104 has been proven in mice xenograft models of Philadelphia-positive ALL, where it resulted in a significant decrease in blast counts in the bone marrow along with increased survival [65]. LS104 also showed a synergistic enhancement of apoptosis in JAK2 V617F-positive cells when used in combination with an ATP-competitive JAK2 [64]. Based on these positive findings LS104 has recently entered clinical trials for treatment of patients with hematological malignancies and myeloproliferative disorders [64, 67].

6.3.5 ON044580

ON044580 is another non-ATP-competitive kinase inhibitor with activity toward both BCR-ABL and JAK2 with many similar properties to LS104 [68, 69]. This compound was able to induce apoptosis in primary cells from leukemic patients expressing the JAK2 V617F mutation and from CML patients regardless of the stage of disease or imatinib sensitivity. Furthermore, when tested on bone marrow cells from patients with monosomy 7 myelodysplastic syndrome (MDS), the cytotoxic effects were limited to cells with aneuploidy [69]. Thus, ON044580 also appears to have considerable potential to treat a range of MPDs, such as CML and MDS, particular as an alternative for patients who develop resistance to current therapies. However, the clinical safety and efficacy of this inhibitor have yet to be demonstrated.

6.4 Conclusion

JAK inhibitors represent some of the most promising agents for mitigating the effects of STAT hyperactivation in neoplasia. The multi-kinase inhibitors that target JAKs and other tyrosine kinases represent particularly attractive agents in this regard, since they are likely to affect several upstream pathways that converge at the level of STAT activation.

Acknowledgments The authors recognize the support of a Faculty of Health Postdoctoral Research Fellowship (PR) from Deakin University.

References

1. Levine RL, Wadleigh M, Cools J et al (2005) Activating mutation in the tyrosine kinase JAK2 in polycythemia vera, essential thrombocythemia, and myeloid metaplasia with myelofibrosis. Cancer Cell 7:387–397
2. Scott LM, Tong W, Levine RL et al (2007) JAK2 exon 12 mutations in polycythemia vera and idiopathic erythrocytosis. N Engl J Med 356:459–468
3. Barrio S, Gallardo M, Arenas A et al (2013) Inhibition of related JAK/STAT pathways with molecular targeted drugs shows strong synergy with ruxolitinib in chronic myeloproliferative neoplasm. Br J Haematol 161:667–676
4. Hu Y, Hong Y, Xu Y et al (2014) Inhibition of the JAK/STAT pathway with ruxolitinib overcomes cisplatin resistance in non-small-cell lung cancer NSCLC. Apoptosis 19:1627–1636
5. Cleeland CS, Dantzer R, Sloan J et al (2013) Cytokine profile changes in 309 myelofibrosis patients: comparison of JAK1/JAK2 inhibitor therapy vs. placebo-correltive analysis from the Comfort-I trial. Blood 122:4074a
6. Verstovsek S, Kantarjian H, Mesa RA et al (2010) Safety and efficacy of INCB018424, a JAK1 and JAK2 inhibitor, in myelofibrosis. N Engl J Med 363:1117–1127
7. Verstovsek S, Mesa RA, Gotlib J et al (2012) A double-blind, placebo-controlled trial of ruxolitinib for myelofibrosis. N Engl J Med 366:799–807
8. Harrison C, Kiladjian JJ, Al-Ali HK et al (2012) JAK inhibition with ruxolitinib versus best available therapy for myelofibrosis. N Engl J Med 366:787–798
9. Harrison C, Mesa R, Ross D et al (2013) Practical management of patients with myelofibrosis receiving ruxolitinib. Expert Rev Hematol 6:511–523
10. Cervantes F, Vannucchi AM, Kiladjian JJ et al (2013) Three-year efficacy, safety, and survival findings from COMFORT-II, a phase 3 study comparing ruxolitinib with best available therapy for myelofibrosis. Blood 122:4047–4053
11. Verstovsek S, Passamonti F, Rambaldi A et al (2014) A phase 2 study of ruxolitinib, an oral JAK1 and JAK2 Inhibitor, in patients with advanced polycythemia vera who are refractory or intolerant to hydroxyurea. Cancer 120:513–520
12. Vannucchi AM, Kiladjian JJ, Griesshammer M et al (2015) Ruxolitinib versus standard therapy for the treatment of polycythemia vera. N Engl J Med 372:426–435
13. An HJ, Choi EK, Kim JS et al (2014) INCB018424 induces apoptotic cell death through the suppression of pJAK1 in human colon cancer cells. Neoplasma 61:56–62
14. Hurwitz HI, Uppal N, Wagner SA et al (2015) Randomized, double-blind, phase II study of ruxolitinib or placebo in combination with capecitabine in patients with metastatic pancreatic cancer for whom therapy with gemcitabine has failed. J Clin Oncol 33:4039–4047
15. Wernig G, Kharas MG, Okabe R et al (2008) Efficacy of TG101348, a selective JAK2 inhibitor, in treatment of a murine model of JAK2V617F-induced polycythemia vera. Cancer Cell 13:311–320

16. Lasho TL, Tefferi A, Hood JD et al (2008) TG101348, a JAK2-selective antagonist, inhibits primary hematopoietic cells derived from myeloproliferative disorder patients with JAK2V617F, MPLW515K or JAK2 exon 12 mutations as well as mutation negative patients. Leukemia 22:1790–1792

17. Pardanani A, Tefferi A, Jamieson C et al (2015) A phase 2 randomized dose-ranging study of the JAK2-selective inhibitor fedratinib (SAR302503) in patients with myelofibrosis. Blood Cancer J 5:e335

18. Pardanani A, Gotlib JR, Jamieson C et al (2011) Safety and efficacy of TG101348, a selective JAK2 inhibitor, in myelofibrosis. J Clin Oncol 29:789–796

19. Jamieson C, Hasserjian R, Gotlib J et al (2015) Effect of treatment with a JAK2-selective inhibitor, fedratinib, on bone marrow fibrosis in patients with myelofibrosis. J Transl Med 13:294

20. Pardanani A, Lasho T, Smith G et al (2009) CYT387, a selective JAK1/JAK2 inhibitor: in vitro assessment of kinase selectivity and preclinical studies using cell lines and primary cells from polycythemia vera patients. Leukemia 23:1441–1445

21. Tyner JW, Bumm TG, Deininger J et al (2010) CYT387, a novel JAK2 inhibitor, induces hematologic responses and normalizes inflammatory cytokines in murine myeloproliferative neoplasms. Blood 115:5232–5240

22. Pardanani A, Laborde RR, Lasho TL et al (2013) Safety and efficacy of CYT387, a JAK1 and JAK2 inhibitor, in myelofibrosis. Leukemia 27:1322–1327

23. Olcaydu D, Harutyunyan A, Jager R et al (2009) A common JAK2 haplotype confers susceptibility to myeloproliferative neoplasms. Nat Genet 41:450–454

24. Liew SH, Nichols KK, Klamerus KJ et al (2012) Tofacitinib (CP-690,550), a Janus kinase inhibitor for dry eye disease: results from a phase 1/2 trial. Ophthalmology 119:1328–1335

25. Fleischmann R, Kremer J, Cush J et al (2012) Placebo-controlled trial of tofacitinib monotherapy in rheumatoid arthritis. N Engl J Med 367:495–507

26. van Vollenhoven RF, Fleischmann R, Cohen S et al (2012) Tofacitinib or adalimumab versus placebo in rheumatoid arthritis. N Engl J Med 367:508–519

27. Boy MG, Wang C, Wilkinson BE et al (2009) Double-blind, placebo-controlled, dose-escalation study to evaluate the pharmacologic effect of CP-690,550 in patients with psoriasis. J Invest Dermatol 129:2299–2302

28. Tanaka Y, Suzuki M, Nakamura H et al (2011) Phase II study of tofacitinib (CP-690,550) combined with methotrexate in patients with rheumatoid arthritis and an inadequate response to methotrexate. Arthritis Care Res (Hoboken) 63:1150–1158

29. Sandborn WJ, Ghosh S, Panes J et al (2012) Tofacitinib, an oral Janus kinase inhibitor, in active ulcerative colitis. N Engl J Med 367:616–624

30. Manshouri T, Quintas-Cardama A, Nussenzveig RH et al (2008) The JAK kinase inhibitor CP-690,550 suppresses the growth of human polycythemia vera cells carrying the JAK2V617F mutation. Cancer Sci 99:1265–1273

31. Bilori B, Thota S, Clemente MJ et al (2015) Tofacitinib as a novel salvage therapy for refractory T-cell large granular lymphocytic leukemia. Leukemia 29:2427–2429

32. Xin H, Herrmann A, Reckamp K et al (2011) Antiangiogenic and antimetastatic activity of JAK inhibitor AZD1480. Cancer Res 71:6601–6610

33. Ioannidis S, Lamb ML, Wang T et al (2011) Discovery of 5-chloro-N2-[(1S)-1-(5-fluoropyrimidin-2-yl)ethyl]-N4-(5-methyl-1H-pyrazol-3-yl)pyrimidine-2,4-diamine (AZD1480) as a novel inhibitor of the JAK/STAT pathway. J Med Chem 54:262–276

34. Hedvat M, Huszar D, Herrmann A et al (2009) The JAK2 inhibitor AZD1480 potently blocks Stat3 signaling and oncogenesis in solid tumors. Cancer Cell 16:487–497

35. Yan S, Li Z, Thiele CJ (2013) Inhibition of STAT3 with orally active JAK inhibitor, AZD1480, decreases tumor growth in neuroblastoma and pediatric sarcomas in vitro and in vivo. Oncotarget 4:433–445

36. McFarland BC, Ma JY, Langford CP et al (2011) Therapeutic potential of AZD1480 for the treatment of human glioblastoma. Mol Cancer Ther 10:2384–2393

37. Houghton PJ, Kurmasheva RT, Lyalin D et al (2014) Initial solid tumor testing (stage 1) of AZD1480, an inhibitor of Janus kinases 1 and 2 by the pediatric preclinical testing program. Pediatr Blood Cancer 61:1972–1979

38. Plimack ER, Lorusso PM, McCoon P et al (2013) AZD1480: a phase I study of a novel JAK2 inhibitor in solid tumors. Oncologist 18:819–820
39. Verstovsek S, Hoffman R, Mascarenhas J et al (2015) A phase I, open-label, multi-center study of the JAK2 inhibitor AZD1480 in patients with myelofibrosis. Leuk Res 39:157–163
40. Ma L, Clayton JR, Walgren RA et al (2013) Discovery and characterization of LY2784544, a small-molecule tyrosine kinase inhibitor of JAK2V617F. Blood Cancer J 3:e109
41. Mesa RA, Salama ME, Giles JL et al (2013) Phase I study of LY2784544, a JAK2 selective inhibitor, in patinets with myelofibrosis (MF), polycythemia vera (PV), and essential thrombo-cythemia (ET). Blood 122:665a
42. Forsyth T, Kearney PC, Kim BG et al (2012) SAR and in vivo evaluation of 4-aryl-2-aminoalkylpyrimidines as potent and selective Janus kinase 2 (JAK2) inhibitors. Bioorg Med Chem Lett 22:7653–7658
43. Verstovsek S, Tam CS, Wadleigh M et al (2014) Phase I evaluation of XL019, an oral, potent, and selective JAK2 inhibitor. Leuk Res 38:316–322
44. Nakaya Y, Shide K, Niwa T et al (2011) Efficacy of NS-018, a potent and selective JAK2/Src inhibitor, in primary cells and mouse models of myeloproliferative neoplasms. Blood Cancer J 1:e29
45. Nakaya Y, Shide K, Naito H et al (2014) Effect of NS-018, a selective JAK2V617F inhibitor, in a murine model of myelofibrosis. Blood Cancer J 4:e174
46. Verstovsek S, Talpaz M, Ritchie EK et al (2014) A phase 1/2, open-label, dose escalation, multi-center study to assess the safety, tolerability, pharmacokinetics and pharmacodynamics of orally administered NS-018 in patients with primary myelofibrosis (PMF), post-polycythemia vera myelofibrosis (postPV MF) or post-essential thrombocythemia myelofibro-sis (postET MF). Blood 124:1839a
47. Purandare AV, McDevitt TM, Wan H et al (2012) Characterization of BMS-911543, a func-tionally selective small-molecule inhibitor of JAK2. Leukemia 26:280–288
48. Pomicter AD, Eiring AM, Senina AV et al (2015) Limited efficacy of BMS-911543 in a murine model of Janus kinase 2 V617F myeloproliferative neoplasm. Exp Hematol 43:537–545
49. Pardanani A, Roberts AW, Seymour JF et al (2013) BMS-911543, a selective JAK2 inhibitor: a multicenter phase 1/2a study in myelofibrosis. Blood 122:664a
50. Liu PC, Caulder E, Li J et al (2009) Combined inhibition of Janus kinase 1/2 for the treatment of JAK2V617F-driven neoplasms: selective effects on mutant cells and improvements in mea-sures of disease severity. Clin Cancer Res 15:6891–6900
51. Koppikar P, Abdel-Wahab O, Hedvat C et al (2010) Efficacy of the JAK2 inhibitor INCB16562 in a murine model of MPLW515L-induced thrombocytosis and myelofibrosis. Blood 115:2919–2927
52. Li J, Favata M, Kelley JA et al (2010) INCB16562, a JAK1/2 selective inhibitor, is efficacious against multiple myeloma cells and reverses the protective effects of cytokine and stromal cell support. Neoplasia 12:28–38
53. Baffert F, Regnier CH, De Pover A et al (2010) Potent and selective inhibition of polycythemia by the quinoxaline JAK2 inhibitor NVP-BSK805. Mol Cancer Ther 9:1945–1955
54. Hart S, Goh KC, Novotny-Diermayr V et al (2011) SB1518, a novel macrocyclic pyrimidine-based JAK2 inhibitor for the treatment of myeloid and lymphoid malignancies. Leukemia 25:1751–1759
55. Komrokji RS, Seymour JF, Roberts AW et al (2015) Results of a phase 2 study of pacritinib (SB1518), a JAK2/JAK2(V617F) inhibitor, in patients with myelofibrosis. Blood 125:2649–2655
56. Younes A, Romaguera J, Fanale M et al (2012) Phase I study of a novel oral Janus kinase 2 inhibitor, SB1518, in patients with relapsed lymphoma: evidence of clinical and biologic activity in multiple lymphoma subtypes. J Clin Oncol 30:4161–4167
57. Hexner EO, Serdikoff C, Jan M et al (2008) Lestaurtinib (CEP701) is a JAK2 inhibitor that suppresses JAK2/STAT5 signaling and the proliferation of primary erythroid cells from patients with myeloproliferative disorders. Blood 111:5663–5671

58. Santos FP, Kantarjian HM, Jain N et al (2010) Phase 2 study of CEP-701, an orally available JAK2 inhibitor, in patients with primary or post-polycythemia vera/essential thrombocythemia myelofibrosis. Blood 115:1131–1136

59. Hexner E, Roboz G, Hoffman R et al (2014) Open-label study of oral CEP-701 (lestaurtinib) in patients with polycythaemia vera or essential thrombocythaemia with JAK2-V617F mutation. Br J Haematol 164:83–93

60. Carter TA, Wodicka LM, Shah NP et al (2005) Inhibition of drug-resistant mutants of ABL, KIT, and EGF receptor kinases. Proc Natl Acad Sci USA 102:11011–11016

61. Harrington EA, Bebbington D, Moore J et al (2004) VX-680, a potent and selective small-molecule inhibitor of the Aurora kinases, suppresses tumor growth in vivo. Nat Med 10:262–267

62. Giles FJ, Swords RT, Nagler A et al (2013) MK-0457, an Aurora kinase and BCR-ABL inhibitor, is active in patients with BCR-ABL T315I leukemia. Leukemia 27:113–117

63. Giles FJ, Cortes J, Jones D et al (2007) MK-0457, a novel kinase inhibitor, is active in patients with chronic myeloid leukemia or acute lymphocytic leukemia with the T315I BCR-ABL mutation. Blood 109:500–502

64. Lipka DB, Hoffmann LS, Heidel F et al (2008) LS104, a non-ATP-competitive small-molecule inhibitor of JAK2, is potently inducing apoptosis in JAK2V617F-positive cells. Mol Cancer Ther 7:1176–1184

65. Grunberger T, Demin P, Rounova O et al (2003) Inhibition of acute lymphoblastic and myeloid leukemias by a novel kinase inhibitor. Blood 102:4153–4158

66. Kasper S, Breitenbuecher F, Hoehn Y et al (2008) The kinase inhibitor LS104 induces apoptosis, enhances cytotoxic effects of chemotherapeutic drugs and is targeting the receptor tyrosine kinase FLT3 in acute myeloid leukemia. Leuk Res 32:1698–1708

67. Jatiani SS, Baker SJ, Silverman LR et al (2010) Jak/STAT pathways in cytokine signaling and myeloproliferative disorders: approaches for targeted therapies. Genes Cancer 1:979–993

68. Reddy MV, Pallela VR, Cosenza SC et al (2010) Design, synthesis and evaluation of (E)-alpha-benzylthio chalcones as novel inhibitors of BCR-ABL kinase. Bioorg Med Chem 18:2317–2326

69. Jatiani SS, Cosenza SC, Reddy MV et al (2010) A non-ATP-competitive dual inhibitor of JAK2 and BCR-ABL kinases: elucidation of a novel therapeutic spectrum based on substrate competitive inhibition. Genes Cancer 1:331–345

Chapter 7
Inhibitors of Upstream Inducers of STAT Activation

Janani Kumar

Abstract Activation of STATs, especially STAT3 and STAT5, is commonly observed in solid tumors and hematological malignancies. In several instances the key upstream signaling molecules responsible for STAT activation have been identified. Many of these proteins are able to be targeted with specific antibodies or small molecules and so represent attractive candidates for therapeutic development. This chapter details several promising agents that target receptors — both receptor tyrosine kinases and cytokine receptors — and downstream kinases that activate STATs in cancer, including EGFR, VEGFR, IL-6R, SRC and ABL.

Keywords EGFR • VEGFR • IL-6R • SRC • ABL • STAT3 • RTK • Inhibitor • Cancer

7.1 Introduction

A number of molecules that mediate STAT activation have been identified in a range of malignancies, several of which are involved in the hyperactivation of STATs observed. These include receptor tyrosine kinases (RTKs), non-receptor tyrosine kinases (non-RTKs) and cytokine receptors, which represent attractive targets for treatment. This has led to the development of a variety of specific inhibitors of these molecules, several of which have shown clinical efficacy. This chapter describes the most important of these inhibitors (Fig. 7.1).

7.2 Epidermal Growth Factor Receptor Inhibitors

Epidermal growth factor receptor (EGFR) and related receptors are known to be active in multiple cancers — where downstream STAT3 activation plays a key role — and have been shown to be validated therapeutic target in several solid tumors [1].

J. Kumar (✉)
School of Biomedical Sciences and Pharmacy, University of Newcastle,
Callaghan, NSW 2308, Australia
e-mail: kumarjanani17@gmail.com

© Springer International Publishing Switzerland 2016   177
A.C. Ward (ed.), *STAT Inhibitors in Cancer*, Cancer Drug
Discovery and Development, DOI 10.1007/978-3-319-42949-6_7

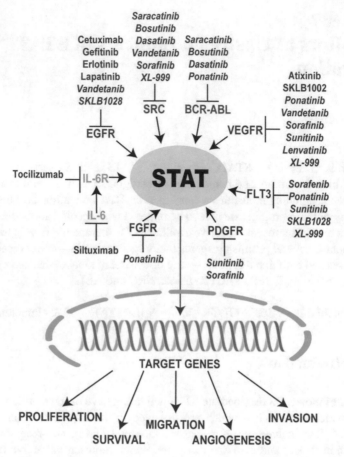

Fig. 7.1 Targeting molecules upstream of STAT activation. Schematic representation of STAT activation by representative RTKs (*red*), cytokine receptors (*green*), and non-RTKs (*brown*), and the downstream phenotypes affected. Inhibitors that target each are indicated (antibodies: *purple*; small chemicals: *blue*), with those with multiple targets in italics

7.2.1 Cetuximab

Cetuximab is a humanized mouse monoclonal antibody against epidermal growth factor receptor (EGFR) that acts by interacting with the EGFR ligand-binding domain thereby blocking EGF binding [2], the efficacy of which directly correlated with STAT3 inhibition [3]. The effectiveness of cetuximab was initially demonstrated in colon cancer cells, including suppressed tumor growth in a mouse xenograft model of the disease [4], and has been approved for use in colon cancer with wildtype K-RAS [5]. Cetuximab has also been shown to be effective in inhibiting EGFR-mediated signalling in a variety of other cancers, including head and neck squamous epithelial cell cancer, pancreatic cancer, renal cancer, prostate cancer and bladder cancer [2, 3], Importantly, the compound has proven to act synergistically with other treatment modalities, including various chemotherapeutic regimes [6, 7], which has led to its approval in head and neck squamous epithelial cell cancer in combination with platinum-based chemotherapy [6]. Cetuximab also induces radio-sensitivity that has recently been demonstrated to be augmented by concurrent inhibition of JAK1 [8]. Common side effects include skin blemishes, swelling of the face, arms, hands, lower legs, feet, body aches or pain, chills, congestion and cough.

7.2.2 Gefitinib

Gefitinib is a specific inhibitor of the tyrosine kinase activity of EGFR by targeting the ATP-binding pocket [1]. It has demonstrated effectiveness in non-small cell lung cancer (NSCLC) patients expressing mutant forms of EGFR [9], and has been approved for use in this clinical setting. Variable results have been obtained in the treatment of acute myeloid leukemia (AML) [10, 11], but there remains potential for use of this agent in chronic lymphocytic leukemia, although its effects in this cancer type may be due to its action on other kinases [12]. Interestingly, gefitinib resistance has been shown to be typically mediated by the pro-survival effects of STAT3 [13], as described for several other EGFR inhibitors [14]. This has led to the successful use of gefitinib in combination with JAK/STAT3 inhibitors, including in ovarian cancer [15]. Side effects of treatment include dark urine, headache, fatigue and decreased appetite.

7.2.3 Erlotinib

Erlotinib is also a tyrosine kinase inhibitor that targets the ATP-binding pocket of the EGFR kinase domain and thereby inhibits downstream signaling including via the JAK/STAT pathway [1]. It has proven efficacious in several cancer settings, notably including NSCLC [16], and has been approved for therapy in NSCLC and pancreatic cancer. Erlotinib has also demonstrated effectiveness in other cancers, including in chemically induced mouse model of oral squamous cell carcinoma [17], as well as AML, where it enhances chemosensitivity in vitro [18], leading to synergistic effects in combination with a DNA methyltransferase inhibitor [19]. Erlotinib has shown promise in AML [20], which has seen its evaluation in AML and myelodysplastic syndrome (MDS) [21, 22]. It has also been shown to inhibit JAK V617F activity and growth of polycythemia vera cells [23], suggesting it may also be applicable to myeloproliferative disorders. Some of the reported side effects include nausea, stomach upset, vomiting, loss of appetite, weight loss, diarrhea, mouth sores, dry skin, acne, eye irritation, or fatigue.

7.2.4   Lapatinib

Lapatinib is another tyrosine kinase inhibitor that is specific for EGFR as well as the closely-related ERBB2/HER2 [24], which is able to block downstream signalling via STAT3, as well as AKT and MAPKs [25, 26]. It has demonstrated clinical effectiveness against a range of carcinomas [27] and has approval for use in breast cancer [28, 29], where it has been shown to specifically reduce breast cancer stem cells [28]. Lapatinib has also shown effectiveness in pre-clinical studies on other cancers, blocking tumor growth in an orthotopic model of human testicular germ cell cancer [30] and inducing apoptosis in chronic myelogenous leukemia (CML) cell lines and patient blasts [31, 32]. Common side effects reported include nausea, vomiting, mouth sores, rash, hair loss, and sleep disturbance.

7.2.5   PKI166

PKI166 is also a dual EGFR and ERBB2 tyrosine kinase inhibitor, which blocks downstream signaling cascades including the JAK2/STAT3 pathway [33]. It has been shown to suppress growth of pancreatic carcinoma xenografts concomitant with induction of apoptosis in endothelial cells [34], as well as inhibit angiogenesis in a human renal cell carcinoma xenograft model via its effects on STAT3 [35]. This drug has undergone phase I clinical trials in patients with advanced solid malignancies and was shown to be well tolerated [36], with minor side effects such as diarrhoea, skin rash and fatigue.

7.3   Vascular Epithelial Growth Factor Receptor Inhibitors

Vascular epithelial growth factor receptor (VEGFR) family members play critical roles in angiogenesis, an essential part of tumor growth, as well as vasculature integrity, important in effective chemotherapy, making these useful targets for cancer therapy [37].

7.3.1   Axitinib

Axitinib is an inhibitor of VEGFR1-3, with weaker activity toward other kinases that inhibits downstream signaling cascades including STAT3 [38]. It has been shown to inhibit growth of tumors *in vivo*, including in a breast cancer xenograft model by decreasing vascular permeability [39]. Following favorable clinical trials, atixinib has been approved for use in refractory renal cell carcinoma [38], while it has also shown clinical efficacy in pancreatic cancer patients [40]. Axitinib has been demonstrated to exert other effects, inhibiting JAK2/STAT3-dependent epithelial-to-mesenchymal transition and metastasis of cervical cancer cells [41], and by ameliorating accumulation of myeloid-derived suppressor cells via a STAT3-dependent mechanism to enhance anti-tumor activity in renal cell carcinoma [42]. More recently, its application has been demonstrated potential for the treatment of imatinib-resistant BCR-ABL positive CML [43]. Side effects include diarrhea, hypertension, weight loss, nausea and asthenia.

7.3.2   SKLB1002

SKLB1002 is a novel VEGFR2 inhibitor that has been shown to be very effective at inhibiting angiogenesis and tumor growth *in vivo* [44]. In addition, it has been shown to normalize the vasculature thereby increasing retention of chemotherapeutic agents to enhance their effectiveness [45]. Synergistic antitumor effects have been observed with SKLB1002 and both hyperthermia and chemotherapy [45, 46]. This drug is yet to be tested in clinical trials.

7.4   Non-RTK Inhibitors

Several intracellular kinases also play an important role in STAT activation in cancer, notably including JAKs, SRCs and BCR-ABL [47–49]. JAK inhibitors are detailed in Chap. 6, and so are not mentioned further here.

7.4.1   Saracatinib

Saracatinib (AZD0530) is an oral tyrosine kinase inhibitor targeting both SRC and BCR-ABL kinases [50]. It has shown strong activity in a variety of pre-clinical cancer models. Thus, saracatinib inhibited the growth and migration of gastric cancer cells with increased apoptosis due to reduction of STAT3-mediated anti-apoptotic genes, leading to a decreased tumor burden in xenograft models [51]. It was also able to reduce cell-cycle progression of estrogen receptor-positive primary ovarian cancer cells in culture and as xenografts, and induced autophagy in combination with fulvestrant [52]. Saracatinib is being trialled in several clinical settings [53], but efficacy in published clinical trial has so far been poor [54]. Common side effects reported include fatigue, nausea, cough, and adrenal insufficiency.

7.4.2   Bosutinib

Bosutinib (SKI-606) is an orally administered ATP-competitive inhibitor specific for BCR-ABL and members of the SRC family of kinases [55]. Bosutinib has been shown to decrease the migration and invasion of breast cancer cells by inhibiting multiple signaling pathway including STAT3 [56], and was also able to reduce tumor burden in xenograft models of colon cancer [57]. Bosutinib showed efficacy against CML, including in xenograft models of the disease, along with variable hematological toxicity [58]. In comparison to imatinib, bosutinib showed similar effectiveness in CML patients, with gastrointestinal and liver-related side effects observed [59], and has subsequently been approved for use in resistant/intolerant BCR-ABL positive CML.

7.4.3   Dasatinib

Dosatinib (BMS-354825) is another oral ATP-competitive inhibitor of BCR-ABL that also acts on SRC and other tyrosine kinases [60]. Hepatocellular carcinoma cells treated with dasatinib showed decreased proliferation, adhesion, migration and invasion as well as inhibition of downstream pathways [61]. In human AML cells, dasatinib induced cell differentiation that correlated with inhibition of STAT1 signalling [62]. Dasatinib also enhanced cisplatin sensitivity in esophageal squamous cell carcinoma (ESCC) cells through suppression of PI3K/AKT and STAT3 signaling [63]. This agent similarly inhibited STAT3 phosphorylation in glioma and prostate cancer cells leading to decreased cell growth and metastasis, as well as increased apoptosis [64, 65]. Dasatinib has demonstrated efficacy in BCR-ABL-positive CML patients, including those resistant to imatinib [66], and has been approved for clinical use in CML, although further investigation is needed with regards to solid tumors. Side effects include neutropenia, myelosuppression and pleural effusion.

7.5   Multi-TK Inhibitors

An exciting recent development has been the success of inhibitors that target multiple tyrosine kinases (TKs).

7.5.1   Ponatinib

Ponatinib represents a tyrosine kinase inhibitor originally designed to target BCR-ABL, but also acts on various RTKs, including VEGFRs, FGFRs, FLT3 and TIE2, with downstream effects on STAT3 and STAT5 activation demonstrated in several cases [67, 68]. This compound has been used to treat patients with refractory CML and BCR-ABL positive acute lymphoblastic leukemia (ALL) [67]. Posatinib has also demonstrated effectiveness in imatinib-resistant chronic eosinophilic leukemia (CEL), concomitant with reduced activation of both STAT3 and STAT5 [69], as well as in a rhabdosarcoma xenograft model, where it blocked STAT3 activation from both wildtype and mutant forms of FGFR [68]. Common side effects include peripheral edema and neuropathy, dizziness, headache, gastrointestinal haemorrhage and hyperesthesia.

7.5.2 Vandetanib

Vandetanib (ZD6474) is an oral tyrosine kinase inhibitor of the RTKs VEGFR, EGFR and RET, as well as SRC [70, 71]. This compound has been approved for treatment of medullary thyroid cancer [72] and has undergone a clinical trial for NSCLC (#NCT00687297), showing similar side effects to gefitinib. Other studies have shown vandetanib was effective in inducing apoptosis of CML cells by blocking SRC-mediated STAT3 activation [71], as well as eliciting both anti-proliferative and anti-angiogenic effects in a head and neck squamous cell carcinoma (HNSCC) xenograft model through inhibition of VEGFR and EGFR signals [73].

7.5.3 Sorafenib

Sorafenib is a multi-TK inhibitor, which targets the RTKs VEGFR, PDGFR and FLT3, as well as SRC and RAF, impacting on downstream STAT3 activation in several cases [74–76]. This agent has been shown to be efficacious in several clinical settings, including advanced hepatocarcinoma [77], renal cell carcinoma (RCC) [78] and thyroid carcinoma [79], where it is approved for clinical use. Sorafenib has also been demonstrated to be effective in MDS/AML cell models and patient samples, largely due to its effects on mutant FLT3 [75], through induction of apoptosis [80]. Common side effects include acne, dry skin, nausea, diarrhoea, patchy hair loss/thinning, loss of appetite, dry mouth, hoarseness, or tiredness.

7.5.4 Sunitinib

Sunitinib (SU11248) is a TK inhibitor active against the RTKs VEGFR, c-KIT, PDGFR and FLT3 [81–83]. This compound has shown clinical efficacy on imatinib-resistant gastrointestinal stromal tumors [84] and RCCs [85]. It is also been trialled in AML with activating FLT3 mutations [86]. Side effects include jaundice, pigmentation defects, fatigue, nausea, vomiting, mouth sores and pain.

7.5.5 SKLB1028

SKLB1028 is a novel oral inhibitor of the RTKs EGFR and FLT3, as well as the intracellular BCR-ABL [87]. This compound elicited reduced tumor burden in a K562 leukemic mouse xenograft models, and is destined for clinical trials for leukemic patients in combination with chemotherapy [87].

7.5.6 Lenvatinib

Lenvatinib (also known as E7080) is an oral inhibitor of VEGFR2, RET and c-KIT that inhibits multiple signalling pathways including STAT3 [88]. Through its action on VEGFR2, lenvatinib acts to decrease vascular endothelial cell migration and proliferation, and augment vascular endothelial cell apoptosis [88]. Lenvatinib has successfully passed phase I trials on patients with a variety of solid tumors [89], and following successful phase II and III clinical trials has been approved for use in refractory thyroid cancer [90] and in combination with mTor inhibitors in metastatic RCC [91]. Common side effects include high blood pressure, fatigue, diarrhea, joint and muscle pain.

7.5.7 Other Multi-TK Inhibitors

A few alternate SRC inhibitors that act, at least in part, by inhibiting STAT3 signaling are at various stages of clinical evaluation in solid tumour. For example, XL999 is a new chemical entity that inhibits a spectrum of RTKs, including, PDGFR, VEGFR, KIT and FLT3, as well as SRC. It induces a cell-cycle block that provides broad antitumor activity in xenograft models. XL999 has shown efficacy in several cancer settings, but has been hampered by cardiotoxicity [92].

7.6 Interleukin-6 Receptor (IL-6R) Inhibitors

Interleukin-6 (IL-6) signaling through its specific receptor (IL-6R) plays a pivotal role in the proliferation, differentiation, survival, and angiogenesis of malignant cells, largely via activation of the downstream JAK2/STAT3 pathway [93], which makes it an attractive therapeutic target in cancer [94].

7.6.1 Tocilizumab

Tocilizumab is a humanized monoclonal antibody inhibitor targeting IL-6R, which blocks ligand-induced activation [95]. It was able to block IL-6–mediated STAT3 activation and inhibited tumor progression in a xenograft model of oral squamous carcinoma, as well as lead to a significant impairment of tumor angiogenesis [96]. Tocilizumab also inhibited proliferative signalling via STAT3 in MCF7 breast cancer cells in a dose-dependent manner [97]. In chronic lymphocytic leukemia (CLL) cells, it blocked constitutive activation of STAT3 via IL-6R and decreased expression of the key downstream genes MCL-1 and BCL-xL to overcome chemoresistance [98]. Tocilizumab was also able to inhibit IL-6R-mediated proliferative responses in NSCLC cells [99]. Several clinical studies have shown tocilizumab as a promising drug for the treatment of chronic inflammatory diseases, although clinical trials testing the efficacy of tocilizumab in cancer are yet to be performed.

7.6.2 Siltuximab

Siltuximab (or CNTO328) is a potent antibody that targets IL-6 thereby limiting its bioactivity [100]. Siltuximab has been shown to inhibit IL-6R-mediated STAT3 activation, exerting an anti-tumor effect in various pre-clinical studies, such as lung cancer [101] and prostate cancer [102], in the latter case impacting on the stem cell pool. Promising clinical trial results have been obtained in prostate cancer [103], RCC [104], multiple myeloma [105, 106] and non-Hodgkin's lymphoma [106]. Siltuximab is safe, but has side effects of increased weight, rash, pruritus, hyperuricemia, and upper respiratory tract infection.

7.7 Conclusion

Inhibition of receptors and tyrosine kinases lying upstream of STATs represent some of the most promising agents for mitigating the effects of STATs — particularly STAT3 — in cancer. Several of these have progressed to successful clinical trials for specific malignancies. However, most remain unexplored in many cancer types, but provide an ongoing avenue for therapeutic development in cancers in which STAT activation has been identified.

References

1. Ji H, Sharpless NE, Wong KK (2006) EGFR targeted therapy: view from biological standpoint. Cell Cycle 5:2072–2076
2. Waksal HW (1999) Role of an anti-epidermal growth factor receptor in treating cancer. Cancer Metastasis Rev 18:427–436
3. Ung N, Putoczki TL, Stylli SS et al (2014) Anti-EGFR therapeutic efficacy correlates directly with inhibition of STAT3 activity. Cancer Biol Ther 15:623–632
4. Goldstein NI, Prewett M, Zuklys K et al (1995) Biological efficacy of a chimeric antibody to the epidermal growth factor receptor in a human tumor xenograft model. Clin Cancer Res 1:1311–1318

5. Messersmith WA, Ahnen DJ (2008) Targeting EGFR in colorectal cancer. N Engl J Med 359:1834–1836
6. Licitra L, Storkel S, Kerr KM et al (2013) Predictive value of epidermal growth factor receptor expression for first-line chemotherapy plus cetuximab in patients with head and neck and colorectal cancer: analysis of data from the EXTREME and CRYSTAL studies. Eur J Cancer 49:1161–1168
7. Inoue K, Slaton JW, Perrotte P et al (2000) Paclitaxel enhances the effects of the anti-epidermal growth factor receptor monoclonal antibody ImClone C225 in mice with metastatic human bladder transitional cell carcinoma. Clin Cancer Res 6:4874–4884
8. Bonner JA, Trummel HQ, Bonner AB et al (2015) Enhancement of cetuximab-induced radiosensitization by JAK-1 inhibition. BMC Cancer 15:673
9. Lynch TJ, Bell DW, Sordella R et al (2004) Activating mutations in the epidermal growth factor receptor underlying responsiveness of non-small-cell lung cancer to gefitinib. N Engl J Med 350:2129–2139
10. Williams R (2005) Treatment of acute myeloid leukemia with gefitinib: clinical trials recommended. Nat Clin Pract Oncol 2:540
11. Deangelo DJ, Neuberg D, Amrein PC et al (2014) A phase II study of the EGFR inhibitor gefitinib in patients with acute myeloid leukemia. Leuk Res 38:430–434
12. Dielschneider RF, Xiao W, Yoon JY et al (2014) Gefitinib targets ZAP-70-expressing chronic lymphocytic leukemia cells and inhibits B-cell receptor signaling. Cell Death Dis 5:e1439
13. Wu K, Chang Q, Lu Y et al (2013) Gefitinib resistance resulted from STAT3-mediated Akt activation in lung cancer cells. Oncotarget 4:2430–2438
14. Sen M, Joyce S, Panahandeh M et al (2012) Targeting Stat3 abrogates EGFR inhibitor resistance in cancer. Clin Cancer Res 18:4986–4996
15. Wen W, Wu J, Liu L et al (2015) Synergistic anti-tumor effect of combined inhibition of EGFR and JAK/STAT3 pathways in human ovarian cancer. Mol Cancer 14:100–104
16. Petty TL (2003) Determinants of tumor response and survival with erlotinib in patients with non-small-cell lung cancer. J Clin Oncol 1:3–4
17. Leeman-Neill RJ, Seethala RR, Singh SV et al (2011) Inhibition of EGFR-STAT3 signaling with erlotinib prevents carcinogenesis in a chemically-induced mouse model of oral squamous cell carcinoma. Cancer Prev Res 4:230–237
18. Lainey E, Sebert M, Thepot S et al (2012) Erlotinib antagonizes ABC transporters in acute myeloid leukemia. Cell Cycle 11:4079–4092
19. Lainey E, Wolfromm A, Marie N et al (2013) Azacytidine and erlotinib exert synergistic effects against acute myeloid leukemia. Oncogene 32:4331–4342
20. Chan G, Pilichowska M (2007) Complete remission in a patient with acute myelogenous leukemia treated with erlotinib for non small-cell lung cancer. Blood 110:1079–1080
21. Sayar H, Czader M, Amin C et al (2015) Pilot study of erlotinib in patients with acute myeloid leukemia. Leuk Res 39:170–172
22. Thepot S, Boehrer S, Seegers V et al (2014) A phase I/II trial of Erlotinib in higher risk myelodysplastic syndromes and acute myeloid leukemia after azacitidine failure. Leuk Res 38:1430–1434
23. Li Z, Xu M, Xing S et al (2007) Erlotinib effectively inhibits JAK2V617F activity and Polycythemia vera cell growth. J Biol Chem 282:3428–3432
24. Nelson MH, Dolder CR (2006) Lapatinib: a novel dual tyrosine kinase inhibitor with activity in solid tumors. Ann Pharmacother 40:261–269
25. Xia W, Bacus S, Hegde P et al (2006) A model of acquired autoresistance to a potent ErbB2 tyrosine kinase inhibitor and a therapeutic strategy to prevent its onset in breast cancer. Proc Natl Acad Sci U S A 103:7795–7800
26. Geyer CE, Forster J, Lindquist D et al (2006) Lapatinib plus capecitabine for HER2-positive advanced breast cancer. N Engl J Med 355:2733–2743
27. Burris HA, Hurwitz HI, Dees EC et al (2005) Phase I safety, pharmacokinetics, and clinical activity study of lapatinib (GW572016), a reversible dual inhibitor of epidermal growth

factor receptor tyrosine kinases, in heavily pretreated patients with metastatic carcinomas. J Clin Oncol 23:5305–5313

28. Alvarez RH, Valero V, Hortobagyi GN (2010) Emerging targeted therapies for breast cancer. J Clin Oncol 28:3366–3379

29. Sambade MJ, Camp JT, Kimple RJ et al (2009) Mechanism of lapatinib-mediated radiosensitization of breast cancer cells is primarily by inhibition of the Raf>MEK>ERK mitogen-activated protein kinase cascade and radiosensitization of lapatinib-resistant cells restored by direct inhibition of MEK. Radiother Oncol 93:639–644

30. Juliachs M, Castillo-Avila W, Vidal A et al (2013) ErbBs inhibition by lapatinib blocks tumor growth in an orthotopic model of human testicular germ cell tumor. Int J Cancer 133:235–246

31. Lainey E, Thepot S, Bouteloup C et al (2011) Tyrosine kinase inhibitors for the treatment of acute myeloid leukemia: delineation of anti-leukemic mechanisms of action. Biochem Pharmacol 82:1457–1466

32. Huang HL, Chen YC, Huang YC et al (2011) Lapatinib induces autophagy, apoptosis and megakaryocytic differentiation in chronic myelogenous leukemia K562 cells. PLoS One 6:e29014

33. Ranson M (2004) Epidermal growth factor receptor tyrosine kinase inhibitors. Br J Cancer 90:2250–2255

34. Bruns CJ, Solorzano CC, Harbison MT et al (2000) Blockade of the epidermal growth factor receptor signaling by a novel tyrosine kinase inhibitor leads to apoptosis of endothelial cells and therapy of human pancreatic carcinoma. Cancer Res 60:2926–2935

35. Kedar D, Baker CH, Killion JJ et al (2002) Blockade of the epidermal growth factor receptor signaling inhibits angiogenesis leading to regression of human renal cell carcinoma growing orthotopically in nude mice. Clin Cancer Res 8:3592–3600

36. Hoekstra R, Dumez H, Eskens FA et al (2005) Phase I and pharmacologic study of PKI166, an epidermal growth factor receptor tyrosine kinase inhibitor, in patients with advanced solid malignancies. Clin Cancer Res 11:6908–6915

37. Rapisarda A, Melillo G (2012) Role of the VEGF/VEGFR axis in cancer biology and therapy. Adv Cancer Res 114:237–267

38. Escudier B, Gore M (2011) Axitinib for the management of metastatic renal cell carcinoma. Drugs R D 11(2):113–126

39. Wilmes LJ, Pallavicini MG, Fleming LM et al (2007) AG-013736, a novel inhibitor of VEGF receptor tyrosine kinases, inhibits breast cancer growth and decreases vascular permeability as detected by dynamic contrast-enhanced magnetic resonance imaging. Magn Reson Imaging 25:319–327

40. Spano JP, Chodkiewicz C, Maurel J et al (2008) Efficacy of gemcitabine plus axitinib compared with gemcitabine alone in patients with advanced pancreatic cancer: an open-label randomised phase II study. Lancet 371:2101–2108

41. Zhang RR (2013) Enhanced antitumor effect of axitinib synergistic interaction with AG490 via VEGFR2/JAK2/STAT3 signaling mediated epithelial–mesenchymal transition in cervical cancer in vitro. Asian Biomed 7:39–49

42. Yuan H, Cai P, Li Q et al (2014) Axitinib augments antitumor activity in renal cell carcinoma via STAT3-dependent reversal of myeloid-derived suppressor cell accumulation. Biomed Pharmacother 68:751–756

43. Killock D (2015) Haematological cancer: BCL-ABL1 resistance mutation—breakthrough with axitinib. Nat Rev Clin Oncol 12:252

44. Zhang S, Cao Z, Tian H et al (2011) SKLB1002, a novel potent inhibitor of VEGF receptor 2 signaling, inhibits angiogenesis and tumor growth in vivo. Clin Cancer Res 17:4439–4450

45. Shen G, Li Y, Du T et al (2012) SKLB1002, a novel inhibitor of VEGF receptor 2 signaling, induces vascular normalization to improve systemically administered chemotherapy efficacy. Neoplasma 59:486–493

46. Nie W, Ma XL, Sang YX et al (2014) Synergic antitumor effect of SKLB1002 and local hyperthermia in 4T1 and CT26. Clin Exp Med 14:203–213

47. James C, Ugo V, Le Couédic J-P et al (2005) A unique clonal JAK2 mutation leading to constitutive signalling causes polycythaemia vera. Nature 434:1144–1148
48. Shuai K, Halpern J, ten Hoeve J et al (1996) Constitutive activation of STAT5 by the BCR-ABL oncogene in chronic myelogenous leukemia. Oncogene 13:247–254
49. Bromberg JF, Horvath CM, Besser D et al (1998) Stat3 activation is required for cellular transformation by v-src. Mol Cell Biol 18:2553–2558
50. Hennequin LF, Allen J, Breed J et al (2006) N-(5-chloro-1,3-benzodioxol-4-yl)-7-[2-(4-methylpiperazin-1-yl)ethoxy]-5-(tetrahydro-2H-pyran-4-yloxy)quinazolin-4-amine, a novel, highly selective, orally available, dual-specific c-Src/Abl kinase inhibitor. J Med Chem 49:6465–6488
51. Nam HJ, Im SA, Oh DY et al (2013) Antitumor activity of saracatinib (AZD0530), a c-Src/Abl kinase inhibitor, alone or in combination with chemotherapeutic agents in gastric cancer. Mol Cancer Ther 12:16–26
52. Simpkins F, Hevia-Paez P, Sun J et al (2012) Src Inhibition with saracatinib reverses fulvestrant resistance in ER-positive ovarian cancer models in vitro and in vivo. Clin Cancer Res 18(21):5911–5923
53. Puls LN, Eadens M, Messersmith W (2011) Current status of SRC inhibitors in solid tumor malignancies. Oncologist 16:566–578
54. Gucalp A, Sparano JA, Caravelli J et al (2011) Phase II trial of saracatinib (AZD0530), an oral SRC-inhibitor for the treatment of patients with hormone receptor-negative metastatic breast cancer. Clin Breast Cancer 11:306–311
55. Puttini M, Coluccia AM, Boschelli F et al (2006) In vitro and in vivo activity of SKI-606, a novel Src-Abl inhibitor, against imatinib-resistant Bcr-Abl+neoplastic cells. Cancer Res 66:11314–11322
56. Vultur A, Buettner R, Kowolik C et al (2008) SKI-606 (bosutinib), a novel Src kinase inhibitor, suppresses migration and invasion of human breast cancer cells. Mol Cancer Ther 7:1185–1194
57. Golas JM, Lucas J, Etienne C et al (2005) SKI-606, a Src/Abl inhibitor with in vivo activity in colon tumor xenograft models. Cancer Res 65:5358–5364
58. Boschelli F, Arndt K, Gambacorti-Passerini C (2010) Bosutinib: a review of preclinical studies in chronic myelogenous leukaemia. Eur J Cancer 46:1781–1789
59. Cortes JE, Kim DW, Kantarjian HM et al (2012) Bosutinib versus imatinib in newly diagnosed chronic-phase chronic myeloid leukemia: results from the BELA trial. J Clin Oncol 30(28):3486–3492
60. Lombardo LJ, Lee FY, Chen P et al (2004) Discovery of N-(2-Chloro-6-methyl-phenyl)-2-(6-(4-(2-hydroxyethyl)-piperazin-1-yl)-2-methylpyrimidin-4- ylamino)thiazole-5-carboxamide (BMS-354825), a dual Src/Abl kinase inhibitor with potent antitumor activity in preclinical assays. J Med Chem 47:6658–6661
61. Chang AY, Wang M (2013) Molecular mechanisms of action and potential biomarkers of growth inhibition of dasatinib (BMS-354825) on hepatocellular carcinoma cells. BMC Cancer 13:267
62. Fang Y, Zhong L, Lin M et al (2013) MEK/ERK dependent activation of STAT1 mediates dasatinib-induced differentiation of acute myeloid leukemia. PLoS One 8:e66915
63. Chen J, Lan T, Zhang W et al (2015) Dasatinib enhances cisplatin sensitivity in human esophageal squamous cell carcinoma (ESCC) cells via suppression of PI3K/AKT and Stat3 pathways. Arch Biochem Biophys 575:38–45
64. Premkumar DR, Jane EP, Agostino NR et al (2010) Dasatinib synergizes with JSI-124 to inhibit growth and migration and induce apoptosis of malignant human glioma cells. J Carcinog 9:1477
65. Rice L, Lepler S, Pampo C et al (2012) Impact of the SRC inhibitor dasatinib on the metastatic phenotype of human prostate cancer cells. Clin Exp Metastasis 29:133–142
66. Talpaz M, Shah NP, Kantarjian H et al (2006) Dasatinib in imatinib-resistant Philadelphia chromosome-positive leukemias. N Engl J Med 354(24):2531–2541
67. O'Hare T, Shakespeare WC, Zhu X et al (2009) AP24534, a pan-BCR-ABL inhibitor for chronic myeloid leukemia, potently inhibits the T315I mutant and overcomes mutation-based resistance. Cancer Cell 16:401–412

68. Li SQ, Cheuk AT, Shern JF et al (2013) Targeting wild-type and mutationally activated FGFR4 in rhabdomyosarcoma with the inhibitor ponatinib (AP24534). PLoS One 8:e76551
69. Jin Y, Ging K, Li H et al (2014) Ponatinib efficiently kills imatinib-resistant chronic eosinophilic leukemia cells harboring gatekeeper mutant T674I FIP1L1-PDGFRalpha: roles of Mcl-1 and beta-catenin. Mol Cancer 13:17
70. Sathornsumetee S, Rich JN (2006) Vandetanib, a novel multitargeted kinase inhibitor, in cancer therapy. Drugs Today (Barc) 42:657–670
71. Jia HY, Wu JX, Zhu XF et al (2009) ZD6474 inhibits Src kinase leading to apoptosis of imatinib-resistant K562 cells. Leuk Res 33:1512–1519
72. Dadu R, Hu MN, Grubbs EG et al (2015) Use of tyrosine kinase inhibitors for treatment of medullary thyroid carcinoma. Recent Results Cancer Res 204:227–249
73. Sano D, Kawakami M, Fujita K et al (2007) Antitumor effects of ZD6474 on head and neck squamous cell carcinoma. Oncol Rep 17:289–295
74. Wilhelm SM, Adnane L, Newell P et al (2008) Preclinical overview of sorafenib, a multikinase inhibitor that targets both Raf and VEGF and PDGF receptor tyrosine kinase signaling. Mol Cancer Ther 7:3129–3140
75. Zhang W, Konopleva M, Shi YX et al (2008) Mutant FLT3: a direct target of sorafenib in acute myelogenous leukemia. J Natl Cancer Inst 100:184–198
76. Zhao W, Zhang T, Qu B et al (2011) Sorafenib induces apoptosis in HL60 cells by inhibiting Src kinase-mediated STAT3 phosphorylation. Anticancer Drugs 22:79–88
77. Keating GM, Santoro A (2009) Sorafenib: a review of its use in advanced hepatocellular carcinoma. Drugs 69:223–240
78. Escudier B, Eisen T, Stadler WM et al (2007) Sorafenib in advanced clear-cell renal-cell carcinoma. N Engl J Med 356:125–134
79. Pitoia F, Jerkovich F (2016) Selective use of sorafenib in the treatment of thyroid cancer. Drug Des Devel Ther 10:1119–1131
80. Zhang W, Konopleva M, Ruvolo VR et al (2008) Sorafenib induces apoptosis of AML cells via Bim-mediated activation of the intrinsic apoptotic pathway. Leukemia 22:808–818
81. Sun L, Liang C, Shirazian S et al (2003) Discovery of 5-[5-fluoro-2-oxo-1,2- dihydroindol-(3Z)-ylidenemethyl]-2,4- dimethyl-1H-pyrrole-3-carboxylic acid (2-diethylaminoethyl) amide, a novel tyrosine kinase inhibitor targeting vascular endothelial and platelet-derived growth factor receptor tyrosine kinase. J Med Chem 46:1116–1119
82. O'Farrell AM, Abrams TJ, Yuen HA et al (2003) SU11248 is a novel FLT3 tyrosine kinase inhibitor with potent activity in vitro and in vivo. Blood 101:3597–3605
83. Hartmann JT, Kanz L (2008) Sunitinib and periodic hair depigmentation due to temporary c-KIT inhibition. Arch Dermatol 144:1525–1526
84. Demetri GD, van Oosterom AT, Garrett CR et al (2006) Efficacy and safety of sunitinib in patients with advanced gastrointestinal stromal tumour after failure of imatinib: a randomised controlled trial. Lancet 368:1329–1338
85. Motzer RJ, Hutson TE, Tomczak P et al (2007) Sunitinib versus interferon alfa in metastatic renal-cell carcinoma. N Engl J Med 356:115–124
86. Fiedler W, Kayser S, Kebenko M et al (2015) A phase I/II study of sunitinib and intensive chemotherapy in patients over 60 years of age with acute myeloid leukaemia and activating FLT3 mutations. Br J Haematol 169:694–700
87. Cao ZX, Liu JJ, Zheng RL et al (2012) SKLB1028, a novel oral multikinase inhibitor of EGFR, FLT3 and Abl, displays exceptional activity in models of FLT3-driven AML and considerable potency in models of CML harboring Abl mutants. Leukemia 26:1892–1895
88. Matsui J, Funahashi Y, Uenaka T et al (2008) Multi-kinase inhibitor E7080 suppresses lymph node and lung metastases of human mammary breast tumor MDA-MB-231 via inhibition of vascular endothelial growth factor-receptor (VEGF-R) 2 and VEGF-R3 kinase. Clin Cancer Res 14:5459–5465
89. Glen H, Boss D, Evans TR et al (2007) A phase I dose finding study of E7080 in patients (pts) with advanced malignancies. J Clin Oncol 25:14073a
90. Ferrari SM, Fallahi P, Politti U et al (2015) Molecular targeted therapies of aggressive thyroid cancer. Front Endocrinol (Lausanne) 6:176

91. Motzer RJ, Hutson TE, Glen H et al (2015) Lenvatinib, everolimus, and the combination in patients with metastatic renal cell carcinoma: a randomised, phase 2, open-label, multicentre trial. Lancet Oncol 16:1473–1482

92. Cripe L, McGuire W, Wertheim M et al (2007) Integrated report of the phase 2 experience with XL999 administered IV to patients (pts) with NSCLC, renal cell CA (RCC), metastatic colorectal CA (CRC), recurrent ovarian CA, acute myelogenous leukemia (AML), and multiple myeloma (MM). J Clin Oncol 25(18S):3591a

93. Sansone P, Bromberg J (2012) Targeting the interleukin-6/Jak/Stat pathway in human malignancies. J Clin Oncol 30:1005–1014

94. Tanaka T, Narazaki M, Kishimoto T (2012) Therapeutic targeting of the interleukin-6 receptor. Annu Rev Pharmacol Toxicol 52:199–219

95. Nishimoto N, Kishimoto T (2008) Humanized antihuman IL-6 receptor antibody, tocilizumab. Handb Exp Pharmacol 181:151–160

96. Shinriki S, Jono H, Ota K et al (2009) Humanized anti-interleukin-6 receptor antibody suppresses tumor angiogenesis and in vivo growth of human oral squamous cell carcinoma. Clin Cancer Res 15:5426–5434

97. Jiang XP, Yang DC, Elliott RL et al (2011) Down-regulation of expression of interleukin-6 and its receptor results in growth inhibition of MCF-7 breast cancer cells. Anticancer Res 31:2899–2906

98. Wang P, Farren T, Agrawal SG (2013) Tocilizumab overcomes chemo-resistance of CLL cells. Blood 122:5305

99. Kim NH, Kim SK, Kim DS et al (2015) Anti-proliferative action of IL-6R-targeted antibody tocilizumab for non-small cell lung cancer cells. Oncol Lett 9:2283–2288

100. Chen R, Chen B (2015) Siltuximab (CNTO 328): a promising option for human malignancies. Drug Des Devel Ther 9:3455–3458

101. Song L, Smith MA, Doshi P et al (2014) Antitumor efficacy of the anti-interleukin-6 (IL-6) antibody siltuximab in mouse xenograft models of lung cancer. J Thorac Oncol 9:974–982

102. Kroon P, Berry PA, Stower MJ et al (2013) JAK-STAT blockade inhibits tumor initiation and clonogenic recovery of prostate cancer stem-like cells. Cancer Res 73:5288–5298

103. Karkera J, Steiner H, Li W et al (2011) The anti-interleukin-6 antibody siltuximab down-regulates genes implicated in tumorigenesis in prostate cancer patients from a phase I study. Prostate 71:1455–1465

104. Rossi JF, Négrier S, James ND et al (2010) A phase I/II study of siltuximab (CNTO 328), an anti-interleukin-6 monoclonal antibody, in metastatic renal cell cancer. Br J Cancer 103:1154–1162

105. Voorhees PM, Chen Q, Kuhn DJ et al (2007) Inhibition of interleukin-6 signaling with CNTO 328 enhances the activity of bortezomib in preclinical models of multiple myeloma. Clin Cancer Res 13:6469–6478

106. Kurzrock R, Voorhees PM, Casper C et al (2013) A phase I, open-label study of siltuximab, an anti-IL-6 monoclonal antibody, in patients with B-cell non-Hodgkin lymphoma, multiple myeloma, or Castleman disease. Clin Cancer Res 19:3659–3670

Index

© Springer International Publishing Switzerland 2016
A.C. Ward (ed.), *STAT Inhibitors in Cancer*, Cancer Drug
Discovery and Development, DOI 10.1007/978-3-319-42949-6

Printed in the United States
By Bookmasters